Clayton's Electrotherapy

Clayton's Electrotherapy

10th Edition

Edited by

SHEILA KITCHEN PhD
MSc Course Coordinator,
Physiotherapy Group,
King's College, London, UK

SARAH BAZIN MCSP
Director of Therapy Services,
Department of Physiotherapy,
Solihull Hospital, Solihull, UK

WB Saunders Company Ltd

London • Philadelphia • Toronto • Sydney • Tokyo

WB Saunders Company Ltd
An imprint of Harcourt Publishers Limited

© 1996 WB Saunders Company Ltd
© 1999 Harcourt Publishers Limited

This book is printed on acid free paper

First published 1948 as *Clayton's Electrotherapy and Actinotherapy*
Eighth edition 1981
Ninth edition 1985
Third printing 1992
Fourth printing 1994
Reprinted 1997
Reprinted 1999

A catalogue record for this book is available from the British Library

ISBN 0–7020–1762–0

Design by Landmark Design Associates

Editorial and Production Services by Fisher Duncan
10 Barley Mow Passage, London W4 4PH

Typeset by J&L Composition Ltd, Filey, North Yorkshire

Printed and bound in Great Britain by The Bath Press, Bath

Contents

Contributors

David Baxter DPhil MCSP
Professor of Rehabilitation Sciences
University of Ulster at Jordanstown
Room 14J15
Newtownabbey
County Antrim BT37 0QB

Sarah Bazin MCSP
Director of Therapy Services
Department of Physiotherapy
Solihull Hospital
Solihull
West Midlands B91 2JL

Robert Charman FCSP DipTP MCSP (Retired)
Formerly: Senior Lecturer
School of Physiotherapy
Institute of Health Care Studies
University Hospital of Wales
Cardiff

Kenneth J Collins DPhil MB BS FRCP (Retired)
Formerly: Honorary Senior Clinical Lecturer
(University College Hospital)
Member of MRC Staff
MRC Unit
Dept of Geriatric Medicine
St Pancras Hospital
London NW1 0PE

Brian L Diffey PhD CPhys FInstP FIPSM
Professor and Consultant Medical Physicist
Regional Medical Physics Department
Durham Unit
Dryburn Hospital
Durham DH1 5TW

Mary Dyson PhD CBiol MIBiol FAIUM FCSP
Head of Tissue Repair Research Unit
Division of Anatomy and Cell Biology
Guy's Hospital
London SE1 9RT

Peter M Farr MD MB ChB MRCP
Consultant Dermatologist
Royal Victoria Infirmary
Newcastle upon Tyne NE1 5LP

Victoria Frampton SRP MCSP
Therapy Manager
Thanet Healthcare Trust
Physiotherapy Department
Thanet General Hospital
St Peters Road
Margate
Kent CT9 4AN

Tracey Howe PhD MSc GradDipPhys MCSP
Cert Ed
The University of Manchester
School of Nursing Studies
Director, Centre for Habilitation
and Muscle Performance
Ladywell Hospital
Eccles New Road
Manchester M5 2AA

Lorna Johnson MSc MCSP
Physiotherapy Group
Biomedical Sciences Division
King's College

Kensington Campus
Campdel Hill Road
London W8 7AH

Sheila Kitchen PhD MSc MCSP DipTP
MSc Course Coordinator
Physiotherapy Group
Biomedical Sciences Division
King's College
Kensington Campus
Campus Hill Road
London W8 7AH

Denis Martin PhD MCSP
Physiotherapy Department
Queen Margaret's College
Leith Campus
Duke Street
Edinburgh EH6 8HF

Joan McMeeken PhD Dip Phty MSC MAPA
Professor & Head of School of Physiotherapy
Faculty of Medicine, Dentistry and
Health Sciences
University of Melbourne
Parkville
Victoria 3052
Australia

Shona Scott MSc MCSP
Physiotherapy Department
Queen Margaret's College
Leith Campus
Duke Street
Edinburgh EH6 8HF

Oona Scott PhD MCSP
Reader
Department of Rehabilitation Sciences
University of East London
Romford Road
London E15 4LZ

Barry Stillman FACP DipPhty MAPA MCSP
School of Physiotherapy
Faculty of Medicine, Dentistry and
Health Sciences
University of Melbourne
Parkville
Victoria 3052
Australia

Gail ter Haar PhD
The Institute of Cancer Research
Royal Cancer Hospital
Joint Department of Physics
The Royal Marsden NHS Trust
Downs Road
Sutton
Surrey SM2 5PT

Tim Watson PhD MCSP DipTP
Senior Lecturer
Dept of Health Studies
Brunel University College
Borough Road
Isleworth
Middlesex TW7 5DU

Leslie Wood PhD
Senior Lecturer in Physiology
Glasgow Caledonian University
Southbrae Campus
Southbrae Drive
Jordanhill
Glasgow G13 1PP

Steve Young PhD
Guy's Hospital
Tissue Repair Research Unit
Division of Anatomy and Cell Biology
Guy's Hospital
London SE1 9RT

Introduction

SARAH BAZIN

After 47 years as a standard electrotherapy textbook the tenth edition of *Clayton's Electrotherapy* has been totally redesigned and rewritten with the aim to provide information about the latest advances and to reflect current research. It is now a multicontributor book with sections written by experts in the area of each electrophysical modality. The authors include physicists, physiotherapists, and biologists, who are either clinicians, researchers or teachers.

The book begins by setting out the physical foundations. It looks at electrical properties of biological tissues and the physiology of tissue repair, pain, sensory and motor nerve activation. It describes the electrophysical effects of thermal, athermal and stimulating applications.

Conductive methods of heating and cooling have a section to themselves. Electromagnetic radiations cover infrared, shortwave (both pulsed and continuous), microwave, laser therapy and ultraviolet radiation. Ultrasound stands alone in the fifth section, whilst motor stimulation includes TENS, interferential and electrical investigations. The final chapter is concerned with electrical stimulation for wound healing.

For completeness, modalities that are currently less popular in Britain are also included. Infrared is an effective method of surface heating, and microwave, which is unfashionable in the UK at the present time, supplies an effective mode of deep heating.

The book does not set out to provide information on methods of operating the equipment as this is provided with the machine when it is supplied and must be read by each practitioner prior to use.

Electrotherapy is one of the core skills of the physiotherapist, though it is also used by other clinical groups such as veterinarians and chiropodists. As with other modes of treatment, the practice of electrotherapy is subject to changes in thinking and is affected by technological advancement and research. Recent years have seen a rapid increase in the number and quality of studies which have been conducted to examine the physical behaviour of many agents, their biostimulative effects upon tissue and their clinical efficiency.

This latest edition of *Clayton's Electrotherapy* attempts to take account of the most recent findings and present an up-to-date and readable account of our knowledge at the present time.

The editors wish to thank the authors for their commitment to this project and to all those who have been associated with it, from publishers to clerical staff and including members of family.

A

Scientific Background

1

Electrophysical Principles

GAIL TER HAAR

Introduction
•
Wave Motion
•
Electricity and Magnetism
•
Mechanical Waves

Introduction

Electrophysical agents are used by physiotherapists to treat a wide variety of conditions. These agents include both electromagnetic and sound waves, in addition to muscle and nerve stimulating currents. This chapter contains, in simple terms, the basic physics necessary for the understanding of the remainder of the book.

An understanding of wave motion is central to getting to grips with the physics of any form of therapy that uses either electrical or mechanical energy. A general description of wave motion therefore precedes more detailed treatment of electricity and magnetism, and of ultrasound.

Wave Motion

Wave motion transfers energy from one place to another. We are familiar with waves in our everyday lives. Think of a cork floating in a pond into which a stone is dropped. Ripples move out from where the stone enters the water, and some of the stone's energy is transferred to the pond's edge. The cork bobs up and down, but does not move within the pond.

An easy way to demonstrate wave motion is to use a Slinky spring toy. Two types of wave exist: *transverse waves* which can be mimicked by raising and lowering one end of the spring rapidly, as shown in Figure 1.1, and *longitudinal waves* which can be demonstrated by extending the spring

Figure 1.1   If a spring that is attached at one end is flicked up and down, a transverse wave is produced.

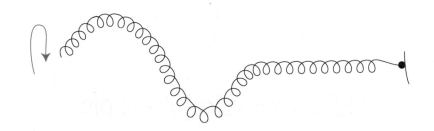

Transverse wave

along its length, and then letting it go (Figure 1.2). Water waves, the motion of a violin string, and electromagnetic waves as in shortwave diathermy, infrared and interferential are examples of transverse waves. Sound, as used in ultrasound therapy, propagates mainly as longitudinal waves.

It is much more difficult to picture a longitudinal wave than a transverse wave. If we compare our spring with the wave travelling down it (Figure 1.2) to an unstretched spring, you can see regions where the coils are closer together, and regions where the coils are further apart. We call the part of the spring where the coils are closely spaced a region of *compression*, and the region where they are separated further than they were at rest, a region of *rarefaction*.

We are used to describing waves on the sea in terms of peaks and troughs. The movement up to a wave crest, down to a trough, and back up to the crest again is known as a *cycle of oscillation*. A cork floating in the sea bobs up and down as the waves go past. The height difference of the cork between a crest and a trough is twice the *amplitude*. Perhaps a simpler way of visualizing the amplitude is as the difference in water height above the sea bed between a flat, calm sea and the crest of the wave. The number of wave crests passing the cork in a second is the wave *frequency* (f). Frequency is measured in *hertz* (Hz), where 1 Hz is 1 cycle/second. The time that elapses between two adjacent wave crests passing the cork is the *period* (τ) of the oscillation. This has units of time. If each cycle therefore takes τ

Figure 1.2   Extending a spring along its length and letting it go again produces a longitudinal wave.

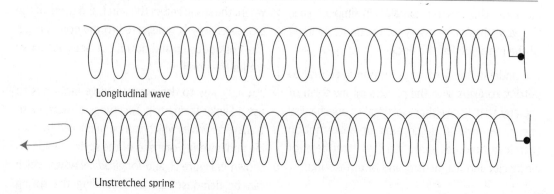

Longitudinal wave

Unstretched spring

Figure 1.3   (a) and (b) show the position of two points A and C in the path of a wave as it passes through. The displacements shown in (a) and (b) are frozen at two different times, between which the wave has moved on a fraction of a wavelength. (c) shows the displacement of the point during two cycles.

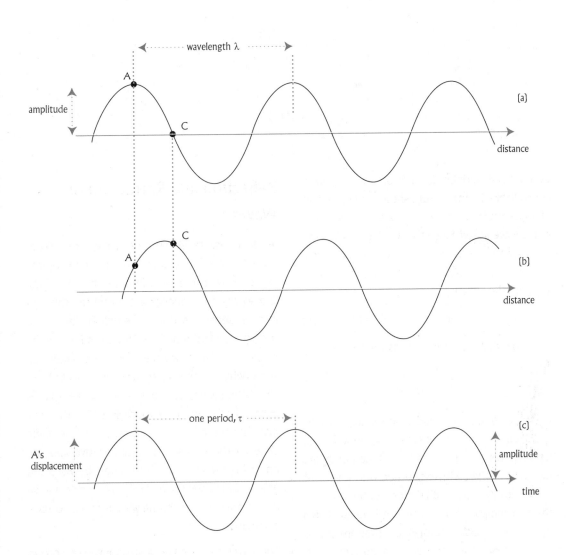

seconds, there must be $1/\tau$ cycles in each second. The number of cycles that occur in a second has already been defined as the frequency, and so we can write:

$$f = 1/\tau, \text{ or} \tag{1}$$

$$\tau = 1/f. \tag{2}$$

The distance between two adjacent wave crests is the *wavelength* (λ).

Figures 1.3a and b shows a wave frozen at two moments, a short time apart. It can be seen that the different points on the wave have changed position relative to the central line, but have not moved in space. In fact, if you tracked A's motion

Figure 1.4 Points A and B, and also A' and B', are always in the same relative position in the wave. They are in phase. Points A and C are out of phase.

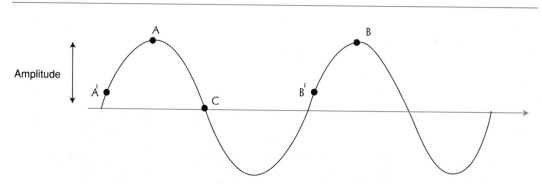

over several periods, its motion up and down would look like the picture shown in Figure 1.3c. The speed at which the wave crests move is known as the wave *speed*. Since the wave moves a wavelength (λ) in one cycle, and one cycle takes a time equal to the period τ, then the wave speed (c) is given by the equation:

$$c = \lambda/t. \qquad (3)$$

We know that $1/t$ is the same as the frequency f, and so

$$c = f\lambda \qquad (4)$$

In Figure 1.4, points A and B on the wave (or A' and B') are moving in the same way and will reach the crest (or trough) together. These points are said to be *in phase* with each other. The movement from A to B (or A' to B') represents one *cycle* of the wave motion. A and C are not in phase; C is a quarter of a cycle ahead of A and they are said to have a *phase difference* (ϕ) of a quarter cycle. Phase is usually expressed as an angle, where a complete cycle is 2π radians (or 360°). A quarter cycle therefore represents a phase difference of $\pi/2$ radians (90°). This is illustrated in Figure 1.5.

Reflection and Refraction of Waves

When waves travelling through a medium arrive at the surface of a second medium some of the energy is reflected back into the first medium, and some of the energy is transmitted through into the second medium. The proportion of the total energy that is reflected is determined by the properties of the two media involved. Figure 1.6 shows what happens when waves are reflected by a flat (plane) surface. An imaginary line that is perpendicular to the surface is called the *normal*. The *law of reflection* states that the angle between the incident (incoming) wave and the normal is always equal to the angle between the reflected wave and the normal. If the incident wave is at normal incidence, the wave is reflected back along its path.

The waves that are transmitted into the second medium may undergo *refraction*. This is the bending of light towards the normal when it travels from one medium into one in which the wave speed is lower, or away from the normal when the wave speed in the second medium is higher. This is shown in Figure 1.7. For example, light bends towards the normal as it enters water from air since it travels more slowly in water than

Figure 1.5 Phase angle can be likened to the turning of a water wheel. Imagine two wheels, A and B, both with a mark on their rim. A does not move, but B turns, and as it does, the rim mark executes the circles, each complete turn representing one *cycle*. The angle through which the mark turns in one cycle is 360° (2π radians). Thus, for example, if compared with A, when the mark on B's rim has moved around a quarter of a turn (*cycle*), the angle between the two marks is a quarter of 360° (90° or π/2 radians), whereas, after half a turn, the angle between the two marks is 180° or π radians. This angle between the two marks is analagous to the phase *difference*. As B rotates, the height of the mark above the wheel's hub varies. If the wheel turns at a constant speed, then the mark's height traces out a *sine wave* when plotted against time.

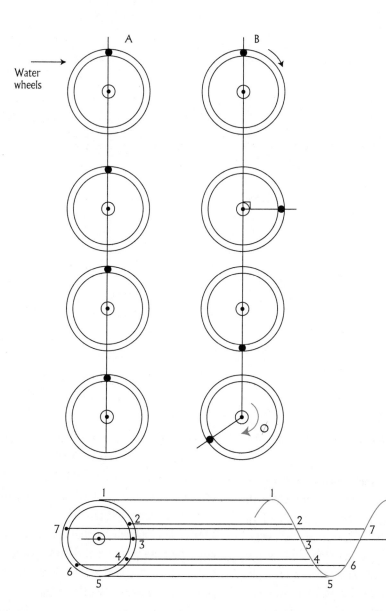

Figure 1.6　The law of reflection states that the angle of incidence equals the angle of reflection.

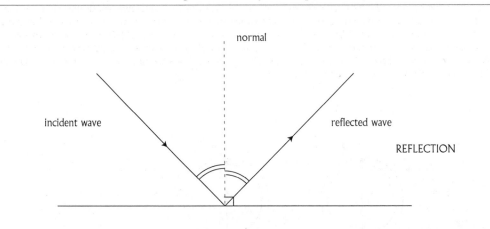

Figure 1.7　When a beam passes from one medium to another, it may be refracted, i.e. it changes its direction.

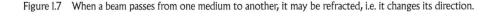

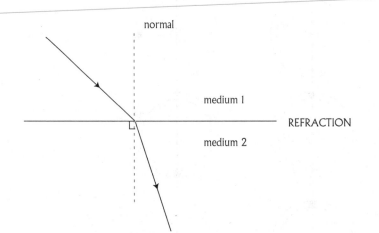

in air, and so a swimming pool may appear shallower than it really is.

As has been discussed earlier, waves carry energy. There are conditions, however, under which the transport of energy can be stopped, and the energy can be localized. This happens in a *standing (stationary) wave*. A standing wave is produced when an incident wave meets a returning reflected wave with the same amplitude. When the two waves meet, the total amplitude is the sum of the two individual amplitudes. Thus, as can be

seen in Figure 1.8a, if the trough of one wave coincides with the crest of the other, the two waves cancel each other out. If, however, the crest of one meets the crest of the other, the wave motion is reinforced (Figure 1.8b) and the total amplitude doubles. In the reinforced standing wave there are points that always have zero amplitude; these are called *nodes*. Similarly, there are points that always have the greatest amplitude, and these are called *antinodes*. Nodes and antinodes are shown in Figure 1.8b. The distance

Figure 1.8 A standing wave is formed when two waves of equal amplitude, travelling in opposite directions, meet. (a) the two waves cancel each other out. (b) The two waves add to reinforce each other.

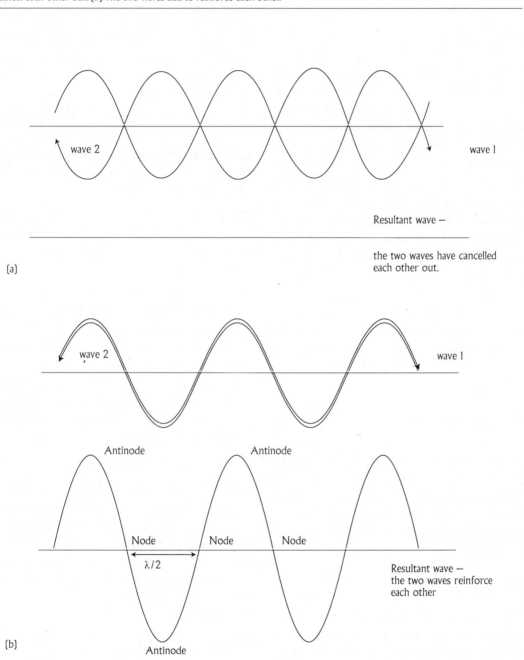

between adjacent nodes, or adjacent antinodes is one half wavelength.

Polarization

In flicking the Slinky spring up and down to produce a transverse wave, one has an infinite number of choices as to which direction to move it, so long as the motion is at right angles to the line of the spring. If the spring is always moved in a fixed direction, the wave is said to be *polarized* – the waves are in that plane only. However, if the waves (or directions in which the spring is moved) are in a number of different directions, the waves are *unpolarized*. It is possible to polarize the waves by passing them through a filter that allows only waves that are in one plane to pass through. This can be visualized by envisaging a piece of card with a long narrow slit in it. This will allow the waves formed in the plane of the slit to go through, but no others – the card therefore acts as a polarizing filter.

Electricity and Magnetism

We are all familiar with effects of electrical charges even if we are not all aware of their causes. The 'static' experienced when brushing newly-washed hair or undressing, and the electrical discharge obvious in lightning are examples of the effects of charges.

Electricity

Matter is made up of atoms, an atom being the smallest particle of an element that can be identified as being from that element. The atom is made up of a positively charged central nucleus (made up of positively charged *protons* and uncharged *neutrons*), with negatively charged particles (*electrons*) orbiting around it, resembling a mini-ature solar system. An atom contains as many protons as there are electrons, and so has no net charge. If this balance is destroyed, the atom has a non-zero net charge and is called an *ion*. If an electron is removed from the atom it becomes a *positive ion*, and if an electron is added the atom becomes a *negative ion*.

Two particles of opposite charge attract each other, and two particles of the same charge repel each other (push each other away). Hence, an electron and a proton are attracted to each other, while two electrons repel each other.

The unit of charge is a *coulomb* (C). An electron has a charge of 1.6×10^{-19} C, so it takes a very large number (6.2×10^{18}) of electrons to make up one Coulomb.

The force between two particles of charge q_1 and q_2 is proportional to the product of q_1 and q_2 ($q_1 \times q_2$), and inversely proportional to the distance between them (d) squared (Figure 1.9). Thus, the force is proportional to $q_1 q_2 / d^2$. The constant of proportionality (i.e. the invariant number) necessary to allow one to calculate the force between two charges is $1/4\pi\varepsilon$, where ε is the *permittivity* of the medium containing the two charges:

$$F = q_1 q_2 / 4\pi\varepsilon d^2 \qquad (5)$$

If one of the charges is negative, then the force is attractive. If the particles are in a vacuum, the permittivity used is ε_0, this is known as the *permittivity of free space*. For a medium other than a vacuum, the permittivity is often quoted as a multiple of ε_0, where the multiplying factor, κ, is known as the *relative permittivity* or *dielectric constant*. So:

Figure 1.9   Two particles of charge q_1 and q_2 a distance of d apart experience a force between them that is proportional to $q_1 q_2 / d^2$.

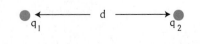

$$\varepsilon = \kappa \varepsilon_0, \text{ or} \qquad (6a)$$

$$\kappa = \varepsilon / \varepsilon_0. \qquad (6b)$$

Electric Fields

An *electric field* exists around any charged particle. If a smaller charge that is free to move is placed in the field, the paths it will move along are called *lines of force* (or *field lines*). Examples of fields and their patterns are shown in Figure 1.10.

The *electric field strength*, E, is defined as the force per unit charge on a particle placed in the field. A little thought shows that $E = F/q$, where F is the force and q is the particle's charge. The units used to describe E are newtons/coulomb (N/C).

Figure 1.10   Examples of electric fields near charged particles and plates. (a) Field between two particles of equal and opposite charges. (b) Field between two positively charged particles. (c) Field between a charged particle and an oppositely charged plate. (d) Field between two oppositely charged plates.

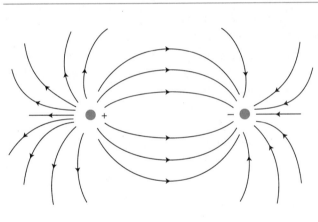

(a)

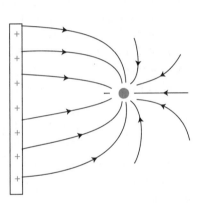

(c)

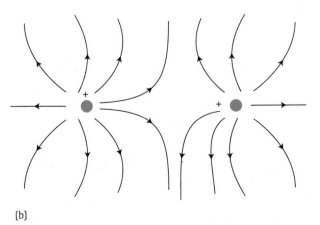

(b)

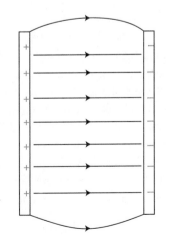

(d)

If E is the same throughout a field, it is said to be uniform. In this case, the field lines are parallel to each other as shown in Figure 1.10d. If a charged particle is moved in this field, work is done on it, unless it moves perpendicular to the field lines. This is somewhat analogous to moving a ball around on earth. If the ball is always kept at the same height, and moved horizontally, its potential energy remains constant. If the ball is raised, or lowered, its potential energy is changed. The ball has no potential energy when it lies on the ground. In a non-uniform field where the lines are not parallel, moving a charged particle always results in a change of potential energy. The *electric potential*, V, is defined as the potential energy per unit charge of a positively charged particle placed at that point. Electric potential is measured in units of *volts*. Since the position at which the electric potential energy is zero is taken as infinity, another way of thinking of the electrical potential at a point is as the work done in moving the charge to that point from infinity. In practice it is easier to compare the electrical potential at two points in the field than to consider infinity. The difference in the work required to move a charge from infinity to a point, A, and that required to move it to another point, B, is called the *potential difference* (p.d.) between the two points; this is also measured in *volts*. The p.d. is best thought of as a kind of pressure difference. Between the two points there will be a gradient in potential (just as there is a pressure gradient between the top and bottom of a waterfall). This gradient is described in units of volts/metre. In a uniform field between parallel plates with potential difference V, and separation d, the potential gradient is given by V/d. If a particle of charge q is moved from one plate to another, the work done is qV. Work is force × distance, and so the force, F, is given by:

$$F = qV/d. \tag{7}$$

Since the electric field strength, E, is given by:

$$E = F/q, \tag{8}$$

it follows that:

$$E = V/d. \tag{9}$$

Remember that V/d is the potential gradient. From this equation we can see that the electric field strength can be increased by bringing the two plates closer together. Although the derivation is more complicated, the electric field strength at any point in a non-uniform field can also be shown to be the same as the potential gradient at that point.

Any electric circuit needs a supply of power to drive the electrons around the conductors. A source has one positive and one negative terminal, and the source forces the electrons out from its negative terminal. Electrical energy can be produced within the source by a number of means. Dynamos convert mechanical energy into electrical energy, solar cells convert the sun's energy into electrical energy, and batteries convert chemical energy into electrical energy. The force acting on the electrons is called the *electromotive force* (e.m.f.). This is defined as the electrical energy produced per unit charge inside the source. The unit in which e.m.f. is measured is the volt, because 1 volt is 1 joule/coulomb.

Electric Current

An *electric current* is the flow of electric charge (usually electrons). In some materials (for example, metals) where the atoms are bound into a lattice structure, the charge is carried by electrons. In materials in which the atoms are free to move, the charge is carried by ions. A liquid in which the ions are the charge carriers is called an *electrolyte*. An *insulator* is a material that has no free charge carriers, and so is unable to carry an electric current. Current is measured using an ammeter, and the unit in which it is given is the *ampere*. An ampere represents 1 coulomb of charge flowing through a point in 1 second.

There are two types of electric current. A *direct current* (DC) is one in which the flow of electrons is in one direction only, and an *alternating current* (AC) is one in which the current flows first one way and then another. In considering electric circuits, it is easiest to think first of direct currents. A later section points to the differences between AC and DC circuits.

Resistance and Ohm's Law

The flow of electric charge through a conductor is analogous to the flow of water through pipes. If water is pumped round the system, narrow pipes put up more resistance to flow than wide ones. Electrical conductors also put up a *resistance* to the flow of charge. As the charged particles move through a conductor they collide with other charge carriers and with the resident atoms; the current flow is thus impeded by the constituents of the conductor.

Georg Ohm was able to demonstrate that the current flowing in a circuit is proportional to the potential difference across it. His law (*Ohm's Law*), formally stated, is:

The current flowing through a metallic conductor is proportional to the potential difference that exists across it, provided that all physical conditions remain constant.

So, $I \propto V$; this could also be written as $V \propto I$, where the constant of proportionality is the *resistance*. The equation resulting from Ohm's Law is therefore:

$$V = IR. \qquad (10)$$

R is measured in ohms (Ω). The Ohm is defined as the resistance of a body such that a one volt potential difference across the body results in a current of 1 ampere through it.

The resistance of a piece of wire increases with its length, and decreases as its cross-sectional area increases. A property called *resistivity* is defined which is a property of the material only, and not of the material's shape. The resistance R of a piece of wire with resistivity ρ, length L and area A is given by:

$$R = \rho L / A. \qquad (11)$$

When electrons flow through a conductor, they collide with the atoms in the conductor material and impart energy to those atoms. This leads to heating of the conductor. The unit used for measuring energy is the *joule*. We have seen earlier (see equation 7) that the potential difference measured in volts is the work done in moving unit charge between two points. So it follows from this that since potential difference is work done per unit charge:

$$volt = joule / coulomb, \qquad (12a)$$

$$(joule = volt\ coulomb). \qquad (12b)$$

The unit of power measurement is the *Watt*. Power is the rate of doing work, so a Watt is a joule / second. It follows from the equation above that:

$$1\ watt = 1\ joule / second \qquad (13a)$$

$$= 1\ volt\ coulomb / second. \qquad (13b)$$

We know from the definition given above that a coulomb / second is an ampere. So, we have:

$$1\ watt = 1\ volt.ampere. \qquad (14)$$

In other words, the electrical power developed in a circuit is given by:

$$Power = VI, \qquad (15)$$

where V is in volts, I is in amperes, and the power is in watts.

From Ohm's Law we can make substitutions in this equation to express power in terms of different combinations of V, I and R. So:

$$W = VI, \tag{16a}$$

$$W = I^2R, \tag{16b}$$

$$W = V^2/R, \tag{16c}$$

are equivalent equations, where W is in watts, V is in volts and R is in ohms.

Capacitance

Any passive device capable of storing electric charge is called a *capacitor*. This is the electrical equivalent of a compressed spring, which stores energy until it is allowed to expand. A capacitor stores charge until it can release it by becoming part of a completed electrical circuit. If you apply an electric potential, V, between two plates of a capacitor, one plate becomes positively charged, and the other becomes charged with an equal but opposite negative charge. If an insulating material, known as a *dielectric* is placed between the plates, the capacity to store charge is increased. The *relative permittivity*, or *dielectric constant* we came across earlier has another definition: it is also the ratio of the charge that can be stored between two plates with a dielectric material between them, to that which can be stored without the dielectric.

A capacitor is drawn as a pair of parallel lines. Its *capacitance*, C, is defined as the charge (Q) stored per unit potential difference across its plates.

$$C = Q/V. \tag{17}$$

Since Q is measured in coulombs, and V is measured in volts, the unit for capacitance is the coulomb/volt, known as the *farad*. Commonly, the capacitance of a capacitor found in an electric circuit is a few micro- (10^{-6}) or pico- (10^{-12}) farads.

A capacitor is *charged* by applying a potential difference across its plates. It is *discharged* (the charge is allowed to flow away from the plates) by providing an electrical connection between the plates.

Electric Circuits

The symbols used to denote different components used in electrical circuits are shown in Figure 1.11.

Two electrical components are said to be in *series* if they carry the same current. The potential difference across a series of components is the sum of the potential differences across each one. The components are in *parallel* if they have the same potential difference across them. The current is the sum of the currents flowing through them.

RESISTORS IN SERIES

If several resistors are joined in series with each other, the same current flows through them all since electrons cannot be lost on the way through. From Ohm's Law, the potential, V_i, across each resistance in Figure 11a, is given by:

$$V_i = IR_i. \tag{18}$$

If the total potential across the whole string is V, then:

$$V = V_1 + V_2 + V_3 + \dots + V_i. \tag{19}$$

So:

$$V = IR_1 + IR_2 + IR_3 + \dots + IR_i$$

$$= I(R_1 + R_2 + R_3 + \dots + R_i). \tag{20}$$

Figure 1.11   Symbols used in drawing electrical circuits. (a) Resistor. (b) Variable resistor. (c) Capacitor. (d) DC Source. (e) AC Source. (f) Inductance. (g) Switch. (h) Bulb.

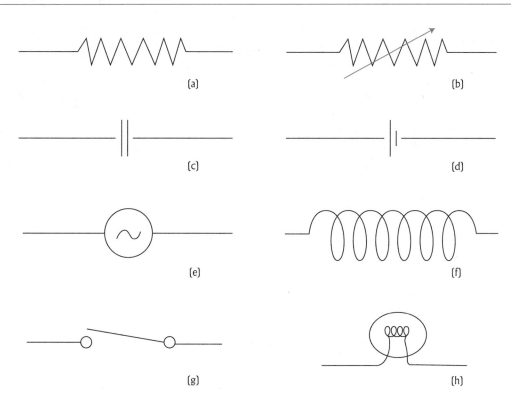

Thus the single resistance needed to have the same effect as the string of resistors, R_{total}, is the sum of all the resistances:

$$R_{total} = R_1 + R_2 + R_3 + ... + R_i. \qquad (21)$$

For example, in the string shown in Figure 1.12b, the total resistance R_{total}, is $2 + 5 + 10 \ \Omega = 17\Omega$.

RESISTORS IN PARALLEL

Resistors may also be wired up in parallel as shown in Figure 1.13a. The total flow of current through all resistors, I, is the same as the sum of the currents through each resistor:

$$I = I_1 + I_2 + I_3 + ... + I_i. \qquad (22)$$

The potential difference across each resistor is the same. Using Ohm's Law in the above equation, we can write:

$$I = V/R_1 + V/R_2 + V/R_3 + ... + V/R_i$$

$$= V(1/R_1 + 1/R_2 + 1/R_3 + ... + 1/R_i). \quad (23)$$

Therefore the single resistance that could replace these parallel resistors has a value:

$$1/R_{total} = 1/R_1 + 1/R_2 + 1/R_3 + ... + 1/R_i. \quad (24)$$

For example, if three resistors of 2, 5 and 10 Ω are in parallel, as shown in Figure 1.13b, the equivalent resistor is $1/(1/2 + 1/5 + 1/10)$, which is $1/(0.5 + 0.2 + 0.1) = 1/0.8 = 1.25 \ \Omega$.

Figure 1.12   Resistors in series.

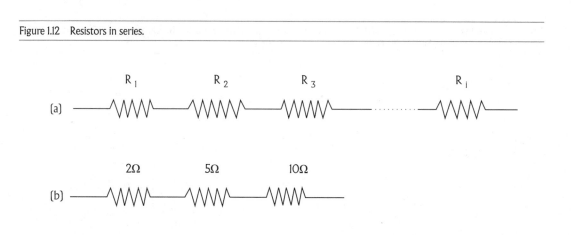

Figure 1.13   Resistors in parallel.

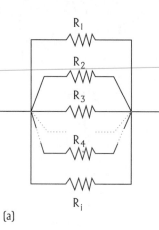

(a)

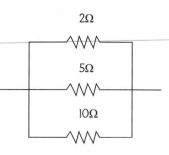

(b)

CAPACITORS IN SERIES

A voltage applied across four capacitors in series induces charges of +Q and -Q on the plates of each (Figure 1.14). Using equation 17 we know that:

$$1/C = V/Q.$$

The potential difference across the row is the sum of the potentials across each capacitor, and so the single capacitance, C, equivalent to the three capacitors C_1, C_2 and C_3 is given by:

$$1/C = (V_1 + V_2 + V_3 + V_4)/Q \tag{25}$$

$$= V_1/Q + V_2/Q + V_3/Q + V_4/Q$$

$$= 1/C_1 + 1/C_2 + 1/C_3 + 1/C_4. \tag{26}$$

If the capacitances are 2, 1, 5 and 10 µF, then C = 0.56 µF.

Figure 1.14   Capacitors in series.

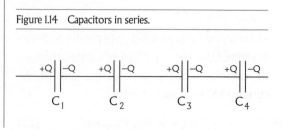

CAPACITORS IN PARALLEL

If capacitors are connected in parallel as shown in Figure 1.15, the total charge developed on them is the sum of the charges on each of them. The current is never negative. The potential difference is the same across all the capacitors.

The effective capacitance of all the capacitors put together is given by the expression:

$$C = Q/V,$$

where

$$Q = Q_1 + Q_2 + Q_3 + Q_4,$$

and so:

$$C = Q_1/V + Q_2/V + Q_3/V + Q_4/V \quad (27)$$

$$= C_1 + C_2 + C_3 + C_4. \quad (28)$$

If the capacitances are 1, 2, 5 and 10 μF, then C is 18 μF.

DIRECT AND ALTERNATING CURRENT

As discussed earlier, two types of electric current exist: direct current and alternating current. The most common type of alternating current has a sinusoidal waveform, such as that found in the electricity mains. For sinusoidal AC, the relationships between frequency and period etc. defined in the first section hold true. The variation of current can be described by the relationship:

$$I = I_0\sin(2\pi ft), \quad (29),$$

and, similarly, the voltage is described by:

$$V = V_0\sin(2\pi ft), \quad (30)$$

where $\sin(2\pi ft)$ is the expression to tell you the wave form is a sine wave of frequency f, and I_0 and V_0 are the maximum values of current and voltage (the amplitude of the oscillation). Clearly, the average current over one cycle in Figure 1.16 is zero – the current is positive as much as it is negative – and the same applies to the voltage.

In some instances, an alternating current may be *rectified* as shown in Figures 1.16b and c. Here, the average current is clearly not zero. For *half wave rectification*, the average current is $0.318I_0$, and for *full wave rectification* the average current is $0.636I_0$.

If an alternating current flows through a resistor the average current is zero, but the heating effect is not. On each pass through the resistor, the electrons heat it slightly, whatever the direction of flow. Clearly, despite the zero net current, some energy is expended in the circuit, and an *effective current* is defined to account for this. The effective current (also known as the *root mean square* (RMS) *current*, I_{RMS}), is the value of the constant current that, if allowed to flow for the same length of time, would expend the same amount of electrical energy for a fixed voltage as the alternating current. An *effective voltage* (root mean square (RMS) voltage, V_{RMS}) is defined, in a similar way, as the constant voltage that,

Figure 1.15   Capacitors in parallel.

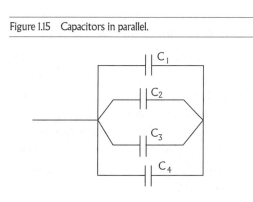

Figure 1.16   Rectification of an alternating current. (a) Unrectified wave. (b) Half wave rectification. (c) Full wave rectification.

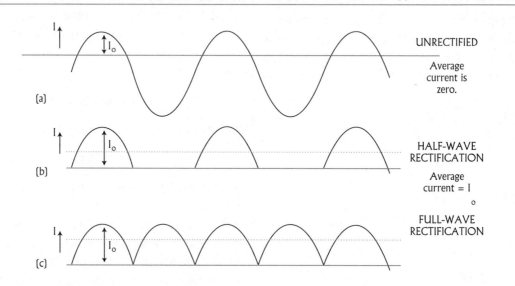

(a) UNRECTIFIED

Average current is zero.

(b) HALF-WAVE RECTIFICATION

Average current = I_o

(c) FULL-WAVE RECTIFICATION

if present for the same length of time, would expend the same amount of electrical energy for a fixed voltage as the alternating voltage.

From equation 16 the power, W, in DC circuits is given by:

$$W = VI,$$

where W is in watts, V is in volts, I is in amperes. Similarly, in an AC circuit:

$$W = V_{RMS}I_{RMS} \qquad (31)$$

Ohm's Law can be used if the effective currents and voltages are used. Thus the power may also be written:

$$W = I_{eff}^2R, \qquad (32)$$

or

$$W = V_{eff}^2/R. \qquad (33)$$

It can be shown that $I_{eff} = I_0/\sqrt{2} = 0.707I_0$ and that $V_{eff} = V_0/\sqrt{2} = 0.707V_0$.

Capacitors allow alternating currents to flow. Instead of talking about resistance across capaci-

tor plates, we talk about *impedance* (Z). This is defined as the ratio of the amplitudes of the voltage and current in the same way as resistance is given by V/R for direct current. It can be shown that:

$$Z = 1/\omega C, \qquad (34)$$

where C is the capacitance and ω (the *angular frequency*) = $2\pi f$.

Magnetism

Most of us have used a compass, and know that the needle swings around to point North-South. The compass is a permanent bar magnet that aligns itself with the earth's magnetic field.

There are two magnetic poles: the North and the South pole. In many ways, the two poles of a magnet act in the same way as opposite electric charges. Like magnetic poles repel each other, and unlike poles attract. There is a force between two magnets a distance d apart from each other, and the equation describing the force is very similar to that in equation 5:

$$F = m_1m_2/4\pi\mu d^2. \qquad (35)$$

Here, μ is the *permeability* of the medium, μ_0 (the permeability of free space) is used when the magnets lie in a vacuum. The strength of a magnet is measured in units of *webers* (Wb). The unit of permeability is the *henry/metre* (H/m). *Relative permeability*, μ_r, is defined by the relationship:

$$\mu_r = \mu/\mu_0. \qquad (36)$$

A *magnetic field* exists at a point if a small magnet put there experiences a force. It will line up along the *magnetic field lines*. The fields around some permanent magnets are shown in Figure 1.17.

The number of magnetic lines of force passing through an area, A, is known as the *magnetic flux* (N). The magnetic flux going through a unit area that is aligned perpendicular to the field is the *magnetic flux density* (B). Magnetic flux density is measured in units of *tesla* (T); 1 tesla = 1 Wb/m^2.

Electromagnetism

Wires carrying an electric current produce magnetic fields around them. The magnetic field around a long straight wire is in the form of concentric circles with the wire at their centre. A solenoid (coil of wire) creates a field somewhat similar to that produced by a permanent bar magnet, with the main difference being that there is a uniform field inside it. This uniformity of field is used to advantage in short wave diathermy applications. Figure 1.18 illustrates these fields.

ELECTROMAGNETIC SPECTRUM

Light is a form of electromagnetic radiation. It can be split up into its different component parts using a prism, with each colour of the 'rainbow' having a different wavelength. Electromagnetic waves are electric and magnetic fields that travel through space without the need for a medium to carry them (Figure 1.19). They travel at a speed of 3 $\times 10^8$ m/s in a vacuum. There is a whole spectrum

Figure 1.17 (a) Magnetic field around a single permanent bar magnet. (b) Magnetic field around two bar magnets.

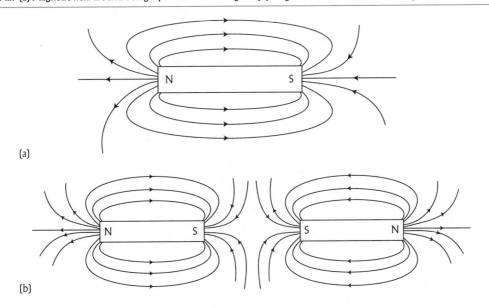

(a)

(b)

Figure 1.18 (a) Magnetic field around a long straight wire carrying an electric current. (b) Magnetic field around a coil carrying an electric current.

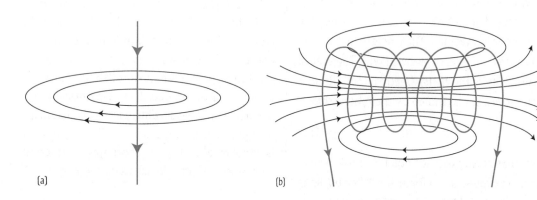

(a)   (b)

of such waves of which light is only a small part. Other radiations in the spectrum include radiowaves, microwaves and x-rays; the spectrum is shown in Figure 1.20. The behaviour of electromagnetic radiation can be usefully described, not only in terms of wave motion, but also in terms of 'particles'. It can be thought of as discrete 'packets' of energy and momentum, sometimes referred to as *quanta*. The energy in joules of a quanta of radiation is determined by its frequency, and is given by the equation:

$$E = h\nu, \qquad (37)$$

where ν is the frequency, and h is *Planck's constant* (h = 6.62×10^{-34} Js). It is more usual to quote electromagnetic energies in *electronvolts* (eV); 1 eV = 1.6×1.10^{-13} J. It can be seen from Figure 1.20 that energies at the long wavelength end of the spectrum are very small. It is generally thought that energies in excess of 30 eV are required to ionize atoms, and so this allows the spectrum to be classified in two bands: ionizing and nonionizing radiations.

The wavelength of the radiation determines the size of objects with which it will interact. A wave

Figure 1.19   An electromagnetic wave. Electric and magnetic fields travel together.

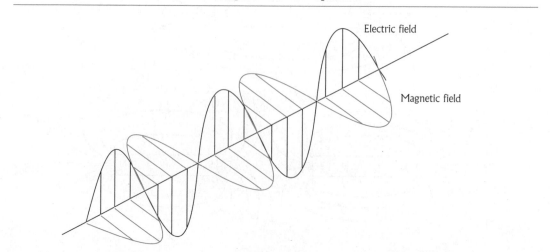

Electric field

Magnetic field

with a wavelength of 100 m (a radio wave) will not 'see' something of the size of an atom and will pass by undisturbed. However, a wave with a wavelength of 10^{-12} m (a γ ray) will interact with the atomic nucleus, to which it has a comparable size. Infrared radiation has a wavelength comparable to the size of an atom or molecule and so can interact with them, imparting kinetic energy (heat).

ELECTROMAGNETIC INDUCTION

The dynamo, on a bicycle wheel, that is used to power the bicycle's lights makes use of electromagnetic induction. Electromagnetic induction is in many ways the reverse of electromagnetism. When a magnet and a conducting wire move relative to one another, a current is induced in the wire. In the bicycle wheel, a magnet is made to rotate near a fixed coil of wire which forms part of

Figure 1.20 The electromagnetic spectrum.

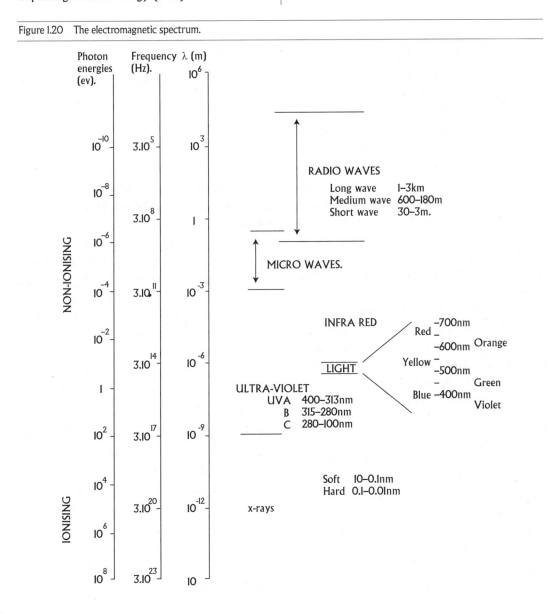

Figure 1.21   LC tuned circuits. (a) Series LC circuit. (b) Parallel LC circuit.

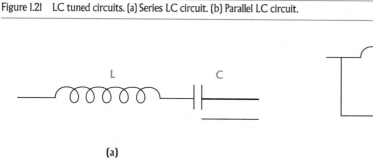

(a)

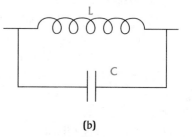

(b)

a circuit that includes the lamp bulb. Current is induced in the wire, and the lamp is lit.

The electrons in the wire approaching (or being approached by) a magnetic field experience a force as they enter the field. All of the electrons are displaced towards one end of the wire, so that end becomes negatively charged. Conversely, the other end takes up a positive charge. Therefore an electromotive force is induced between the two ends, and, if the circuit is completed, a current will flow. If the wire is coiled, the induced current is increased. We call a coil of conducting wire used in this way an *inductor*. The e.m.f. induced in the conductor equals the rate of change of flux linkage – this is *Faraday's Law* of electromagnetic induction. The direction of the induced current is always such that it opposes the change which caused it – *Lenz's Law*. In this sense, an inductor acts as a resistance in the circuit. They are often used to block changing voltages while allowing steady (DC) voltages through.

An inductor (L) and capacitor (C) are sometimes used in series or parallel to produce *LC tuned circuits* (Figure 1.21). It can be shown that these circuits have a resonant frequency, f, such that, for a series LC tuned circuit, it offers very low impedance to waves of that frequency, but has an extremely high impedance to everything else, and for a parallel LC tuned circuit it offers a very high resistance to waves of frequency f and allows other frequencies through. They therefore act as filters. The resonant frequency is given by the equation:

$$f = 1/2\pi\sqrt{(LC)}. \qquad (38)$$

MUTUAL INDUCTION

A changing magnetic field from a current-carrying conductor can induce an e.m.f. and current in a second conductor nearby. This current will vary, and in its turn can produce its own varying magnetic field that induces an e.m.f. and current in the first conductor. Each conductor therefore induces a current in the other (Figure 1.22). This is *mutual inductance*. The mutual inductance is 1 henry if one volt is induced in one conductor by a current change of one ampere per second in the other. An AC transformer makes use of mutual inductance.

SELF INDUCTANCE

When a current is switched into a coil, the growing current in the coil causes a change in magnetic flux in the coil. This, in turn, causes an e.m.f. that opposes the e.m.f. of the battery. This is called a *back* e.m.f. This effect is increased if there is a soft iron core in the coil.

A conductor has a self inductance of 1 henry if a back e.m.f. of 1 volt is induced by a changing current of 1 ampere/second.

Figure 1.22 Mutual induction. The changing magnetic field in one coil can induce a current in a second coil. The magnetic field thus created will create a current in the first coil. A soft iron core enhances this effect.

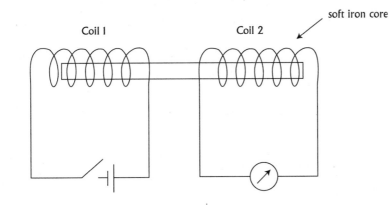

Mechanical Waves

The most important mechanical wave in physiotherapy is ultrasound. Sound waves differ from electromagnetic waves in one major way: the waves are a form of *mechanical energy*, and as such cannot propagate through a vacuum. The energy passes through a medium by the movement of molecules which transfer their momentum in the direction of the wave. Sound is produced by a moving surface; this may be a diaphragm in a loud speaker, for example, or a transducer front face in medical ultrasound. As the surface moves forward, it *compresses* the molecules immediately in front. These molecules in turn push forward against their neighbours in an attempt to restore their former arrangement, and these in turn push their neighbours. The compression therefore moves away from its source. If the surface now moves in the opposite direction, the density of the molecules is reduced next to it (a region of *rarefaction* is created), and so molecules move in to fill the space. This in turn leaves a low density region which is immediately filled by more molecules, and so the rarefaction moves away from the source. This has been illu-

strated in Figure 1.23. This type of wave is called a *longitudinal wave* because the displacement of the molecules is along the direction in which the wave moves.

Ultrasound

The velocity of sound in air is 330 m/s. The human ear can hear frequencies up to about 18 000 Hz (18 kHz). The wavelength of audible sound (calculated using equation 4) where the ear is most sensitive (about 1.6 kHz) is about 20 cm. At ultrasonic frequencies (above 18 kHz), the wavelength becomes so short that the sound does not travel far through air. (At 1.5 MHz, the wavelength is about 0.2 mm.) However, ultrasound will travel through water, a medium for which the sound velocity is 1500 m/s. At 1.5 MHz the wavelength is 1 mm. This fact is used in medicine since most body tissues are comprised mainly of water, and the millimetre wavelengths at the low megahertz frequencies used (0.75–10MHz) is comparable with the size of the tissue structures with which the interaction is required.

Ultrasound is generated from a transducer. A transducer is a device that transforms one form of energy into another. The transducer most

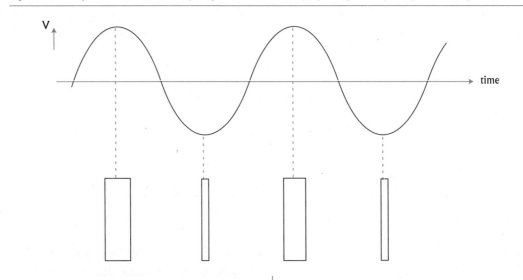

Figure 1.23 The piezoelectric effect. The crystal gets fatter and thinner, depending on the polarity of the voltage.

commonly used in ultrasound changes electrical energy into mechanical energy using the *piezo-electric effect*. A piezoelectric crystal has the property that if a voltage is applied across it, it will change its thickness, and alternatively if the crystal thickness is changed then a voltage develops across the crystal (this is the *inverse* piezoelectric effect). Thus, if an oscillating voltage is applied across the crystal it will alternately get thicker and thinner than its resting thickness, following the polarity of the voltage (Figure 1.23). As the front face of the transducer moves backwards and forwards, regions of compression and rarefaction move out from it, forming an ultrasonic wave. The piezoelectric material most commonly used for physiotherapy transducers is lead zirconate titanate (PZT).

The voltage across the ultrasound transducer may either be applied continuously over the whole treatment time (*continuous wave*, CW), or may be applied in bursts, on for a time, off for a time, and so on; this is known as *pulsed mode*. The wave trains for continuous wave and pulsed mode are shown in Figure 1.24.

In the pulsed mode, the pulsing regime may be described in one of three ways (Figure 1.24b):

1 x seconds on; y seconds off.
2 m:s, where m represents the 'mark' and s represents the 'space', where the ratio represents that of the on time to the off time; this is called the *mark:space ratio*. So, if x is twice y, m:s is 2:1. In order to discover the true pulsing regime, it is also necessary to know the pulse length.
3 The *duty cycle*: this is the pulse length as a percentage of the total on and off time, so it is given by $x/(x + y) \times 100\%$.

Take, for example, a common pulsing regime as shown in Figure 1.25. This may be described as 2 ms on:8 ms off, as 1:4 mark:space ratio, pulse length 2 ms, or as a 20% ($2/10 \times 100\%$) duty cycle. It is worth noting that, at 1 MHz, a pulse of length 2 ms contains 2000 cycles.

Intensity

The energy in an ultrasound wave is characterized by *intensity*. This is the energy crossing a unit area perpendicular to the wave in unit time; the units

Figure 1.24 (a) Continuous wave ultrasound (b) Pulsed ultrasound. In this example, the sound is on for x seconds, and off for y seconds.

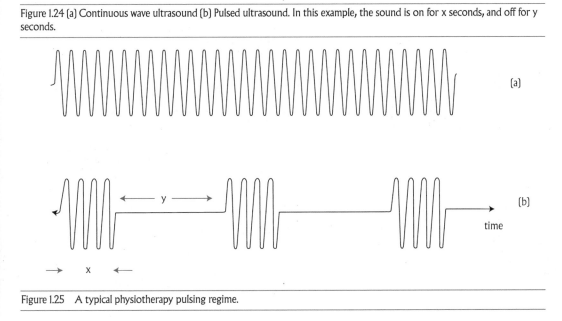

(a)

(b)

time

y

x

Figure 1.25   A typical physiotherapy pulsing regime.

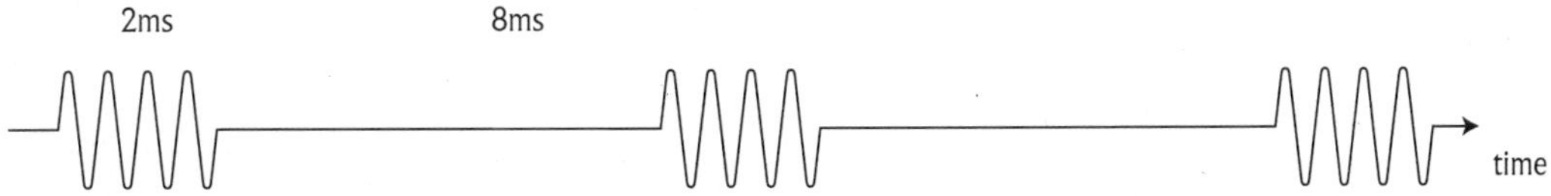

2ms   8ms

time

used are *watts/m²*. However, for medical applications, the square metre is an inappropriately large area in terms of regions of the human body to be treated, and so the unit used in medical ultrasound is watts/cm².

Several types of intensity are used to describe ultrasound exposures. The field from a circular piezoelectric disc is complex. Near the transducer there are many peaks and troughs, but as the beam moves further from the transducer the field pattern becomes more uniform. The region near the transducer is known as the *near field* or *Fresnel zone*; the region beyond that is called the *far field* or *Fraunhoffer zone*. The boundary between the two zones is at a distance given by r^2/λ where r is the transducer radius and λ is the wavelength of the ultrasound. This is the position of the peak of intensity on the beam axis that is furthest from the transducer. Physiotherapy

ultrasound commonly operates at 0.75, 1.0, 1.5 or 3 MHz. The extent of the near field is shown in Table 1.1, p. 29 for a number of frequencies and transducer sizes. This demonstrates that most physiotherapy ultrasound exposures are carried out in the near field, which has many peaks of intensity. It also indicates that a number of intensities need to be identified.

The transverse field profiles shown in Figure 1.27 illustrate the problem. Both profiles have the same peak intensity I_0, but the levels are rather different if they are averaged over the whole beam. Peak levels are the most significant parameter if the beam is held stationary over one tissue volume for a long time, but if the transducer is kept in continuous motion, the average value becomes more important as this is what the tissue will experience. In a continuous wave field therefore, two intensities are defined, the *spatial peak*

Figure 1.26 (a) Transverse intensity distributions at different distances from the transducer. (b) Intensity distribution on axis.

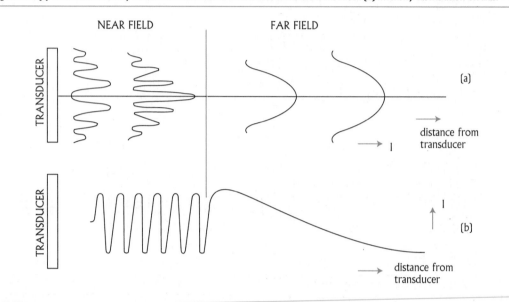

Figure 1.27 (a) Example of a transverse beam profile in the near field. (b) Transverse beam profile in the far field. This has the same peak intensity as the profile in (a).

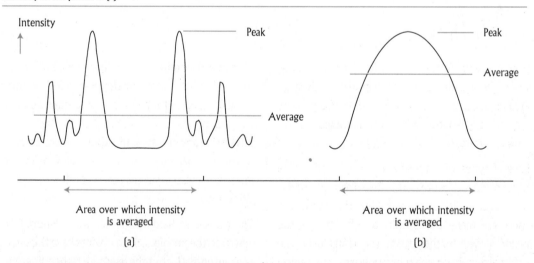

intensity (I_{SP}) and the *spatial average intensity* (I_{SA}). Things become more complicated in a pulsed field. Here, the analogy is of a boy standing up to his ankles in the sea. As the waves come in, the water rises up his legs, and drops again as the wave moves past, only to come up again on the next wave. There is a high water mark on the boy's legs, representing the highest point reached by the wave while he was standing there (the *temporal peak*) and there is an average water level experienced during the paddle (the *temporal average*). In the same way, a *temporal peak intensity* and a *temporal average intensity* can be identified as the highest intensity experienced at a point in tissue over a period of time, and the average intensity experienced at that point over a time, where the averaging is done over both on times and off times. If these temporal intensities are measured at the point in tissue where the spatial peak intensity is found, then a *spatial peak temporal peak intensity* (I_{SPTP}) and a *spatial peak, temporal average intensity* (I_{SPTA}) can be determined. If these temporal intensities are combined with spatial averaging, the *spatial average temporal average* (I_{SATA}) and *spatial average temporal peak intensities* (I_{SATP}) can also be defined. These are demonstrated in Figures 1.27 and 1.28.

For example, take a beam with $I_{SP} = 3\ W/cm^2$ and $I_{SA} = 2\ W/cm^2$ while the sound is on, pulsed 2 ms on, 8 ms off. Whatever the temporal peak, the temporal average will be 20% of this since the sound is only on for a fifth of the time. Thus, $I_{SPTP} = 3\ W/cm^2$, $I_{SPTA} = 0.6\ W/cm^2$, $I_{SATP} = 2\ W/cm^2$, $I_{SATA} = 0.4\ W/cm^2$.

The ultrasound field can also be described in terms of the pressures involved. It can be seen from Figure 1.29 that the pressure oscillates around the ambient level of the medium through which it passes. The field can therefore also be characterized in terms of *pressure amplitude* (usually the *peak positive pressure amplitude*, p_+, and the *peak negative pressure amplitude*, p_-) found anywhere in the field.

Intensity and pressure are related by the expression:

$$I = p^2/2\rho c, \qquad (39)$$

where ρ is the density, and c is the speed of sound in the medium.

Ultrasound interacts with tissue in several ways. The two mechanisms thought to be most important are heat and cavitation. Cavitation is the

Figure 1.28 Diagram to illustrate the different types of intensity. I_{SP}: spatial peak; I_{SA}: spatial average; I_{TP}: temporal peak; I_{SPTP}: spatial peak-temporal peak; I_{SPTA}: spatial peak-temporal average.

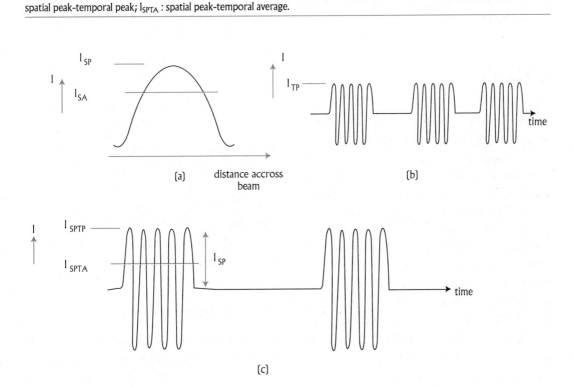

Figure I.29 An ultrasound exposure can be described in terms of pressure. The peak positive pressure amplitude, p_+, and the peak negative pressure amplitude, P_- are shown.

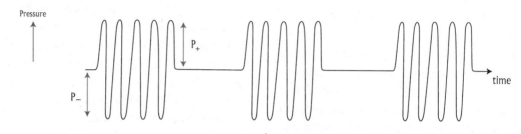

activity of bubbles in an ultrasonic field. The oscillating pressure can cause bubbles to grow, and to oscillate. An oscillating bubble causes the liquids around it to stream, and considerable shear stresses may occur. In some instances they may become *resonant*, in which case they start to oscillate unstably and may undergo violent collapse, causing tissue damage in their vicinity. When the amount of tissue heating is being considered, spatially-averaged intensities are the most relevant parameters. However, when cavitation is considered, it is the peak negative pressure that is the most relevant parameter.

Calibration

Ultrasound fields can be calibrated using a number of methods, depending on the information required. The pressure distribution can be mapped using a pressure sensitive PVDF (polyvinylidene-difluoride) membrane hydrophone which makes use of the inverse piezoelectric effect. Field plotting is a lengthy and detailed process usually undertaken by manufacturers or medical physics departments. It is always advisable to have had transducers calibrated in this way before use, and again when a fault is suspected. It provides an easy way of identifying damaged crystals. The calibration method of choice within a physiotherapy department should be a radiation pressure balance. When ultrasound hits a target in water, it exerts a force on the target (radiation

pressure) and tries to move it. If this is suitably counterbalanced, the radiation force can be calculated. This device averages over the target area, and allows a rapid assessment of reproducibility of output from day to day. This is an important check that should be incorporated into any treatment routine.

Reflection of ultrasound waves

Tissue offers resistance to the passage of ultrasound. This resistance is called the *acoustic impedance*, Z, and may be calculated from the expression:

$$Z = \rho c, \qquad (40)$$

where ρ is the density and c is the velocity of sound. The unit in which Z is measured is the *rayl*.

The amount of sound reflected from a plane surface between two materials of impedance Z_1 and Z_2 is $(Z_2 - Z_1)/(Z_2 + Z_1)$, and the amount of sound transmitted is $2Z_2/(Z_2 + Z_1)$. Water has an impedance of 1.5×10^6 rayl, fat has an impedance of 1.4×10^6 rayl, muscle of 1.7×10^6 rayl and bone of 7×10^6 rayl.

Attenuation

As ultrasound passes through tissue, some of the energy is reflected by the structures in the path (*scattering*), and some of the energy is

Figure 1.30   Ultrasound energy is attenuated exponentially as it travels through tissue. Bone attenuates most strongly.

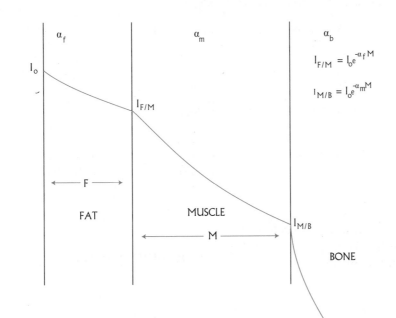

absorbed by the medium itself, leading to local heating (*absorption*). *Attenuation* (the loss of energy from the beam) is due to these two mechanisms, with absorption accounting for 60–80% of the energy loss. If the intensity incident on tissue is I_O, and the intensity after travelling through x cm of tissue is I, these are related by the expression:

$$I = I_0 \, e^{-ax}. \qquad (41)$$

The way in which the intensity drops as it goes through tissue is shown in Figure 1.30; this is known as *exponential decay*.

Attenuation coefficient values are often quoted in dB/cm/MHz or nepers/cm (1 dB/cm = 4.34 nepers/cm). The decibel (dB) represents a ratio of intensity levels such that the intensity level quoted in decibels is $10\log_{10} I_0/I$. It can be shown that when the intensity level is 3 dB, the ratio of

Table 1.1

Extent of near field for different ultrasound transducers.

Frequency MHz	r cm	$r^{2/\lambda}$ cm
0.75	0.5	1.25
	1.0	5
	1.5	11.25
1.0	0.5	0.6
	1.0	6.7
	1.5	15
1.5	0.5	2.5
	1.0	10
	1.5	22.5
3.0	0.5	5
	1.0	20
	1.5	45

r is the transducer radius; λ is the ultrasonic wavelength

Table 1.2
Tissue ultrasound attenuation coefficients and half value layers.

Tissue	Attenuation dB/cm/MHz	Half value layer at 1 MHz	Half value layer at 3 MHz
Blood	0.2	15 cm	5 cm
Fat	0.6	5 cm	1.6 cm
Liver	1.0	3 cm	1 cm
Muscle	1.3–3.3	1–2 cm	3–6 mm
Bone	20	1.5 mm	0.5 mm
Lung	41	0.7 mm	0.2 mm
Air	342 (1 MHz)	0.02 mm	
Water	0.002	1500 cm	500 cm

intensities is 2. The attenuation coefficient is quoted as a function of frequency, since they are approximately linearly related.

Table 1.2 shows relative attenuation coefficients for different biological tissues. Also shown are half-value thicknesses. This is the thickness of tissue needed to reduce the intensity by a factor two. It can be seen that bone and lung attenuate the sound very rapidly and very little energy gets into them. They are therefore not suited to physiotherapy ultrasound treatments. In fact, care should be taken when treating over such regions because the lost energy goes into heating the tissue locally. It can also be seen that the half-thickness layer decreases with increasing frequency and so, where deep treatments are required, low frequencies should be used.

Coupling Agents

It can be seen from Table 1.2 that megahertz frequency sound does not travel through air. Therefore, when a patient is being treated, it is essential for an effective treatment that no air comes between the transducer and the skin. There are a number of methods by which ultrasound is applied. The most common method is to use a 'contact' application, where a thin layer of oil or gel is applied to the skin prior to treatment. The requirement for the coupling medium is that it has a similar acoustic impedance to skin. Mineral oils and water-based gels are most commonly used. Awkward geometries can most readily be treated in a water bath, with both the limb to be treated and the transducer being immersed.

2

Electrical Properties of Cells and Tissues

ROBERT A CHARMAN

Introduction
•
Cells as Electrical Systems
•
The Cell as an Electrified System
•
The Electrical Properties of Tissues
•
The Electrical Cell and Electrotherapy

Introduction

Chapter 1 has introduced the basic concepts, units and laws of electrical theory and electromagnetism and explained how the construction and properties of common components of electrical and electronic circuitry, such as conductors, insulators, switches, semiconductors, resistors and capacitors are designed and connected in accordance with the appropriate theory.

Biological tissues seem so different in their wet and salty nature compared, for example, to the metallic wiring of a television set, that they would appear to have nothing in common. Yet the astonishing fact is that living cells are dependent upon electrical activity for their very existence and the tissues that they make, such as bone and fascia, exhibit a wide range of electrical properties. The same theory applies to their use of electrical components. They obey the same laws and use the same units of, for example, voltage, capacitance, current flow, and resistance.

As will be seen, the main difference between electricity in biological tissues and electricity in equipment is that cells and tissues use charged atoms, or *ions*, for the movement of charge whereas electrical and electronic systems use electrons.

With this relationship between biological tissues and electrical circuitry in mind, the rest of this chapter will be devoted to biological electricity, or *bioelectricity*.

Cells as Electrical Systems

Living cells employ many of the properties of electrical systems. For example, they generate electromotive force (e.m.f.), maintain a required potential difference (p.d.) between two points, increase or decrease that p.d. as necessary, use varying resistances in series and in parallel, switch current on and off, control current flow, rectify current flow, possess impedance and, of crucial importance, store charge (i.e. exhibit capacitance).

The average body cell, with all of its ordered complexity and function (Figure 2.1), is between 10 and 50 μm in diameter (μm = 1 micrometer = 1 millionth, or 10^{-6} of a metre). This means that it is some 5–20 times smaller than the smallest particle that the eye can see — a scale

Figure 2.1   Composite diagram of main cell structures which will vary according to cell type. Named structures are discussed in text. (After Gray's Anatomy.)

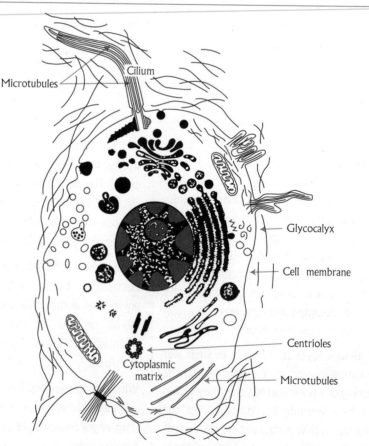

of miniaturization approached only by very advanced microchip construction.

Cells are *wet circuits* that operate in a salty, conductive, medium. In electrical terms, cells have the great advantage of being very compact and thus having extremely short conducting pathways (about 10–20 nanometres; 1 nm = 10^{-9}m) but, against that, they work under some major disadvantages when compared to ordinary electrical and electronic circuitry, they must:

- Continually make and replace all of their electrical components;
- Continually work to generate and maintain regions of differing electrical properties against continual leakage of charge;
- Continually control rates of desired current flow against possible shorting of current;
- Continually work to prevent unwanted current flow when a pathway is switched off.

The ceaseless work involved in achieving and maintaining these essential electrical needs consumes some 50–60% of the metabolic activity of a cell (Alberts *et al.*, 1989).

In marked contrast, ordinary circuits are *dry circuits*, so there is a clear distinction between conducting and non-conducting components. They carry the advantages that:

- The components need only occasional replacement;
- They can store and move charge without leakage;
- Energy is required only when the circuit is in use. For example, no work is required to resist an externally applied e.m.f. (such as the mains supply) when the circuit is switched off because the e.m.f. is passively resisted by the non-conducting properties of the 'off' switch insulator. In contrast, cells have to use active electrical pumps against

the e.m.f. in order to maintain the desired p.d. and prevent current leakage.

Another major difference lies in the type of charge used: ordinary circuits use electrons, which have negligible mass, are highly mobile, and have a diameter some 100 000 times smaller than an atom (10^{-15} m compared to 10^{-10} m). Cells use atoms that have become charged as a result of gaining, or losing, valency shell electrons. Compared to an electron, charged atoms (i.e. ions), are very 'heavy', because of the masses of the protons and neutrons found in each ion's nucleus. For example, the single proton nucleus of the hydrogen ion (H^+, mass 1u; u = 1 atomic mass unit) has about 2000 times the mass of an electron, and the two main ions used by cells to store charge and generate e.m.f., namely sodium ions (Na^+, mass 23u) and potassium ions (K^+, mass 39u), are some 46 000 times and 78 000 times, respectively, more massive than an electron, yet possess only the same unit charge as a single electron (as they have each lost only one electron from their outer electron shell).

Another disadvantage for the cell is that all ions in solution are *hydrated* ions. This means that each ion is surrounded by polar water molecules (H_2O) that are attracted to the ion by their own, very weak polarity. For cations (which are positive), such as N^+ and K^+, water molecules orientate themselves so that the weak negativity of their oxygen atoms are closest to the positive ion; for anions (which are negative), the weak positivity of the water molecule's hydrogen atoms lies closest to the negative ion. Thus every hydrated ion, whether positive or negative, is closely surrounded by a cluster of water molecules. When ions pass through the very narrow ion channels in the cell membrane, whether by diffusion along electrochemical gradients or by active transport, the weak hydration bonds of the water cluster are broken as the H_2O molecules are 'scraped off' the ion as it moves through the membrane channel (Alberts *et al.*, 1989).

The relatively unwieldy masses and sizes of ions mean that they require far more energy to control their movement, and accelerate much more slowly along a given p.d. gradient than do electrons. This is one reason why cellular ionic changes tend to have submillisecond to millisecond (10^{-3} s) response times, in contrast to the nanosecond (10^{-9} s) to attosecond (10^{-18} s) response times achievable in electronic circuitry.

Cellular Circuit Components

The main components used by the cell are membranes, ion pumps, and ion diffusion channels.

MEMBRANES AS CAPACITOR PLATES

Cell membranes are between 5 and 7.5 nm thick, and are composed of a highly mobile but closely packed array of proteolipid molecules arranged as a bilayer, with their lipid tails forming a central zone (Figure 2.2) that is resistant to the passage of electricity and can act as an insulator. The plasma membrane forms the surface boundary of the cell, and the intracellular membranes enclose each of the cell's organelles, with a double membrane being present around the nucleus. A cell membrane, by means of selective permeability to Na^+ and K^+ ions (being relatively impermeable to Na^+ ions but more permeable to K^+ ions), causes its outer surface to have a higher positive charge than its inner surface – there are greater numbers, or densities, of Na^+ and other cations per unit area on the outside surface than there are K^+ on the inner surface. This charge separation results in an average p.d. across the membrane of 80 mV, with the inner surface being relatively *negatively* charged in comparison to the outer surface. Figure 2.3 illustrates the relative differences in cation concentrations on either side of the cell membrane; the 80 mV e.m.f. across the membrane as shown by the arrow.

Figure 2.2 Fluid mosaic of cell membrance. Note the transmembrane receptor protein, attached to the branched glycolipid array, and the charged surface. (After Thibodeau, 1987.)

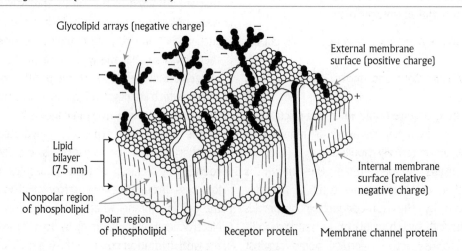

Glycolipid arrays (negative charge)

External membrane surface (positive charge)

Lipid bilayer (7.5 nm)

Nonpolar region of phospholipid

Polar region of phospholipid

Internal membrane surface (relative negative charge)

Receptor protein

Membrane channel protein

Figure 2.3 Schematic diagram illustrating the relative negativity of cations inside the plasma membrane compared to cations on the outside, the resulting transmembrane e.m.f. at a given p.d. in millivolts, and the resistance offered by the central lipid layer acting as an insulator and the Na$^+$ force of the Na$^+$/K$^+$ pump.

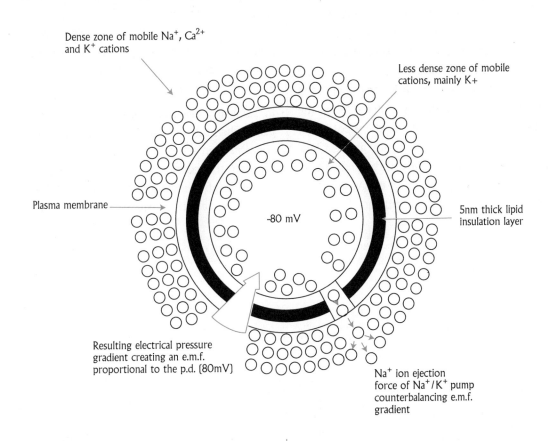

Dense zone of mobile Na$^+$, Ca^{2+} and K$^+$ cations

Less dense zone of mobile cations, mainly K+

Plasma membrane

-80 mV

5nm thick lipid insulation layer

Resulting electrical pressure gradient creating an e.m.f. proportional to the p.d. (80mV)

Na$^+$ ion ejection force of Na$^+$/K$^+$ pump counterbalancing e.m.f. gradient

'Positive' and 'negative' are *relative* terms in electricity. They can mean either a difference of separate positive charge and negative charge concentrations between two points in a circuit, or a *relative* difference in concentration of the same type of charge between two points in a circuit, one point having less charge per unit volume or area than another and therefore being relatively less positive or negative. In ordinary electrical circuits, an e.m.f. is created by a difference of electron (i.e. negative charge) concentration between two points because electrons are the only type of charge that can travel along metal conductors. In cells, the gradient difference is created by separating cations into different concentration strengths either side of a membrane. This separation is also backed up by differences in negatively charged ions inside and outside of the cell.

ION PUMPS

Because fluid filled ion channels are relatively leaky, ion separation across a membrane is controlled by directional ion pumps, such as the Na$^+$/K$^+$ pumps that eject two Na$^+$ ions out of the cell for every K$^+$ ion coming into the cell, to maintain the charge separation across the width of the membrane. Another vitally important ion pump is the Ca^{2+} ion pump that keeps Ca^{2+} ions outside the cell at a concentration some 10 000 greater than inside the cell. Passive ion diffusion channels are controlled by varying the diameter and lining charge of the ion channel as necessary. Figure 2.4 summarizes the activity of these ion channels and pumps and is best read by starting at 'A' on the left-hand side of the diagram, where potassium ions are moving down an electrical gradient into the cell, and moving clockwise through the alphabet to 'K', where representative passive ion channels are shown. The transmembrane 75 mV p.d.

shown here is the resulting average e.m.f. generated by these ionic movements and acts, in effect, as a capacitor's store of charge that is available to do work. The 'bound cations' in the cell form a thin layer of potassium cations that are held to the boundary surface of the negatively charged cytosol by mutual attraction, and do not play any part in membrane ion-pump exchange.

In summary, cell membranes act as capacitor plates when they hold a difference in ion charge concentration across their width. The charge is held on the continuous insulator surface of plasma membranes between the pores of the ion pump channels that help to maintain it. Cell

Figure 2.4 Diagram summarizing plasma membrane K^+ leak channels, ion pumps, and ion channels. Total electrochemical equilibrium acts as an ion battery creating a resting potential across the membrane which is internally negative.

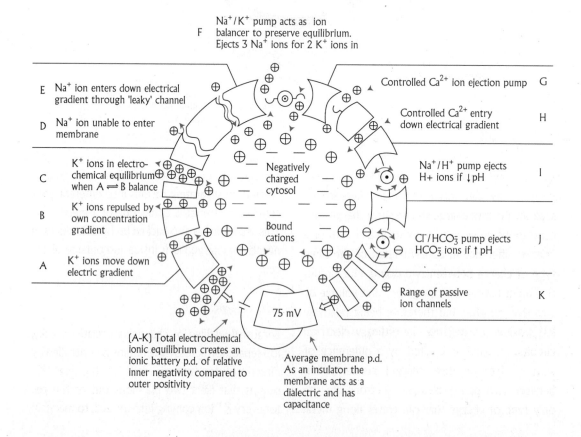

membrane charge is measured in picofarads (1 pF $= 10^{-12}$ F) and/or picocoulombs (pC).

In round figures, the quantity of electrons, or equivalent univalent (single charge) ions, in one coulomb (C) is 6×10^{18}. A farad is the equivalent unit of capacitance where one coulomb of charge creates a p.d. of 1 volt. This is a very large quantity of charge, and capacitors in ordinary circuits are usually rated in microfarads (μF) or picofarads (pF). A quantity of 1 pF is 6×10^6 univalent charges, and cells operate in quantities of a few pC of ions stored upon their membranes, and around 0.01–0.001 pC flowing through individual ion channels. The rate of ion flow (amperage) through individual ion channels is measured in nanoamperes (nA), and the sum rates of ion channel flow across all the membranes of a cell at any given moment, acting as resistances in parallel, is measured in microamperes (μA).

CELL MEMBRANE P.D.

Charge separation creates a p.d. and a resulting e.m.f. between the two areas of charge on either side of the plasma membrane. As this cannot discharge through the middle lipid layer of the membrane, it can be used to create a controlled driving force of ionic flow through the ionic channels. This force can be used as a transport system, and Na^+-ion exclusion from the cell helps to control cytoplasm osmolarity and cell volume. In neurones, the voltage-gated Na^+ pumps are used to transmit impulses. Depending upon the type of cell, membrane p.d.s range from between 10 and 200 mV across their diameter. These are very high voltages to sustain across an incredibly thin membrane of some 7.5 nm width, without breakdown, when the membrane consists only of freely mobile lipid molecules at 37°C undergoing constant thermal agitation. Scaled up into round figures by assuming a central lipid diameter of

5 nm, and an average membrane p.d. of 100 mV, this is the equivalent of an e.m.f. of 2×10^4 V/ mm. One millimetre is the average thickness of the insulation sleeves around the live, neutral and earth wires inside 13 A cabling. At equivalent cell membrane voltages, their sleeve insulator atoms would have to withstand an electron shell deformation force of some 20 000 V without breakdown by shorting, compared to the 230 V mains e.m.f. distortion force that they normally withstand.

The Cell as an Electrified System

This sounds very similar to discussing cells as electrical systems, and the phenomenon is based partly upon active charge separation as discussed in the previous section, but carries a more extended meaning and involves additional components of charge.

To consider the cell as an *electrified system* means considering it as an electrified, or charged, body with a surrounding electrical field that can influence other charged bodies, or objects. It also means looking at cell structure to see whether different components of the cell act as collective wholes that create clearly defined subzones of particular charge, or sign.

Every cell is an electrified resultant of two types of electrical phenomena. One has already been discussed, and this is the active creation by the cell of charged capacitor-like membrane surfaces through selective ion channel diffusion and ion pump maintenance. The second type concerns electrostatics: cell membranes can be considered in terms of electrostatics as their stored charge of inorganic ions creates an electrical field, consisting of an electric flux, or 'lines of force', radiating outwards from their surfaces. To this actively maintained surface charge must be added any organic molecules and compounds, such as proteins, amino acids, polysaccharides and simple sugars in the cytoplasm of the cell, that carry an overall charge and act collectively as an ionic mass. Some organic ions carry a positive charge but the majority are negative (Alberts, 1989). Furthermore, to these must be added those compound molecules that are electrically neutral, but carry charges of opposite sign at their ends – these are *dipoles*. Dipoles tend to rotate about their centre in reponse to an alternating field, and orientate themselves antiparallel to a site of opposite charge, as if pointing at it like a stick.

When the cell is considered in these terms it is found to possess an external charge relative to other charged bodies, and is cross-sectionally divided into four charged zones, two of relatively steady charge strength, and two that vary about a mean value. Figure 2.5 shows the cell as an *electrified system* and should be referred to when

reading the following description as it is a rather unusual way of looking at the cell. From the centre zone outwards, these four electrified zones are as follows:

1 *Central negative zone (steady charge).* This zone is the negatively charged mass of cytoplasm that includes negatively charged proteins, amino acids and other organic molecules, and maintains a steady bulk negativity.
2 *Inner positive zone (variable charge).* This consists of a thin zone of cations, mainly K^+ ions, which both 'coats' the outer surface of the central negative zone with a thin layer of cations (bound cations), and clusters along the inner surface of the plasma membrane as freely mobile cations that are available for transport in and out of the cell as required.
3 *Outer positive zone (variable charge).* This consists of a more extended, and more dense, zone of mobile cations, mainly Na^+ ions and Ca^{2+}

Figure 2.5 Schematic diagram of electrical zones of a cell. The membrane is relatively impermeable to Na^+ and Ca^{2+} ions, so the membrane p.d. has a relative inner negative.

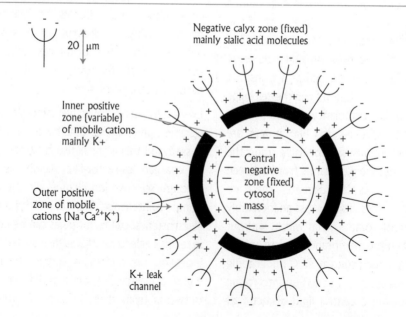

ions, with some K^+ ions, that cluster along the outer surface of the plasma membrane and are therefore extracellular.

4 *Outermost negative calyx zone (steady charge).* This outermost zone of steady negativity is separated from the outer positive zone of the plasma membrane by a distance of some 20 μm. It is created by negatively charged sialic acid molecules that tip many of the glycolipid arrays that project outwards from the surface of the cell like cactus branches. Many of these glycolipid structures are attached through the plasma membrane to the cell's microtubular framework (Figure 2.6). Microtubules are flexible hollow tubes, built from dipole-charged protein blocks like chimney bricks, that have an overall oppositely signed charge at each end, and are, therefore bipolar (i.e. dipoles). They radiate outwards from their centriole base near the central nucleus to the plasma membrane, and sometimes beyond. They help to give the cell shape, provide sites for enzymes, support the membrane, and act as active transport systems throughout the cytoplasm. In neurones they are the channels for axoplasmic flow.

It is this outermost calyx zone of steady negativity that makes each cell act as a negatively charged body; every cell creates a negatively charged field around itself that influences any other charged body close to it. This electrostatic field has important consequences. Although the field is very weak, cell calyx fields repulse each other, thus tending to maintain a 40 μm space between cells, except where there is actual junctional contact. All cellular tissue surfaces, such as the endothelial lining of the vascular system for example, carry a steady negative charge on their surfaces. In this example, the endothelial surface charge repulses the negatively charged blood cells, platelets and plasma proteins so that they are separated from the endothelium by a thin zone of pure plasma fluid. If the endothelium is damaged, the damaged area loses its negativity, allowing the platelets to adhere with consequent risk of thrombus formation (Marino, 1988).

Figure 2.6 Schematic of a cellular cytoskeleton membrane. M – cell membrane potential; GP – glycoprotein extending into extracellular space; MT – microtubule; MF – microfilaments (actin filaments or intermediate filaments); MTL – microtrabecular lattice. Cytoskeletal proteins that connect MT and membrane proteins include spectrin, fodrin, and ankyrin (Hameroff, 1987.)

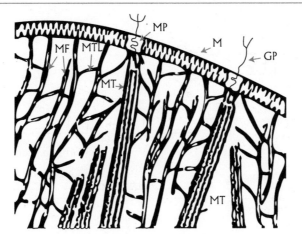

In addition to these four zones, it should be noted that the immediate inner surface of the plasma membrane carries an overall negative charge that holds an important enzyme, protein kinase C, against its surface until it is activated and released by an influx of Ca^{2+} ions to initiate cascade reactions within the cell.

The Electrical Properties of Tissues

All soft tissues include long-chain protein molecules such as collagen, elastin, and keratin in their structure; these molecules have a regular, repeating, subunit structure. Connective tissues, such as capsules, ligaments, fascia and tendon, consist of dense sheets of these molecules, especially collagen. Cartilage consists of collagen and proteoglycans, and bone is a calcified collagenous structure. All such tissue proteins possess one electrical feature in common: when they are mechanically distorted (strained) by an applied mechanical stress they develop *piezoelectric*-type p.d.s upon their external and internal surfaces (Becker and Marino, 1982; Black, 1989). Bone can be taken as a typical example of a tissue developing piezoelectric-like potentials when it is deformed, as shown in Figure 2.7. Surface voltages range from 10–150 mV and are proportional to the degree of strain deformation resulting from a given stress force acting upon the tissue.

Figure 2.7   Apparent piezoelectricity in bone. a) Typical piezocrystal response to momentary deformation; b) Similar transducing response in bone. c) Tension/compression surface potentials of opposite sign to resulting bone cell response. (After Becker and Selden, 1985.)

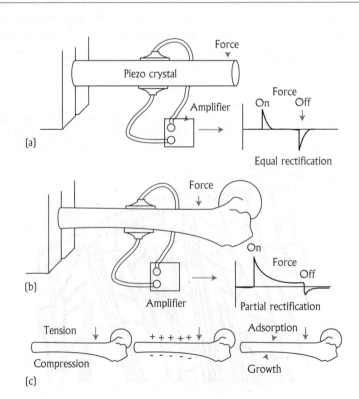

Many regular, lattice-type structures, such as the crystals used in ultrasound equipment and protein molecules, exhibit a piezo (pressure) – electric (surface potential) effect because the mechanical distortion of strain displaces some electrons towards the compressed surfaces (negative) and away from the stretched surfaces (positive). This phenomenon is more fully explained in the chapter on ultrasound therapy, where the crystal transduction of electrical and acoustic energy is discussed. This surface charge exists as long as there is distortion, and disappears when the stress is removed. If the stress force varies over time, so does the strength of the surface charge, so it will be synchronous with it.

Piezoelectric-type Tissue Surface Potentials

These surface p.d.s may either be termed stress- or strain-*related* potentials (SRPs), or stress- or strain-*generated* potentials (SGPs). The terms employed are usually defined in the particular text. Some authorities consider that the applied *stress* force should be considered as the primary cause of these surface p.d.s, whereas others consider that the resulting *strain distortion* is the direct cause. Whichever definition is followed, the p.d. is proportional to the stress or strain within the maximum that can be generated by the tissue. Each individual distorted protein molecule develops a p.d. and the surface tissue p.d. is the resultant sum of these individual contributions (Black, 1989).

Each time a bone, such as the femur, takes a weightbearing load it bends slightly. The compressed concave surface generates a *negative* p.d., and the stretched convex surface generates a *positive* p.d. The point charges are measured in pico coulombs as shown in Figure 2.8. A similar

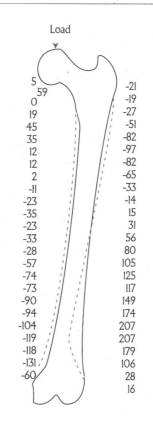

Figure 2.8   Charge distribution (pC/cm^2) along femoral surfaces on loading. Hatched outline is theoretical profile change of growth and resorption proportional to charge strength. (After Becker and Marino, 1982.)

effect occurs within fluid filled channels, such as the Haversian canals, where the surface p.d. is termed a *streaming potential*, as it is the p.d. between the charge generated on the tissue surface and the ionized fluid that is flowing past it. A very thin, electrically neutral, interface develops between the two p.d.s which is called the *slip plane*. In tendons, the tensile stress exerted by muscle contraction against the external load carried by the tendon between the muscle and its skeletal or fascial insertion, generates parallel planes of surface charge along its stretched length, and the same applies to all connective tissue.

The Electrical Cell and Electrotherapy

The first two sections show how basic electrical theory can be applied to cell structure and function by considering the living cell as an electrical system and as an electrified body, respectively. It helps to provide a framework for understanding how the physical effects of various forms of applied electrical, magnetic, electromagnetic and ultrasonic energy may be converted to physiological effects when absorbed by cells. It is particularly relevant to those modalities that evoke a variety of non-thermal cellular responses, such as low-frequency stimulation, and to those modalities that are claimed to possess, and may indeed possess, *non*-thermal effects in addition to any physiological effects resulting from tissue temperature rise following energy absorption from them, for example pulsed and continuous high-frequency fields.

What must always be borne in mind is that cells are functional wholes. To discuss them only in electrical terms is to abstract one aspect of their function, and any consequences arising from such electrical activity must be considered in their physiological context of change in metabolism and function.

The section on the known electrical properties of bone and soft tissues, as distinct from the living cells that manufacture them, is far less familiar. The probable reason for this is that the biological function and significance of these electrical effects are not known for certain, and many claims are hotly disputed. This uncertainty centres upon highly contentious issues concerning cellular responses to various forms of applied direct current, low-frequency currents and fields, high-frequency currents and fields, ultra-

sonic vibration, and pulsed low-energy laser radiation. These issues are discussed in more detail in their relevant chapters.

Leaving aside the *known* and undisputed cellular and body system responses to electrotherapy modalities as a consequence of, for example, heating, cooling, depolarization, mechanical vibration, and photochemical reactions, the unresolved question is whether cells can receive, decode, and act upon, specific frequencies, intensities and waveforms in the same way that they respond to, for example, the arrival of hormone molecules.

There are a number of questions that need to be asked:

- Can cells act as electrical receivers?
- Do they, like radio circuits, have 'frequency windows', which may change according to their metabolic needs during normal function, or when traumatized?
- Can they, in effect, scan incoming frequencies and tune their circuitry to resonate at particular frequencies?
- Can they distinguish between signals that convey *meaning* upon reception compared to random noise?
- Can cells distinguish, amplify, and use, very weak signals, perhaps a hundred to a thousand times weaker than normal membrane p.d.s (measured in microvolts rather than the millivolts of membrane p.d.s), that may be emitted by very active nearby cells in the form of *biophotons* (Kert and Rose, 1989)?
- Can cells respond to oscillatory electrical and/or magnetic fields that are emitted from environmental sources, such as mains cables, high-tension cables, and electronic equipment, which permeate the body by night and day?

If the answer to these questions is 'yes', then it means that particular forms of electrical and/or magnetic energy can act as incoming *first messengers*, like chemical molecules, and the cell will respond to them in a reasonably consistent way, as it does to, say, insulin or growth hormone. If this could be demonstrated beyond reasonable doubt, then *electromagnetic medicine*, as electrotherapy would become, would develop as a recognized specialty. It would be able to deliver measured doses of electrotherapy appropriate to the diagnosis of a wide range of disorders, as, for example, it does now when specific J/cm^2 dosages of UV-A radiation are applied to psoriatic skin in conjunction with psoralen drug therapy (PUVA).

A 'yes' answer also has deep implications concerning the possible role of naturally produced (endogenous) electricity. The *piezoelectric-type* tissue p.d. response to mechanical deformation offers an interesting, and unresolved, test case for discussion.

To those who consider that the evidence supports a working hypothesis that cells can interpret and respond to fluctuating patterns of external e.m.f. impinging upon their charged surfaces, these tissue p.d.s resulting from mechanical deforma-

tion are seen as a self-regulatory command system that instructs tissue cells what to do (Bassett, 1982; Becker and Marino, 1982; Becker and Selden, 1985; Becker, 1991; Black, 1989; Frochlich, 1988; Nordenstrom, 1983). According to this view, mechanical stress and the resulting strain distortion is transduced (a process of energy transformation) into patterns and intensities of surface p.d.s proportional to localized strain deformation. These p.d.s act as a signalling system upon adjacent cells, such as fibrocytes in tendons, chondrocytes in cartilage, and osteoblasts and osteoclasts in bone, *instructing* them to increase/decrease, tissue formation, or increase/decrease tissue absorption, as a response to the imposed mechanical stress. Thus, bone and tendon becomes proportionally thicker with increased load-bearing stress through exercise because the cells have 'read' the proportional intensity and frequency of tissue generated surface p.d.s. Bone, for example, can undergo extensive remodelling in response to sustained changes in load. Figure 2.9 provides a diagrammatic sumary of this hypothesis and should be read clockwise, starting from the initiating agent of mechanical stress.

Figure 2.9 Summary of the role of strain-generated potentials in bone and, by implication, cartilage and connective tissue adaptation to mechanical stress – Wolff's Law control system. (From Becker and Marino, 1982.)

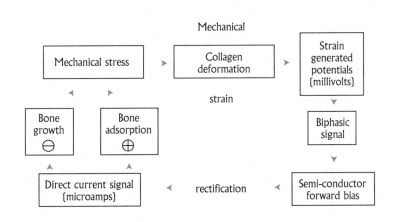

Conversely, the osteoporosis and connective tissue thinning associated with disuse is interpreted from this viewpoint as a lack of stress-induced p.d. stimulus to the cells, with consequent loss of rate of tissue replacement compared to rate of absorption. The late stage of post-fracture remodelling, in this view, is programmed by the intensity distribution of fracture site p.d.s, as shown in Figure 2.10. The important point here is that the remodelling in this case *straightens* the femoral shaft against the compressional forces of weightbearing that should, by mechanical loading, *increase* the deformity of the malleable bone. The argument of those who consider that these tissue p.d.s act as an important information and control system is that the cells, as in this example, are responding to the p.d. intensity gradient created by the stress force and not to the stress force in itself.

Suggested mechanisms whereby tissue p.d.s may act as first messengers are that they may activate ion channels, such as Ca^{2+}, which is an important second messenger that can initiate,

through protein kinase C, specific enzyme cascades within the cell, or be picked up by the charged glycolipid strands that project outwards from the cell, and then conveyed into the cell via connecting microtubule dipoles and 'read off' by enzyme systems attached to the microtubules as shown in Figure 2.6.

A recent theory concerning the possibility that very weak signals, such as electromagnetic fields, or cellular emission of biophotons, can be detected by cells is that the intrinsic random 'noise' energy created by the ceaseless activity of membrane ion channels may be *entrained* by very weak, incoming, oscillatory signals to create strong signals at the same frequency (Wiesenfeld and Moss, 1995). In effect, the random fluctuations of membrane noise energy is converted to strong, regular oscillations that can modify cell behaviour. This random-noise to controlled-signal conversion is known as *stochastic* (random noise) *resonance* (oscillatory frequency), or SR, and its magnitude can be expressed as a signal strength-

Figure 2.10   Adaptive remodelling of fracture mal-union under control of stress-generated potential polarity; concave surface negativity stimulates new bone, and convex surface positivity stimulates bone resorption (postulated feedback control system). (After Black, 1987.)

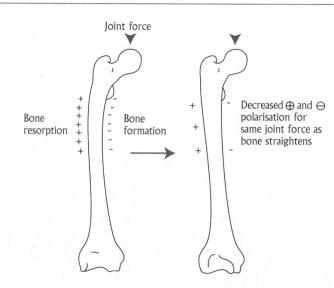

to-noise ratio, or SNR. If, for example, these were shown to be at the same resonant frequency as the mechanical, electroconformational, changes of transmembrane proteins that control the movement of charge across the membrane, then they could act as *first messengers.*

Another contentious example is the undoubted evidence that a wide range of microampere currents ebb and flow through the body along tissue channels connecting areas of differing metabolic activity (Becker, 1991; Borgens *et al.*, 1989; Nordenstrom, 1983). Areas of raised metabolic activity are electrically negative relative to areas of low metabolic activity, and currents flow through, and around, localized areas of tissue trauma and healing. Most standard authorities see these currents, if they recognize their existence at all, as by-products of little significance. Others, as cited above, see them as an essential guiding and regulatory component of body function that works in synergy with the nervous system, vascular system and hormonal system. Nordenstrom (1983), for example, refers to them as a circulatory system that is additional to the former systems. He has modelled the body as an electrical circuit system in which sheets of connective tissue, as in organ capsules, fascial planes, and the vascular system, act as relative insulators, and ionic tissue fluids act as ionic currents that can convey charged substances, such as nutrients and waste products to and fro, and alter tissue osmotic pressures. Nordenstrom considers the enclosed blood circulatory system as at zero electrical potential, analogous to 'earth' in electrical systems, and all other tissues as at a relative positive or negative p.d. to it, according to their level of metabolism. The capillaries are the variable resistance points through which ionic currents between tissues and blood plasma can flow according to their relative difference in potential.

There is considerable evidence (Borgens *et al.*, 1989; O'Connor *et al.*, 1990) to show that electrical tissue gradients during embryonic development act as directional growth markers, that injured tissues generate so called 'injury currents' which stimulate repair processes and that wound healing in skin, as a particular example, is more efficient if the area is kept moist so that microampere currents, driven by e.m.f.s generated by the epidermal layers, can flow across it.

Despite the experimental evidence that seems to support the idea that tissue surface p.d. generation act as a self-regulating control system, most authorities, including, it seems, those who write the standard texts, take a cautious 'non-proven' stance. They are sceptical of theories that equate the properties of recognized cell electrophysiology with ordinary, or solid state, circuitry analogies, and make scant reference to the subject.

References

Alberts B, Bray D, Lewis J, Raff M, Roberts K, Watson D (1989) *Molecular Biology of the Cell*, 2nd edn. Galtand Publishing Inc. New York.

Bassett, CAL (1982) Pulsing electromagnetic fields: a new method to modify cell behaviour in calcified and non calcified tissues. *Calcified Tissue International* 34: 1–8.

Becker, RO, Marino, AA (1982) *Electromagnetism and Life.* State University of New York Press, USA.

Becker, RO, Selden, G (1985) *The Body Electric: Electromagnetism and the Foundation of Life.* W Morrow and Co., New York.

Becker, RO (1991) *Cross Currents.* Bloomsbury, London.

Black, J (1991) *Electrical Stimulation: Its role in growth, repair and remodelling of the musculoskeletal system.* Praeger, New York.

Borgens, RB, Robinson, KR, Vanable, JW, McGinnis, ME (1989) *Electrical Fields in Vertebrate Repair.* Alan R Liss Inc., New York.

Charman, RA (1990) Introduction. Part 1: The electric cell. *Physiotherapy.* 76(9): 502–508.

Charman, RA (1990) Part 2: Cellular reception and emission of electromagnetic signals. *Physiotherapy.* 76(9): 509–516.

Charman, RA (1990) Part 3: Bioelectrical potentials and tissue currents. *Physiotherapy* 76(10): 643–654.

Charman, RA (1990) Part 4: Strain generated potentials in bone and connective tissue. *Physiotherapy* 76(11): 725–730.

Charman, RA (1990) Part 5: Exogenous currents and fields – experimental and clinical applications. *Physiotherapy* 76(12): 743–750.

Charman, RA (1991) Part 6: Environmental currents and fields — the natural background. *Physiotherapy* **77**(1): 8–14.

Charman, RA (1991) Part 7: Environmental currents and fields — man made. *Physiotherapy* **77**(2): 129–140.

Charman, RA (1991) Part 8: Grounds for a new paradigm? *Physiotherapy* **77**(3): 211–216.

Charman, RA (1991) Bioelectromagnetics Bookshelf. *Physiotherapy* **77**(3): 217–221.

Frochlich, H (ed) (1988) *Biological Coherence and Response to External Stimuli.* Springer-Verlag, Heidelberg.

Kert, J, Rose, L (1989) *Clinical Laser Therapy: Low level laser therapy.* Scandinavian Medical Laser Technology, Copenhagen.

Marino, AA (1988) *Modern Bioelectricity.* Marcel Dekker Inc., New York.

Nordenstrom, BEW (1983) *Biologically Closed Circuits: Clinical, experimental and theoretical evidence for an additional circulation.* Nordic Medical Publications, Stockholm, Sweden.

O'Connor, ME, Bentall, RHC, Monahan, JC (eds) (1990) *Emerging Electromagnetic Medicine.* Springer-Verlag, New York.

Thibodeau, GA (1987). *Anatomy and Physiology.* Times Mirror / Mosby College Publishing, St Louis, New York.

Wiesenfield, K, Moss, F (1995) Stochastic resonance and the benefits of noise: from ice ages to crayfish and SQUIBS. *Nature* **373**: 33–36.

3

Tissue Repair

SHEILA KITCHEN AND STEVE YOUNG

Introduction
•
The Principles of Tissue Healing
•
Repair of Specialized Tissues

Introduction

Physiotherapists treat both acute and chronic inflammatory lesions, open and closed wounds, and problems associated with the healing process, such as oedema and haematomas. Use is made of a wide variety of electrophysical agents to initiate or enhance the repair process, including ultrasound, the diathermies, lasers, and low-frequency stimulating currents. In order to understand how electrophysical agents may affect the healing of tissues and the rationale underlying their selection and application, it is essential that the processes underlying healing be considered.

Healing is a complex but essential process without which the body would be unlikely to survive. It involves the integrated actions of cells, matrix and chemical messengers and aims to restore the integrity of the tissue as rapidly as possible. It is a homeostatic mechanism to restore physiological equilibrium, and may be initiated as a result of loss of communication between adjacent cells, between cells and their support, or by cell death. Healing can be described in terms of chemokinesis, cell multiplication and differentiation. A complex series of events occurs, involving the migration of cells of vascular and connective tissue origin to the site of injury. This process is governed by chemotactic substances liberated *in situ*. The healing process, which is common to all body tissue types, may be divided into three overlapping phases:

1 Inflammation;

2 Proliferation;

3 Remodelling.

Healing of all tissue is based upon these phases and normally results in the formation of scar tissue. Limited regeneration of certain tissues such as the epidermis, skeletal muscle and adipose tissue may also occur. The basic principles that underlie repair which lead to scar formation will first be described; subsequently, a brief summary of the regenerative healing of epidermal and muscular tissue is provided.

The Principles of Tissue Healing

Inflammatory Phase

Inflammation is the immediate response to injury. The cardinal signs of inflammation are redness, swelling, heat and pain. The acute, or early, phase of inflammatory response lasts between 24 and 48 hours and is followed by a subacute, or late, phase which lasts between 10 and 14 days. The subacute phase can be extended if there is a continuing source of trauma or if some form of irritation, such as a foreign body or infection, is present.

Tissue injury causes both cell death and blood vessel disruption. The primary purpose of the inflammatory phase of healing is to rid the area of debris and dead tissue and to destroy any invading infection prior to the repair. This phase may be described in terms of vascular and cellular changes which are mediated through the actions of chemical agents.

VASOREGULATION AND BLOOD CLOTTING

The initial vascular reaction involves haemorrhage and fluid loss due to destruction of vessels; vasoconstriction, vessel plugging, and blood coagulation follow, to prevent further blood loss.

These processes lead to the activation of the repair process. Blood loss into the tissues initiates platelet activity and blood coagulation directly, both of which then result in the production of chemical factors which initiate and control the healing process. In addition, the blood clot provides a provisional matrix which facilitates the migration of cells into the wound (Clark, 1991).

Primary vessel constriction occurs, and is due to the release of norepinephrine; this reaction lasts only for a few seconds to a few minutes. During vasoconstriction the opposing cell walls are brought into contact, and adhesion between the surfaces results. Secondary vessel vasoconstriction may follow, due to the action of serotonin, adenosine diphosphate, calcium and thrombin.

Both lymphatics and blood vessels are plugged in order to limit fluid loss. Initial platelet adhesion and aggregation is stimulated by the presence of thrombin (Terkeltaub and Ginsberg, 1988). The platelets adhere to one another, to the vessel walls and to the interstitial extracellular matrix, leading to the build up of relatively unstable platelet plugs (Clark, 1991). The process is continued and consolidated by the release of adhesive proteins such as fibrinogen, fibronectin, thrombospondin and von Willebrand factor by the platelets (Ginsberg *et al.*, 1988).

Coagulation of extravascular blood is thought to be due to the action of platelets and intrinsic and extrinsic clotting mechanisms. Prothrombin is converted to thrombin and thus fibrinogen to fibrin, providing an early wound matrix.

Blood coagulation not only aids haemostasis through clot formation, but adds to the early wound matrix and results in the generation of chemical mediators such as bradykinin (Proud and Kaplan, 1988). These substances affect the local circulation, stimulate the production of further chemical mediators and act as attractants to cells such as neutrophils and monocytes (Clark, 1990a).

Following this period of vasoconstriction, secondary vasodilation and increased permeability of venules occurs due to the effects of histamine, prostaglandins and hydrogen peroxide production (Issekutz, 1981; Williams, 1988). Subsequently, both bradykinin and the anaphylatoxins initiate mechanisms which increase the permeability of undamaged vessels, leading to the release of plasma proteins which contribute to the generation of the extravascular clot.

CELL MIGRATION AND ACTION

Neutrophils and monocytes are the earliest cells to reach the site of injury. They migrate in response to a wide variety of chemical and mechanical stimuli, including the products of the clotting mechanism, the presence of bacteria and cell-derived factors.

The neutrophils' primary action is phagocytosis, and their task is to rid the site of bacteria and of dead and dying materials. Neutrophilic margination within the vascular structures leads to the passage of neutrophils through vessel walls by amoeboid action, enabling them to reach damaged extravascular tissues. Phagocytosis is achieved by neutrophilic lysis. This results in the release of protease and collagenase which begin the lysis of necrotic protein and collagen respectively, as shown in Figure 3.1. Infiltration of the neutrophils into the extravascular tissue ends after a couple of days, marking the end of the early phase of inflammation.

Macrophages are essential to the healing process and can perform the normal function of neutrophils in addition to their other tasks. Monocytes migrate from the vasculature into the tissue space and rapidly differentiate into macrophages; the factors responsible for this change have not been fully identified, but may include the presence of insoluble fibronectin (Hosein *et al.*, 1985), low oxygen tension (Hunt, 1987), chemotactic agents (Ho *et al.*, 1987) and the presence of bacterial lipopolysaccharides and interferons (Riches, 1988). Macrophages phagocytose pathogenic organisms, tissue debris and dying cells (including neutrophils), and release collagenase and proteoglycan, both of which are degrading enzymes that lyse necrotic material (Leibovich and Ross, 1975; Tsukamoto *et al.*, 1981).

CHEMICAL FACTORS

Many factors that influence and control the initial inflammatory process and trigger further developments in the proliferative phase are released by cells during the stage of inflammation. Macrophages release factors which attract fibroblasts to the area (Tsukamoto *et al.*, 1981) and enhance collagen deposition (Weeks, 1972; Clark, 1985). Platelets release growth factors which contribute to the control of fibrin deposition, fibroplasia and angiogenesis through their action on a variety of cells (Clark, 1991). Platelets also release fibronectin, fibrinogen, thrombospondin and von Willebrand factor (Ginsberg *et al.*, 1988); these are necessary for the aggregation of platelets and for their binding to tissue structure. In addition, serotonin, adenosine diphosphate, calcium and thromboxin are released; these are necessary for blood vessel constriction to prevent haemorrhage (Clark, 1991).

Dead and dying cells release substances which influence the development of the neomatrix;

Figure 3.1 Phagocytosis. (a) In phagocytosis, cells such as neutrophils and macrophages ingest large solid particles such as bacteria and dead and dying material. (b) Folds of the plasma membrane surround the particle to be ingested, forming a small vacuole around it which then pinches off inside the cell. (c) Lysosomes may fuse with the vacuole and pour their digestive enzymes (such as protease and collagenase) onto the digested / ingested material.

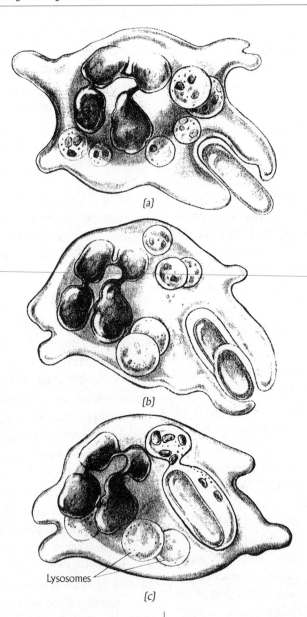

[a]

[b]

Lysosomes

[c]

these include a variety of tissue factors, lactic acid, lactate dehydrogenase, calcium, lysosomal enzymes and fibroblast growth factor (Clark, 1990a). In addition, prostaglandins (PG) are produced by almost all cells of the body following damage, due to alterations in the phospholipid content of the cell walls (Janssen *et al.*, 1991); some types of PG are proinflammatory, increasing vascular permeability, sensitizing pain receptors and attracting leucocytes to the area. Other classes of PG may be anti-inflammatory. Both may be involved in early stages of repair.

Proliferative Phase

Granulation tissue is formed during the proliferative phase. This is a temporary structure that evolves after a period of a couple of days and comprises neomatrix, neovasculature, macrophages and fibroblasts. Granulation tissue precedes the development of mature scar tissue. 'Fibroplasia' is a term that encompasses the processes of fibroblast proliferation and migration, and the development of the collagenous and non-collagenous matrices.

FIBROPLASIA

Fibroblasts produce and organize the major extracellular components of the granulation tissue. They appear to originate from resting fibrocytes situated in the wound margins, and migrate into the wound in response to both chemical and physical attractants (Repesh *et al.*, 1982; McCarthy *et al.*, 1988; Clark, 1990b).

The fibroblast is primarily responsible for the deposition of the new matrix. Once present within the wound, fibroblasts synthesize hyaluronic acid, fibronectin and types I and III collagen — these form the early extracellular matrix. As the matrix matures, certain changes take place: the presence of hyaluronic acid and fibrinogen is gradually reduced, type I collagen becomes the predominant component, and proteoglycans are deposited.

Hyaluronic acid, present only in early wound healing, appears to facilitate cell motility and may be important in fibroblast proliferation (Toole, 1981; Lark *et al.*, 1985). Fibronectin has many functions within a wound; these include action as a chemoattractant to cells such as fibro-

blasts and endothelial cells, augmentation of the attachment of fibroblasts to fibrin, facilitation of the migration of fibroblasts, and possibly provision of a template for collagen deposition (Clark, 1988). Proteoglycans contribute to tissue resilience and help to regulate cell motility and growth, and the deposition of collagen.

Collagen is a generic term covering a number of different types of glycoprotein found in the extracellular matrix. Collagen provides a rigid network which facilitates further healing. The types of collagen within a wound and their quantities are gradually modified with time. Type III (embryonic collagen) is gradually absorbed and replaced by type I collagen, which is mature fibrilar collagen. Type IV collagen may be produced as a part of the basement membrane when skin damage occurs, and type V collagen is deposited around cells, forming a structural support.

Two primary factors affect collagen metabolism and, therefore, production. The first is the effect of the cytokines; Table 3.1 lists some of the cytokines believed to affect collagen metabolism. There appears to be a balance between the stimulatory and inhibitory effects of the these substances, leading to optimal healing with neither over- nor under-production of collagen.

The second factor influencing collagen metabolism is the nature of the extracellular matrix (Mauch *et al.*, 1988; Kulozik *et al.*, 1991). The extracellular matrix provides both a structural scaffold for the tissue and signalling for the cells. Reduced collagen synthesis results from cell contact with mature, type I collagen, upon which the production of collagenase is activated.

ANGIOGENESIS

An extensive vascular system is required to provide for the needs of the proliferative phase.

Table 3.1

Cytokines controlling collagen production

TGF-β	induces collagen synthesis	(Ignotz and Massague, 1986)
IL-1	induces collagen synthesis	(Postlethwaite *et al.*, 1988)
TNF	induces collagen synthesis	(Duncan and Berman, 1989)
IFN (a, β, γ)	decreases collagen synthesis	(Czaja *et al.*, 1987)
TNF-α	decreases collagen synthesis	(Scharffetter *et al.*, 1989)
PGE$_2$	decreases collagen synthesis	(Nicholas *et al.*, 1991)

Key: TGF-β, transforming growth factor β; IL-1, intereukin 1; TNDF, tumour necrosis factor; IFN, interferons; PGE$_2$, prostaglandin E$_2$

Angiogenesis is thought to be initiated by the presence of multiple stimuli. The process initially involves capillary budding, which involves the disruption of the basement membrane of the venule at a point adjacent to the angiogenic stimulus. Endothelial cells migrate towards the stimulus as a cord of cells surrounded by a provisional matrix (Ausprunk *et al.*, 1981; Clark *et al.*, 1982b). Individual sprouts link to form capillary loops, which may in turn develop further sprouts. Lumina appear within the arched cords and blood flow is gradually established, initially in immature, permeable vessels, and later in more mature capillary beds having developed basement membrane components (Ausprunk *et al.*, 1981; Hashimoto and Prewitt, 1987).

The anastomosis of existing vessels and the coupling or recoupling of vessels within the wound space also occurs, leading to a well-developed blood supply within the granulation tissue. However, this state is not retained, as the granulation tissue is later remodelled into scar tissue. Capillary regression occurs, possibly in response to a loss of angiogenic stimuli, and is characterized by changes in the mitochondria of the endothelial cells, their gradual degeneration and necrosis, and final ingestion by macrophages.

Angiogenesis is stimulated and controlled through the action of many substances; these have been reviewed by Folkman and Klagsburn (1987), Madri and Pratt (1988) and Zetter (1988). Effects may be both direct and indirect, and arise from stimuli generated both at the time of injury and during the early stages of repair.

WOUND CONTRACTION

Contraction, which is due to the centripetal movement of pre-existing tissue (Montadon *et al.*, 1977), is the process that reduces the size of a wound. Wound contraction is a major form of wound closure in loose-skinned animals such as rabbits and rats, and rarely leads to loss of function of the involved tissue. In humans, however, it is a 'double-edged sword': if there is too little contraction then wound closure is slow, allowing excess bleeding and possible infection, but too much contraction may lead to tissue contractures, possibly causing deformity and dysfunction. Alone, wound contraction rarely closes a human wound.

Wound contraction begins soon after injury and peaks at two weeks. Many theories have been posited as to the mechanisms involved. Recent work suggests that material within the wound may pull the wound margins inwards. Two theories are currently postulated for this process: they are the cell contraction theory, based on the actions of myofibroblasts (Gabbiani *et al.*,

1971), and the cell traction theory, based on the action of fibroblasts (Ehrlich and Rajaratnam, 1990).

The cell contraction theory suggests that the contractile activity of myofibroblasts draws the edges of the wound together against the constant centrifugal tension of the surrounding tissues. Both actin and myosin have been identified in myofibroblasts, and it is suggested that the myofibroblasts attach themselves to collagen fibres and then retract, holding the collagen in place until it has stabilized its position. The theory suggests that the synchronized activity of the many myofibroblasts will lead to wound shrinkage (Skalli and Gabbiani, 1988).

The cell traction theory suggests that fibroblasts act as the agents of closure by exerting 'traction forces' on the extracellular matrix fibres to which they are attached; the process is analogous to the traction exerted by wheels on a surface. Traction forces are shear, tangential forces that are generated during cell activity. This process brings to mind the action of a traction engine (Figure 3.2).

Much argument surrounds these two theories. Current evidence suggests that wound contraction is cell mediated, and that the cells involved are of fibroblastic origin. Other studies suggest that wound contraction appears to start before many myofibrocytes are present in the area, again implicating fibroblastic activity (Ehrlich and Hembry, 1984; Darby et al., 1990). However, this does not preclude the suggestion that both mechanisms may be involved in the process in a sequential fashion (Hart, 1993).

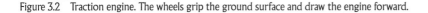

Figure 3.2   Traction engine. The wheels grip the ground surface and draw the engine forward.

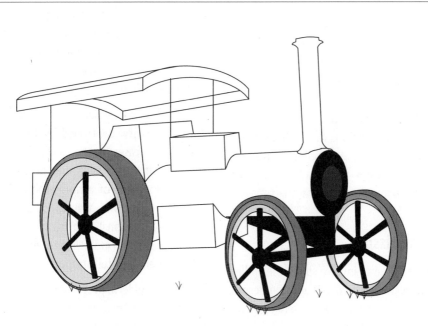

Remodelling

Remodelling of the immature tissue matrix commences at about the same time as new tissue formation, although for clarity it is normally regarded as forming the third phase of healing. The matrix that is present at this stage is gradually replaced and remodelled over the subsequent months and years as the scar tissue matures.

Collagen is immature and gel-like in construction in the early stages of wound healing, and exhibits little tensile strength. Remodelling occurs over a period ranging from several months to years, with type III collagen being partly replace by type I. Fibres reorientate themselves along the lines of stress applied to the lesion, thus resulting in greater tensile strength of the tissue. Wound breaking strength increases with the deposition of collagen, reaching approximately 20% of the normal strength by day 21. The final strength attained will be in the region of 70–80% of the normal value.

Repair of Specialized Tissues

The repair of certain specialized tissues may result in a number of modifications or additions to the normal healing process. A brief description is given of the processes that may occur when epidermal tissue, muscle, and bone are damaged.

Epidermal Tissue

Injuries to the skin may involve either the epidermis alone or both the epidermis and the dermis. When the skin is broken, rapid coverage of the surface is essential to reduce the hazards associated with environmental stress and contamination. While dermal healing is proceeding as described above, re-epithelialization of the surface occurs to repair damage to the epidermis.

Re-epithelialization is initiated within 24 hours of injury. Epidermal basal cells undergo changes which allow them to migrate toward the site of the lesion; they loosen their intercellular attachments (desmosomes), lose their cellular rigidity, and develop actinic pseudopodia – all of which facilitate cell mobility.

Epidermal cells migrate rapidly towards the base of a wound, travelling across the remaining viable basal lamina or the fibrin scaffolding of the blood clot formed in deeper lesions. Cells move across the wound surface in response to a number of substances in the wound matrix, including fibronectin, fibrin and collagen (type IV) which provide a structural network for migration (Hunt and Dunphy, 1980).

There is a certain lack of clarity about the factors that initiate and promote the restructuring process. However, they include chemotactic factors, structural macromolecules, degradative enzymes, tissue geometry (such as the free-edge effect), fibrin, collagen, fibronectin, thrombospondin and growth factors.

Epidermal differentiation follows migration. Mitotic activity, controlled by the cyclic AMP system, increases in the newly formed epithelium, resulting in thickening of the tissue and the development of a normal stratified appearance (Matolsty and Viziam, 1970; Odland and Ross, 1977). Normal keratinization follows, initially in the uppermost layers, followed by the development of a full stratum corneum.

Finally, the epidermis returns to normal. When the basement membrane is present and the re-epithelialization complete, the cells resume their normal appearance and the hemidesmosomes re-form to link the basement membrane and the epidermal layer of cells. Where deficient, the basal lamina is synthesized by the epidermal cells over a infrastructure of newly formed collagen (Clark *et al.*, 1982a).

Muscle Tissue

The degree to which regeneration takes place in muscle appears to depend both on the degree to which the basement membranes of the original fibres have been retained, and on the vascular and

Figure 3.3   Muscle repair. (a) Damaged cellular components are digested by cellular infiltration and inflammation. (b) Satellite cells proliferate and then, (c) fuse into myotubes to form new myofibrils. (d) Myofibrillar proteins are synthesized to 'fill' new fibre resulting in (e) regenerated muscle fibre.

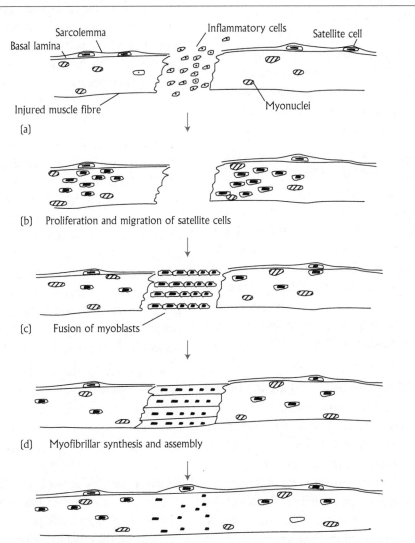

(a)

(b)   Proliferation and migration of satellite cells

(c)   Fusion of myoblasts

(d)   Myofibrillar synthesis and assembly

(e)   Regenerated muscle fibre

nerve supply to the area (Carlson and Faulkner, 1983).

Muscle repair involves the removal of damaged cell components, the proliferation of satellite cells to form new muscle fibre building materials, and the fusion of satellite cells to form new myotubes and muscle fibres (Figure 3.3).

The processes involved in the early degenerative phase have been reviewed by Carpenter and Karpati (1984). Myofibrils lose their regularity and disorganization of the Z disc occurs. Mitochondria become more rounded and lose their regular distribution within the cell. Actin and myosin filaments lose their regularity, glycogen particles disappear, and tissue no longer stains positive for the enzymes, such as phosphorylase, which are used in glycogenolysis.

Proliferation of skeletal muscle satellite cells (or presumptive myoblasts) follows, and these provide a source of myonuclei for the regenerating muscle cells. Bischoff (1986, 1990) hoped to identify the factors which might initiate this process; he suggested that under normal conditions the sarcolemma exerted a negative control on satellite cells to prevent proliferation. This inhibition was removed following structural damage. Positive control through the action of mitogenic factors was also suggested by Bischoff (1990), although the nature of this is as yet unclear.

Regeneration subsequently follows the normal pattern of muscle development, with satellite cells aligning themselves along the basal lamina and fusing into myotubes. The presence of the basal lamina appears to influence this process, providing a substrate upon which alignment can occur, and expressing a number of extracellular matrix components. It is not, however, essential to the process, as reduced levels of regeneration occur in the absence of an intact lamina.

As the myotubules mature and differentiate they synthesize myofibrillar proteins and deposit them in the outer subsarcolemmal region. During this process, the muscle nuclei are normally pushed to the periphery, although a few remain centrally as testimony to the repair process.

Nervous Tissue

When a peripheral axon is damaged it is sometimes possible for it to undergo repair which allows normal conduction to resume. In mammals, however, repair of central axons is not possible, possibly due to the absence of definite endoneurial tubes and the proliferation of macroglia cells. Considerable research is currently being conducted in this area to clarify matters.

When an axon is subject to trauma, changes occur on both sides of the injury. Distally, the axon swells and then disintegrates, with total degeneration and removal of the cytoplasmic matter occurring within the membrane of the axon. A similar process occurs in the proximal direction, gradually progressing toward the cell body. This normally leads to effects in the cell body such as changes in cytoplasmic RNA, dispersion of Nissl granules, production of protein synthesizing organelles, and positional reorganization of both nucleoli and ribosomes (Figure 3.4).

When regrowth of the axon is possible, as in the peripheral nervous system when the cell body has not been destroyed, an intact endoneurial sheath at or near the site of damage helps to establish satisfactory contact with the peripheral receptors and end organs. Following degeneration of the myelin sheath, the Schwann cells proliferate and occupy the endoneurial tube. In addition, they form a bridge across any gap in the continuity of the axon. The proximal part of the axon develops a swelling which gives rise to a large number of

Figure 3.4   Repair of nervous tissue. (a) Both antegrade and retrograde changes occur following damage to a neurone. (b) Wallerian changes, which include generation for the myelin sheath and axon, occur in the antegrade direction. Cell body changes include movement of the nucleus to the periphery, removal of the protein synthesis apparatus and dispersion of Nissl granules.

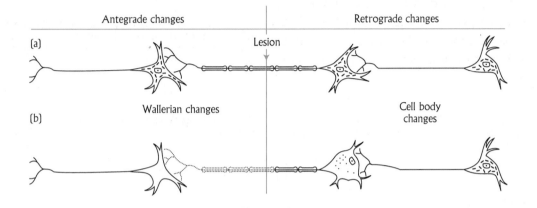

axonal 'sprouts', and these spread out within the tissue surrounding the wound. Though many ultimately serve no useful purpose, one will enter the tube and grow distally, accompanied by the Schwann cells. When the axon finally makes successful contact with the end organs, the Schwann cells begin to synthesize a myelin sheath. Finally, the axonal diameter and the myelin-sheath thickness increase, leading to near-normal conduction behaviour.

Bone Tissue

The repair of bone tissue follows the same basic pattern as that described in the section on the principles of healing, with an added osteogenic component. The process is described in full detail in many texts (for example, Heppenstall, 1980; and Williams *et al*, 1989.

Haemorrhage occurs immediately following injury. A clot forms, and the acute inflammatory phase of repair is initiated. Mast cells, polymorphonuclear leucocytes and macrophages move into the area and appear to be responsible for the release of factors which stimulate tissue repair. Dead and dying tissues are removed by macrophages and osteoclasts and a gradual ingrowth of granulation tissue occurs to replace the clot. This is completed normally by about four days.

Osteoblasts, whether derived from osteocytes, fibroblasts or a number of other sources, become active. They are stimulated into activity by a number of factors, including mast-cell factors, decreased oxygen levels, and bone-morphogenic substances. In addition, chondroblasts may become active under certain conditions, especially when oxygen levels are particularly poor. Small groups of cartilaginous cells appear within this early tissue, chiefly in the region of the periosteum. Osteoblasts deposit calcium both directly in the tissue matrix and in the islands of cartilage. The fracture is now united by a firm but pliable material known as *provisional* (or *soft*) *callus*.

Subsequently, both subperiosteal and endochondral ossification continues and, after about two months, the bone ends become united by primitive (or *woven*) bone, which is known as *hard callus*.

Finally, this woven bone is remodelled to form mature lamellar bone. Both osteoblasts and osteoclasts are involved in this process. The marrow cavity is restored, the contour of the bone smoothed, and the internal structure of the bone reorganized as the type of bone changes and the tissue responds to the normal external forces to which it is again submitted. Figure 3.5 illustrates the process of repair.

References

Ausprunk, DH, Boudreau, CL, Nelson, DA (1981) Proteoglycans in the microvasculature II. Histochemical localization in proliferating capillaries in the rabbit cornea. *American Journal of Pathology* 103: 367–375.

Figure 3.5   Repair of bone. (a) Fracture leads to bleeding and blood clot. (b) Granulation tissue forms. (c) Calcification gradually occurs, leading to, (d) new bone, and (e) remodelling. (After Grays Anatomy)

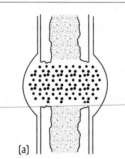

(a)

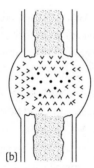

(b)

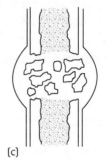

(c)

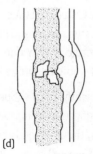

(d)

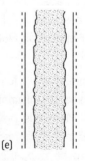

(e)

Bischoff, R (1986) A satellite cell mitogen from crushed adult muscle. *Developmental Biology* 115: 140–147.

Bischoff, R (1990) Interaction between satellite cells and skeletal muscle fibres. *Development* 109: 943–952.

Carlson, BM, Faulkner, JA (1983) The regeneration of skeletal muscle fibres following injury: a review. *Medicine and Science in Sport and Exercise* 15: 187–198.

Carpenter, S, Karpati, G (1984) *Pathology of Skeletal Muscle.* Churchill Livingstone, New York.

Clark, RAF (1985) Cutaneous tissue repair: basic biological considerations. *Journal of the American Academy of Dermatology* 13: 701–725.

Clark, RAF (1988) Over view and general considerations of wound repair, in Clark, RAF, Henson, PM (eds) *The Molecular and Cellular Biology of Wound Repair.* Plenum Press, New York.

Clark, RAF (1990a) Cutaneous wound repair, in Goldsmith, LE (ed) *Biochemistry and Physiology of the Skin* Oxford University Press, Oxford.

Clark, RAF (1990b) Fibronectin matrix deposition and fibronectin receptor expression in healing and normal skin. *Journal of Investigative Dermatology* 94, 6 (supplement): 128S–134S.

Clark, RAF (1991) Cutaneous wound repair: a review with emphasis on integrin receptor expression, in Jansen, H, Rooman, R, Robertson, JIS (eds) *Wound Healing.* Wrightson Biomedical Publishing Ltd, Petersfield.

Clark, RAF, Della Pelle, P, Manseau, E, Lanigan, JM, Dvorak, HF, Colvin, RB (1982a) Fibronectin and fibrin provide a provisional matrix for epidermal cell migration during wound re-epithelialization. *Journal of Investigative Dermatology* 79: 264–269.

Clark, RAF, Della Pelle, P, Manseau, E, Lanigan, JM, Dvorak, HF, Colvin, RB (1982b) Blood vessel fibronectin increases in conjunction with endothelial cell proliferation and capillary ingrowth during wound healing. *Journal of Investigative Dermatology* 79: 269–276.

Czaja, MJ, Weiner, FR, Eghbali, M, Giambrone, MA, Eghbali, M, Zern, M (1987) Differential effects of interferon-gamma on collagen and fibrinectin gene expression. *Journal of Biological Chemistry* 262: 13348–13351.

Darby, I, Skalli, O, Gabbiani, G (1990) A smooth muscle actin is transiently expresses by myofibroblasts during experimental wound healing. *Laboratory Investigation* 63: 21–29.

Duncan, MR, Berman, B (1989) Differential regulation of collagen, glycosaminoglycan, fibronectin and collagenase activity production in cultured human adult fibroblasts by interleukin-1 alpha and beta and tumour necrosis factor alpha and beta. *Journal of Investigative Dermatology* 92: 699–706.

Ehrlich, HP, Hembry, RH (1984) A comparative study of fibroblasts in healing freeze and burn injuries in rats. *American Journal of Pathology* 117: 288–294.

Ehrlich, HP, Rajaratnam, JBM (1990) Cell locomotion forces versus cell contraction forces for collagen lattice contraction: an *in vitro* model of wound contraction. *Tissue and Cell* 22: 407–417.

Folkman, J, Klagsburn, M (1987) Angiogensic factors. *Science* 235: 442–447.

Gabbiani, G, Ryan, GB, Manjo, G (1971) Presence of modified fibroblasts in granulation tissue and their possible role in wound contraction. *Experientia* 27: 549–550.

Ginsberg, MH, Loftus, JC, Plow, EF (1988) Cytoadhesions, intigrins and platlets. *Thrombosis and Haemostasis* 59, 1–6.

Hart, J (1993) *The effect of therapeutic ultrasound on dermal wound repair with emphasis on fibroblast activity.* PhD Thesis, London University, London.

Hashimoto, H, Prewitt, RL (1987) Microvascular changes during wound healing. *International Journal of Microcirculation: Clinical Experiments* 5: 303–310.

Heppenstall, RB (1980) Fracture healing, in Heppenstall RB (ed) *Fracture treatment and healing.* Saunders, Philadelphia.

Ho, Y-S, Lee, WMF, Snyderman, R (1987) Chemoattractant induced activation of *c-fos* gene expression in human monocytes. *Journal of Experimental Medicine* 165: 1524–1538.

Hosein, B, Mosessen, MW, Bianco, C (1985) Monocyte receptors for fibronectin, in van Furth, R (ed) *Mononuclear Phagocytes: Characteristics, Physiology and Function.* Martuus Nijhoff, Dordrecht, Holland.

Hunt, TK (1987) Prospective: a retrospective perspective on the nature of wounds, in Barbul, A, Pines, E, Caldwell, M, Hunt, TK (eds) *Growth Factors and Other Aspects of Wound Healing.* Liss, New York.

Hunt, TK, Dunphy, JE (1980) *Fundamentals of Wound Healing and Wound Infection: Theory and Surgical Practice.* Appleton-Century Croft, New York.

Ignotz, RA, Massague, J (1986) Transforming growth factor β stimulates the expression of fibronectin and collagen and their incorporation into the extracellular matrix. *Journal of Biochemistry* 260: 4337–4342.

Issekutz, AC (1981) Vascular responses during acute neutrophylic inflammation: their relationship to *in vivo* neutrophil emigration. *Laboratory Investigation* 45: 435–441.

Janssen, H, Rooman, R, Robertson, JIS (1991) *Wound Healing.* Wrightson Biomedical Publishing Ltd, Petersfield.

Kulozik, M, Heckmann, M, Mauch, C, Scharffeter, K, Krieg, Th (1991) Cytokine regulation of collagen metabolism during wound healing *in vitro* and *in vivo*, in Jansen, H, Rooman, R, Robertson, JIS (eds) *Wound Healing.* Wrightson Biomedical Publishing Ltd, Petersfield.

Lark, MW, Laterra, J, Culp, LA (1985) Close and focal contact adhesions of fibroblasts to a fibrinectin-containing matrix. *Fed Proc* 44: 394–403.

Leibovich, SJ, Ross, R (1975) The role of macrophages in wound repair. *American Journal of Pathology* 78: 71.

Madri, JA, Pratt, BM (1988) Angiogenesis, in Clark, RAF, Henson, PM (eds) *The Molecular and Cellular Biology of Wound Repair.* Plenum Press, New York.

Matoltsy, AG, Viziam, B (1970) Further observations on epithelialisation of small wounds: an autoradiographic study of incorporation and distribution of ^{3}H-Thymidine in the epithelium covering skin wounds. *Journal of Investigative Dermatology* 55: 20–25.

Mauch, C, Krieg, Th (1990) Fibroblast-matrix interactions and their role in the pathogenesis of fibrosis. *Rheumatic Disease Clinics North America* 16: 93–107.

McCarthy, JB, Sas, DF, Furcht, LT (1988) Mechanism of parenchymal cell migration in wounds, in Clark, RAF, Henson, PM (eds) *The Molecular and Cellular Biology of Wound Repair.* Plenum Press, New York.

Montadon, D, d'Andiran, G and Babbiani, G (1977) The mechanism of wound contraction and epithelialization. *Clinical Plastic Surgery* 4: 325.

Nicolas, JF, Gaycherand, M, Delaporte, E, Hartman, D, Richard, M, Croute, F, Thivolet, J (1991) Wound healing: a result of co-ordinate keratinocyte-fibroblast interactions. The role of keratinocyte cytokines, in Janssen, H, Rooman, R, Robertson, JIS (1991) *Wound Healing*. Wrightson Biomedical Publishing Ltd, Petersfield.

Odland, G, Ross, R (1977) Human wound repair I: epidermal regeneration. *Journal of Cell Biology* **39**: 135–151.

Peacock, EE (1984) Contraction, in Peacock, EE (ed) *Wound Repair*. W B Saunders and Co., Philadelphia.

Prostlethwaite, AE, Raghow, R, Stricklin, GP Poppleton, A, Sayer, JM, Kang, AH (1988) Modulation of fibroblast function by interleukin-I increased steady state accumulation of type I procollagen mRNA and stimulation of other functions but not chemotaxis by human recombinant interleukin-I α and β. *Journal of Cell Biology* **106**: 311–318.

Proud, D, Kaplan, AP (1988) Kinin formation: mechanisms and roles in inflammatory disorders. *Annual Review of Immunology* **6**: 49–83.

Repesh, LA, Fitzgerald, TJ, Furcht, LT (1982) Fibronectin involvement in granulation tissue and wound healing in rabbits. *Journal of Histrochemistry and Cytochemistry* **30**: 351–358.

Riches, DWH (1988) The multiple role of macrophages in wound repair, in Clark RAF, Henson PM (eds) *The Molecular and Cellular Biology of Wound Repair*. Plenum Press, New York.

Scharffetter, K, Heckmann, M, Hatamochi, A, Mauch, C, Stein, B, Riethmuller, G, Ziegler-Heitbrock, HB, Krieg, Th (1989) Synergistic effect of tumour necrosis factor-a and interferon gamma on collagen synthesis in human fibroblasts *in vitro*. *Experimental Cell Research* **181**: 409–419.

Skalli, O, Gabbiani, G (1988) The biology of the myofibroblast: relationship to wound contraction and fibrocontractive diseases, in Clark, RAF, Henson, PM (eds) *The Molecular and Cellular Biology of Wound Repair*. Plenum Press, New York.

Terkeltaub, RA, Ginsberg, MH (1988) Platelets and response to injury, in Clark, RAF, Henson, PM (eds) *The Molecular and Cellular Biology of Wound Repair*. Plenum Press, New York.

Toole, BP (1981) Glycosaminoglycans in morphogenesis, in Hay ED (ed) *Cell Biology of the Extracellular Matrix*. Plenum Press, New York.

Tsukamoto, Y, Helsel, JE, Wahl, SM (1981) Macrophage production of fibronectin, a chemoattractant for fibroblasts. *Journal of Immunology* **127**: 673–678.

Weeks, JR (1972) Prostaglandins. *Annual Review of Pharmacology and Toxicology* **12**: 317.

Williams, PL, Warwick, R, Dyson, M and Bannister, LH (Ed) 1989 *Gray's Anatomy*. Churchill Livingstone. Edinburgh.

Williams, TJ (1988) Factors that affect vessel reactivity and leucocyte emigration, in Clark, RAF, Henson, PM (eds) *The Molecular and Cellular Biology of Wound Repair*. Plenum Press, New York.

Zetter, BR (1988) Angiogenesis: state of the art. *Chest* **93**: 1595–1665.

4

Sensory and Motor Nerve Activation

OONA SCOTT

Introduction
•
Motoneurone to Muscle Activation
•
Muscles – Basic Characteristics, Classification and the Influence of the Motoneurone
•
Afferent Input to the Central Nervous System

Introduction

This section outlines the basics of muscle and peripheral nerve physiology, introduces the concept of nerve–muscle interaction and the effects of electrical stimulation on this interaction.

Brief History

For centuries, people had observed that contact with certain fish gave them a shock and that rubbing certain materials, such as amber, could generate a similar reaction. Luigi Galvani (1791) documented his observation of muscle contracting under the influence of what had been called electricity for over a century (Sir Thomas Browne, 1646). Galvani's observations related to the induction of muscular contraction in frog legs. He came to believe that nerves stimulated muscle electrically.

As the nineteenth century progressed, there was an increasing range of ways in which electricity could be generated, stored and delivered. These included the delivery of alternating current, which was called 'faradic' after Faraday's electromagnetic generator (1831). There were many reports of muscular contraction induced by electricity for the purpose of curing paralysis and other diseases.

In 1833, Duchenne of Boulogne found that he could stimulate muscles electrically without piercing the skin and devised cloth-covered electrodes for percutaneous stimulation. Duchenne called his method of application 'localized currents' and he was the first to use 'faradism' — that is, alternating current — for treatment.

Duchenne observed that there were certain spots — motor points — along the surface of the body whose stimulation gave particularly ample muscle contraction. Differences in response between galvanic and faradic currents were recognized, with denervated muscle responding to galvanic rather than to faradic current. The duration of the current was the deciding factor in eliciting contraction.

During the twentieth century, work with human muscle, which continues alongside work on animal muscle, has become increasingly important. When compared with the brain of other mammals, the human brain seems to have a particularly refined ability to plan and to execute movement. Rothwell (1994), in his recent book reviewing the control of human movement, identified an hierarchical chain running sequentially from the idea of movement through the motor plan into the execution of a programme of commands and on to the movement itself. Such a plan must ensure that different motoneurones are excited and inhibited in the right order, to the correct degree, at the right times.

Definition

Muscle and nerve stimulating currents are electrical currents which are capable of causing the generation of action potentials. They need to be of sufficient intensity and of an appropriate duration to cause depolarization of the nerve or muscle membrane.

Motoneurone to Muscle Activation

Neural Control of Muscle

Smooth, coordinated movement is the output of a complex neuromuscular system. Skeletal muscle is capable of generating varying tensions and, at its very simplest, smooth, coordinated movement depends on the practical issue of contracting the required muscles at the right time. The control of coordinated movement is incredibly complex. Activation of the relevant muscles depends on an appropriate combination of excitation or of inhibition of different motoneurones. These patterns of excitation and inhibition are clearly important and much has still to be learnt about their central control, of how motor units are selected to achieve a particular movement and of how firing patterns are updated as the movement evolves.

The brain uses stereotypical electrical signals — nerve action potentials — to process all of the information which it receives and analyses. The signals themselves consist of potential changes produced by electrical currents flowing across the cell membranes, the currents being carried by ions such as those of sodium, potassium, and chlorine (see *Electrophysiological Properties of Nerve and Muscle* below). The coding of information depends principally on the frequency of impulses transmitted by a nerve fibre, the number of fibres involved and the synaptic connections which the nerve makes. The variability of response occurs at the level of the neuronal synapses and the ability to modify the processes of excitation and inhibition is thought to be the key to changes which occur in the central control mechanisms. It is important to remember that discharge of an action potential down the axon of a motoneurone depends both on the inputs from the periphery and from the rest of the central nervous system.

The Motor Unit

The smallest unit of movement that the central nervous system can control is the *motor unit*, as defined by Sherrington in 1925. This unit consists of the motoneurone, together with its axon and dendrites, the motor end plates and the muscle fibres it supplies. Motoneurones are the largest cells in the ventral horn of the spinal chord. The activity or firing frequency of these cells is dependent on their connections with the afferent inputs from muscles, joints and skin, as well as their connections with the other parts of the central nervous system.

Each motoneurone integrates the excitatory (EPSP) and inhibitory post synaptic (IPSP) potentials from thousands of synapses spread over the cell body or soma, and these influence whether or not it generates an action potential. When an action potential is discharged down the axon of a motoneurone, all the muscle fibres it supplies contract.

Electrical stimulation is used therapeutically to elicit skeletal muscle contraction. In order to understand the way in which external electrical stimulation can be used to supplement or enhance the normal physiological processes, it is important to understand the underlying electrophysiological processes.

Electrophysiological Properties of Nerves and Muscles

Conduction of action potentials along the membranes of nerves and muscles occurs because there is a potential difference between the intracellular fluid and the extracellular fluid (Figure 4.1). The resting potential is of the order of −90 mV for skeletal muscle, and −70 mV for lower motoneurones, the minus sign indicating that the inside of the cell has a negative potential relative to the exterior; this potential difference can be altered by the passage of ions.

In cell membranes of both nerves and muscles, protein molecules are embedded in a double layer of lipid (fat) molecules which are arranged with their hydrophilic heads facing outward and hydrophobic tails extending into the middle of the layer (see Chapter 1). Some protein molecules make contact with both the extracellular and the intracellular fluid. Protein molecules can have control functions with one region being a selectivity filter and another region providing a gate which can be open or closed.

The intracellular and extracellular solutions are in osmotic equilibrium with each other and because

Figure 4.1 The potential difference across a cell membrane measured with an intracellular electrode and an extracellular electrode.

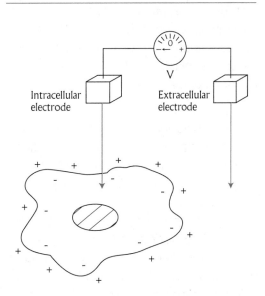

the total number of anions and cations is equal, both are electrically neutral. There is, however, a difference in the proportions of different ions in the two solutions: there is a higher concentration of potassium ions in the intracellular fluid, and higher concentrations of both sodium and chloride ions in the extracellular fluid.

MOVEMENT OF IONS

Ions at high concentration will tend to diffuse to areas of low concentration and their movement is also influenced by voltage gradients, with positive ions being attracted down the negative gradient, and *vice versa*. An outward movement of potassium ions along their concentration gradient would be expected but at the same time the inner surface of the membrane is at a negative potential with respect to the outside, and this tends to restrain the outward movement of positively charged ions.

The equilibrium potential of any ion is proportional to the difference between the logarithms of intracellular concentration and the extracellular concentration and is defined by the *Nernst equation*. The Nernst equation describes the equilibrium potential which is the electric potential necessary to balance a given ionic concentration across a membrane so that the overall passive movement of the ion is zero.

It was proposed originally by Bernstein (1902) that only potassium ions could diffuse across the resting cell membrane. Later work by Hodgkin and Keynes (1955) showed that the cell membrane is permeable to other ions, including sodium ions, and that sodium ions are in a continuous state of flux across the membrane against both the concentration and the electrical gradients. Their findings supported the concept of an active transport system that uses energy supplied by the hydrolysis of adenosine triphosphate (ATP) to pump

sodium ions out of the cell and to accumulate potassium ions within the cell. Evidence suggests that the expulsion of sodium ions to the influx of potassium ions is of the order of 3:2.

GENERATION AND PROPAGATION OF ACTION POTENTIALS

The unequal distribution of ions across the cell membrane of both nerve and muscle cells forms the basis for the generation and propagation of action potentials. Nerve and muscle cells are *excitable* – this means that they are able to produce an action potential after the application of a suitable stimulus (see section *Threshold* below). An action potential is a transient reversal of the membrane potential – a *depolarization*. This lasts for about 1 ms in nerve cells and up to 2 ms in some muscle fibres.

THRESHOLD

An initial opening of a few of the voltage-activated sodium channels occurs, followed by a rapid transient increase in sodium permeability. This allows sodium ions to diffuse rapidly into the cell, causing a sudden accumulation of positive charge on the inside surface of the neural or muscle fibre membrane. The increased permeability to sodium ions is followed by repolarization via the opening of voltage-activated potassium channels; there is some hyperpolarization beyond the resting potential.

The nature of the regenerating mechanism was demonstrated both in terms of the time course of the action potential and in terms of ionic conductance by Hodgkin and Huxley (1952). If the stimulus is below the threshold required to produce an action potential, it reduces but does not reverse the membrane potential. As the stimulus is increased, the potential difference across the cell membrane is reduced until it reaches the critical threshold level. At this level, the stimulus will lead to the automatic generation of an action potential. The level of the threshold varies according to a number of factors which includes how many action potentials the nerve fibre has conducted recently.

After an action potential, two changes occur that make it impossible for the nerve fibre to transmit a second action potential immediately. First, *inactivation* (the *absolute refractory period*) occurs during the falling phase of the action potential during which no amount of externally applied depolarization can initiate a second regenerative response. After the absolute refractory period, there is a *relative refractory period* during which the residual inactivation of the sodium conductance and the relatively high potassium conductance combine to produce an increase in threshold for action potential initiation.

To stimulate a nerve, the stimulus has to be both of sufficient intensity and of sufficient duration to depolarize the nerve membrane. Action potentials can be initiated in peripheral nerves by the application of suitable electrical stimuli (pulses). The rate of change of the stimulus is important. The graph in Figure 4.2 illustrates the relationship between the duration of an electrical stimulus and the intensity of stimulation (see section on *Strength–Duration Curves* in Chapter 20).

If the stimulus is applied very slowly ie the rise time is slow then the rate of depolarization is very slow. There is a steady flow of ions in one direction and no action potential is generated. A slow, steady, unidirectional current and a slow fall is typical of currents used in 'galvanic' treatment or iontophoretic treatments (see Chapter 8), and no stimulation of muscle or nerve occurs. If the stimulus is applied quickly and the duration of the stimulus is long enough, the nerve fibre is rapidly depolarized to the threshold and an action potential is generated. The slower the stimulus is applied, the greater the magnitude of depolarization required to bring the fibre to threshold.

Figure 4.2 The relationship between strength and duration of a stimulus required to generate an action potential in a motor nerve fibre.

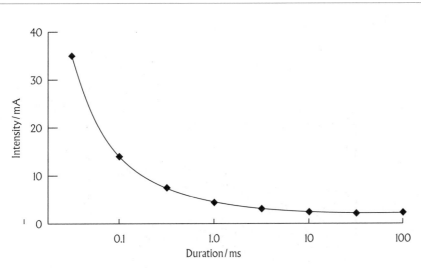

NEURONES AS CONDUCTORS OF ELECTRICITY

Although the permeability properties of cell membranes result in regenerative electrical signals, there are other factors to be considered. Many peripheral motor and sensory nerves are myelinated – myelin being an insulating material formed by Schwann cells and forming as many as 320 membranes in series between the plasma membrane of a nerve fibre and the extracellular fluid. This sheath of membranes is interrupted at regular intervals by the Nodes of Ranvier, which are arranged such that the greater the diameter of the nerve fibre, the greater the internodal distances. Because myelin is an insulator and ions cannot flow easily into and out of the sheathed internodal region, excitation skips from node to node (saltatory conduction), thereby greatly increasing the conduction velocity and, because ionic exchange is limited to the nodal regions, using less energy. While the excitation is progressing from one node to the next on the leading edge of the action potential, many nodes behind are still active. Myelinated nerve fibres exhibit a capability of firing at higher frequencies for more prolonged periods than other nerve fibres.

Table 4.1

Classification of peripheral nerves according to conduction velocity and junction (With permission from *Human Neurophysiology* (2 ed), Chapman and Hall)

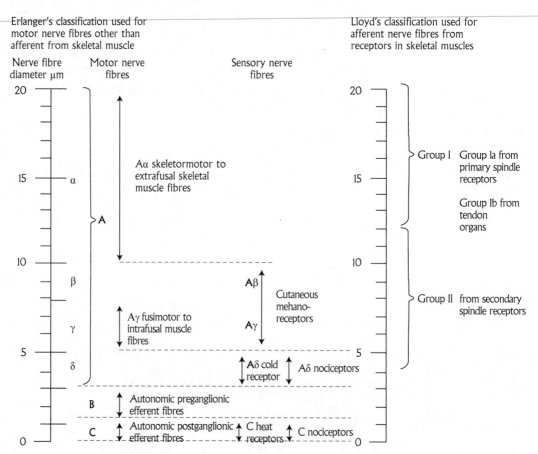

As a general rule, the larger diameter nerves (Group Aα motor nerves) conduct impulses more rapidly and have a lower threshold of excitability than the much smaller Aδ pain fibres. This means that threshold and motor nerve conduction velocities can be tested without exciting the pain fibres. On stimulation, the larger nerve fibres also produce larger signals, their excitatory response lasts for a shorter time, and they have shorter refractory periods (Table 4.1).

Within the muscle, the axon of the motoneurone divides into many branches to inervate muscle fibres that are scattered throughout the muscle and which together make up the motor unit. Each muscle fibre has one neuromuscular junction, lying usually about midway along the fibre.

SYNAPTIC TRANSMISSION

Synapses are points of contact between nerve cells, or between nerves and effector cells such as muscle fibres. At electrical synapses, current generated by an impulse in the presynaptic nerve terminal spreads into the next cell through low-resistance channels. More commonly however, synapses are chemical in action: the gap between the presynaptic and postsynaptic membrane is filled with fluid, and the nerve terminal secretes a chemical, a neurotransmitter, which activates the postsynaptic membrane. The postsynaptic junction or motor end plate is the specialized region on the muscle where the neuromuscular junction comes into close contact with the muscle fibre that it innervates.

Figure 4.3   A section of mammalian skeletal muscle. A single muscle fibre has been cut away to show the individual myofibrils and the thick myosin and thin actin filaments within a sarcomere. The sarcoplasmic reticulum is seen surrounding each myofibril, together with the T system of tubules in which the Ca^{2+} ions are stored and released during muscle contraction.

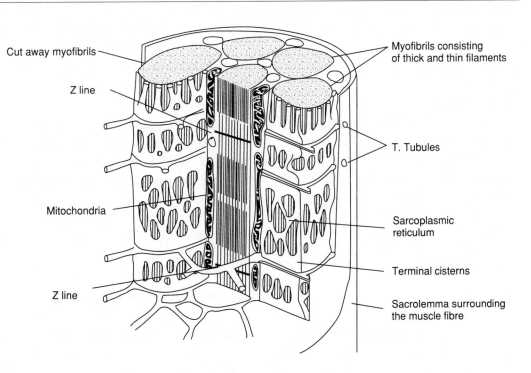

Cut away myofibrils

Z line

Mitochondria

Z line

Myofibrils consisting of thick and thin filaments

T. Tubules

Sarcoplasmic reticulum

Terminal cisterns

Sacrolemma surrounding the muscle fibre

When an action potential arrives at a neuromuscular junction, it causes voltage-dependent calcium channels to open, and allows calcium ions to diffuse into the axon terminal. Acetylcholine from the synaptic vesicles in the nerve terminal diffuse across the synaptic cleft in multimolar packages (or quanta) to combine with the receptor sites on the motor end plate.

This alters the endplate membrane permeability to sodium and potassium and immediately depolarizes the membrane. The endplate potential (EPP) causes a local change in potential of the muscle membrane in close contact with it and propagates a regenerative motor unit action potential (MUAP) in all directions along the adjacent muscle membrane using the mechanism already described for the propagation of action potentials along the axon membrane. The magnitude of a single MUAP is normally sufficient to cause contraction of all muscle fibres belonging to its motor unit – the *all or none principle*.

The action of acetylcholine at the neuromuscular junction is terminated when an enzyme, acetylcholinesterase, is released. The enzyme, which is embedded in the basal lamina of the synaptic cleft of the motor endplate hydrolyses the acetylcholine and thereby prevents prolonged action of the transmitter. Along the length of the muscle fibre, the muscle-cell membrane (the sacrolemma) has numerous infoldings which form a system of membranes called the transverse tubular system or T tubules. As the action potential goes along the sacrolemma, it passes deep into the fibre down the T tubules (Figure 4.3).

CALCIUM RELEASE

Arrival of the action potential in the T tubules depolarizes the sacroplasmic reticulum, another complex membrane system in close contact with the myofibrils. The main function of the sacroplasmic reticulum is to release and take up calcium during contraction and relaxation. Depolarization of the transverse tubular system signals the release of calcium ions from the sacroplasmic reticulum into the sarcoplasm, and allows the actin–myosin cross bridges to bond (see section on *Sliding Filament Hypothesis*). Calcium ions are then actively pumped back into the sacroplasmic reticulum and contraction ceases (Figure 4.4).

Muscles – Basic Characteristics, Classification and the Influence of the Motoneurone

Gross Structure and Function

Muscles vary in shape, size, and in method of attachment to bone or to cartilage. They are often used for more than one function. A single muscle may fulfil stabilizing, power producing and postural roles, as well as a specific controlled movement during a single sequence of movements.

The composition and structure of each muscle is often seen as a compromise between needs for speed of movement, force and economy of energy. There are, however, basic principles governing the mechanical properties of a muscle: the maximum force that can be produced by a muscle is generally proportional to its cross-sectional area; the maximum rate of contraction of a long muscle is greater than that of a short muscle.

As a rule, small muscles with precision tasks such as those in a hand are composed of motor units with few muscle fibres, whereas trunk and proximal limb muscles contain motor units with a large number of muscle fibres. At a simple level, two

Figure 4.4   (a) Sequence of calcium release and uptake during muscle contraction and relaxation. An action potential causes release of calcium ions from the sarcoplasmic reticulum into the sarcoplasm which, in the presence of ATP, causes the interaction of the cross bridges of the myosin filaments with the actin filaments and thus muscle contraction. (b) When calcium is released from the sarcoplasmic reticulum, the myofibril contracts; when calcium is reabsorbed by the sarcoplasmic reticulum, the myofibril relaxes.

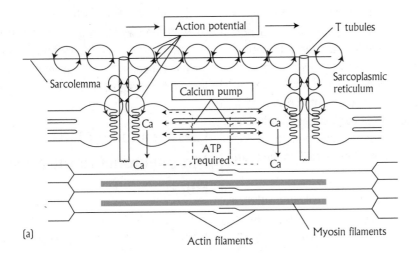

(a)

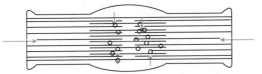

Vesicle of sarcoplasmic reticulum

Calcium from vesicles of sarcoplasmic reticulum into microfibrils

Myofibril shortens

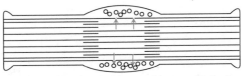

(b)   Calcium actively reabsorbed into vesicles; myofibril relaxes

components are integrated in a single muscle: a contractile component which is altered by stimulation and which can develop an active tension, and an elastic component, connective tissue, through which the contractile component transmits the generated force to the muscle tendon.

The response of a single motor unit to a single action potential is called a *twitch contraction*. (Figure 4.5). The muscle responds with a brief contraction and then returns to its resting state. If more than one impulse is given within an interval that is shorter than the contraction–relaxation cycle time of the motor unit, the muscle does not return to its resting state, and the forces produced by each impulse are said to *summate* or *fuse*.

At a sufficiently high frequency of stimulation, a fused, tetanic or smooth contraction is produced as the force fluctuations of each impulse are indistinguishable in practical terms (Figure 4.6). Because slow-contracting muscle fibres summate and produce a tetanic contraction at lower frequencies of nerve stimulation, investigators realized that slow muscles such as soleus might be more suitable for sustained 'tonic' function at low levels of activation, whereas fast-contracting muscle fibres which fuse at higher frequencies of stimulation may be more appropriate for 'phasic' function, and for generating high forces for short periods of time.

Classification – Matching Motoneurones to the Muscle Fibres

The suggestion that mammalian muscle fibres had diverse functional properties occurred when Ran-

Figure 4.5   The electrical (mv potential change) and mechanical (T, tension) response of a mammalian skeletal muscle fibre to a single action potential resulting in a twitch contraction.

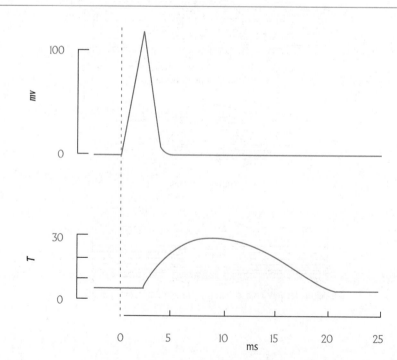

Figure 4.6   The response of human skeletal muscle to different rates of stimulation.

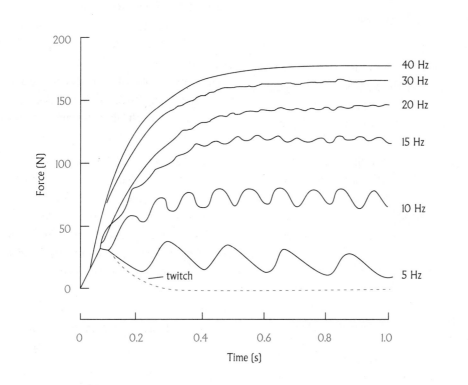

vier (1874) observed that the soleus muscle was a deeper red colour and contracted more slowly than other calf muscles.

Eccles and his coworkers confirmed these observations in 1958 and classified motor units on the basis of the activity patterns of their motoneurones expressed in terms of firing frequency and an ability (or tonicity) to maintain firing. Fast-firing, so-called 'phasic', motoneurones innervated muscle fibres with fast contraction times and slow, 'tonic', motoneurones innervated muscle fibres with slow contraction times.

Edström and Krugelberg (1968) confirmed the similarity of muscle fibres belonging to a single motor unit by a method of glycogen depletion of individual motor units in response to prolonged stimulation of single motor nerve fibres. The finding that muscle fibres of individual motor units were homogeneous and that differences in properties did occur between fibres of different motor units suggested that the activity pattern of the motoneurone was important in determining these properties.

The distribution of muscle fibres that make up a motor unit can be visualized using this method of glycogen depletion. Human muscles can be seen to be heterogeneous in that they are composed of a wide variety of different muscle fibres. Fibres belonging to any one motor unit are spread over a large territory rather than being clustered together. Edström and Krugelberg's finding has recently been modified (Martin *et al.*, 1988) as more sophisticated techniques showed that subtle differences do exist within individual motor units.

Speed of Contraction and Histological Properties

The work of Burke and his colleagues (1973) working on cat gastrocnemius muscle showed a close association between the physiological or mechanical properties and histochemical ('histo' = 'tissue', implying the chemical reaction occurring in the tissues themselves) properties of muscle fibres in each motor unit. They identified three main types of motor units based on the speed of contraction and resistance to fatigue, and stated that each physiological category of muscle unit had a corresponding unique histochemical profile.

1 'FF' motor units, which were fast-contracting with short contraction times, developed relatively high tension, fatigued quickly and possessed high anaerobic glycolytic capacity but low oxidative capacity;

2 'FR' units, which were also fast-contracting, had similarly short twitch-contraction times but developed less tension that the 'FF' units, were less fatiguable , possessed high glycolytic capacity and moderate-to-high oxidative capacity; and

3 'S' units, which were slow contracting with longer twitch-contraction times, developed least tension, and possessed high oxidative and low glycolytic capacity.

This classification by Burke (1973) of motor units by their resistance to fatigue matched that based on enzyme histochemical characteristics of whole muscle fibre populations by Barnard et al. (1971) so that fast glycolytic (FG) fibres probably belong to the 'FF' (most fatigueable) motor units, the fast oxidative glycolytic (FOG) to the 'FR' (less fatiguable) units and the slow oxidative (SO) to the 'S' (fatigue resistant) units.

In human studies, the histological method frequently used to distinguish muscle fibre types is based on staining techniques for myofibrillar actomyosin adenosine triphosphatase (mATPase) activity. The differences in the mATPase activity relate to specific myosin heavy-chain complements and make it possible to distinguish between specific muscle fibre types, called type I and type II for those fibres staining light and dark respectively.

Using differences in pH stability, type II fibres can be further subdivided into two major subgroups: IIa and IIb fibres (see Dubowitz and Brooke, 1973); a further subgroup, IIc, has been identified. Type IIc fibres, which are relatively infrequent, have been found predominantly in foetal and in diseased muscles. Bárány (1967) found that there was a close relationship between myosin ATPase activity and the speed of contraction, indicating that the activity of the myosin molecule correlated with the rate of muscle contraction.

Later work by Garnett and his colleagues (1978), working at St Thomas's Hospital, showed that results with human subjects were comparable to those from other mammals. Using thin wire electrodes in human gastrocnemius, they were able to show that it was possible to measure the time course of contraction of single motor units and to test their twitch-contraction time, using repeated tetani to measure fatiguability. Finally, they were able to deplete the motor unit of glycogen (by stimulating repeatedly for 2 hours), whereupon serial sections of biopsies showed that FF fibres correlated with type IIb fibres, and SO fibres with type I fibres. They also reported that stimulation of sensory nerve endings changed the recruitment order of firing of the motoneurones, causing the larger motoneurones to fire before smaller motoneurones.

Myosin and Actin – Contractile Proteins

At the molecular level, the main elements visible under a light microscope are myofibrils, and these, arranged in parallel, make up a muscle fibre. Each myofibril has longitudinal myofilaments with the alternating light I (isotropic) and dark A (anisotropic) bands, which give skeletal muscle its typical striated or striped appearance (Figure 4.7a).

Under an electron microscope, it becomes

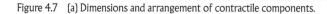

Figure 4.7   (a) Dimensions and arrangement of contractile components.

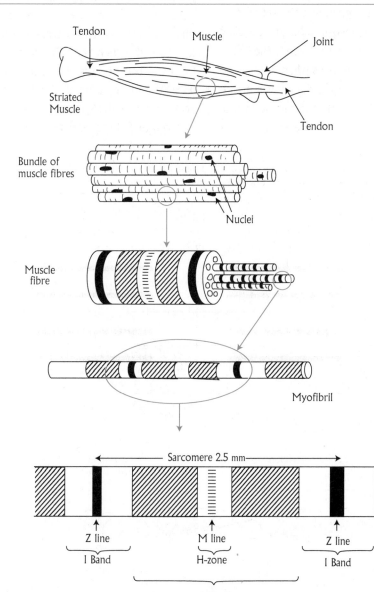

apparent that each myofibril is composed of a series (end to end) of repeating units or sarcomeres, the functional unit of muscle contraction. Within the sarcomere are the myofilaments which are composed mainly of either actin or myosin. Each sarcomere has two sets of thin actin filaments anchored at one end to a network of interconnecting proteins, called the Z line, and, at the other end, interdigitating with a set of thick myosin filaments. The myosin molecules, packed tail to tail, form the wide dark A band. The I band and the H zone are the regions where there is no overlap between the actin and the myosin myofilaments; the I band has only the thin actin molecules and the H zone only the thick myosin myofilaments. Finally, in the centre of the H zone, is the M line, and this is formed by the proteins that bind all the myosin filaments together (Figure 4.7b).

Myosin molecules are relatively large proteins that consist of a globular head or heavy myosin chain portion (HMM) and a light myosin chain tail portion (LMM). Four light chains form the backbone or tail of the myosin molecule and are the thicker filaments in the sarcomere combining end to end with other tails. The portion extending from the backbone is the heavy chain portion (HMM) and consists of the flexible, so-called neck portion – the S_2 portion – and the globular portion, or S_1 head portion, and two associated

Figure 4.7 (b) The layout of the sarcomere and the two contractile proteins, thin (actin) and thick (myosin). (c) The alignment and location of the regulatory proteins, troponin and tropomyosin, on the actin filament.

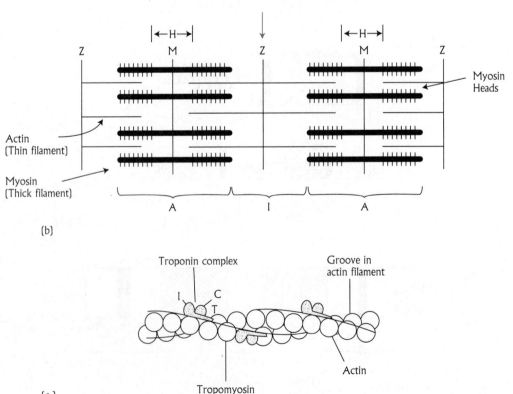

light chains. The composition of these light chains differs in fast and slow muscles, but so far their role has not been established. The globular portion contains the ATP binding site and the actin binding site.

Actin molecules polymerize to form two intertwined helical chains. Each actin monomer is relatively small and roughly spherical in shape. Two regulatory proteins, troponin and tropomyosin, are located on the actin. The two chains of tropomyosin molecules, each about the length of seven actin molecules, fit end to end along the strands of the actin double helix into a groove along the filament length, and they partially cover the myosin binding site (Figure 4.7c).

The Sliding Filament Hypothesis

The force generating mechanism appears to be cyclical, and formation of cross bridges between actin and myosin in the presence of ATP plays an essential role. Both this concept of cross-bridge action and the model of myosin with a head that rotates and stretches a compliant portion of the molecule follow from theories advanced by AF Huxley in 1957, which were then extended by Huxley and Simmons in 1971. They observed no change in length of either the thick myosin or the thin actin filaments and suggested that a sliding motion forces the thin actin filaments at either side of the sarcomere in the A band towards the M line, thereby shortening the sarcomere. Though the exact mechanism is still uncertain, recent work on molecular motors has provided considerable support for the mechanochemical actin-activated myosin–ATPase cycle. One form of this mechanism is illustrated in Figure 4.8.

In step one, the ADP and inorganic phosphate (P_i) are bound to the myosin head. The myosin heads are free to bind to the actin molecules and form an actin–myosin–ADP–P_i complex (step 2). Stored energy is released, the myosin head rotates, and

Figure 4.8 Chemical and physical events occurring during first four steps of the cross-bridge cycle.

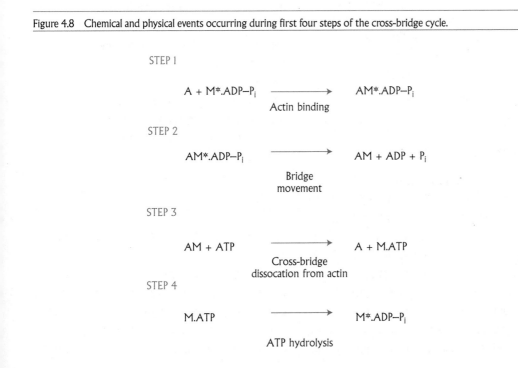

STEP 1

$A + M^*.ADP–P_i \longrightarrow AM^*.ADP–P_i$

Actin binding

STEP 2

$AM^*.ADP–P_i \longrightarrow AM + ADP + P_i$

Bridge movement

STEP 3

$AM + ATP \longrightarrow A + M.ATP$

Cross-bridge dissocation from actin

STEP 4

$M.ATP \longrightarrow M^*.ADP–P_i$

ATP hydrolysis

force is exerted between the two filaments. At this stage, movement occurs between the filaments if they are free to move and, if they are not, an 'isometric contraction' occurs. The link between the myosin and the actin molecules must be broken to allow the myosin cross bridge to reattach to a new actin molecule and repeat the cycle. Binding of a molecule of ATP breaks the link between actin and myosin (step 3). The ATP that is bound to the myosin then splits (step 4) forming the energized state of myosin which can now reattach to a new site on the actin filament.

Role of Calcium in Contraction

At a critical calcium concentration the calcium binds to specific binding sites on troponin, one of the regulatory proteins. Troponin changes its conformation, moving the tropomyosin, and thereby exposing binding sites on the actin molecule (Figure 4.7b). This enables the head of the myosin filament to interact with the binding sites on the actin molecule, forming cross bridges cyclically and so developing force. Removal of calcium reverses this process and tropomyosin moves back into its blocking position.

Recruitment of Motor Units in Voluntary Contractions

In 1929, Adrian and Bronk introduced the concentric-needle electrode and showed that by inserting this electrode directly into the muscle it was possible to record the electrical events that cause contraction of the muscle fibres. They showed that voluntary muscle force could be increased both by increasing the firing frequency of motoneurones and by recruiting additional motor units. In the same year, Denny Brown (1929) found that the smaller motoneurones

which innervate slow-contracting muscle fibres were more readily activated than the larger phasic motoneurones which innervate faster-contracting muscle fibres.

Denny Brown's finding supports the theory (see section *Gross Structure and Function* earlier) that slow muscle fibres are used for sustained activities whereas faster-contracting muscle fibres are used when short bursts of high levels of force are required. As already explained, the frequency of stimulation required to produce a smooth output force or tetanic summation differs; slow muscle fibres having slower contraction and relaxation times summate at lower frequencies of stimulation, whereas faster-contracting muscle fibres generate higher forces and a smooth tetanic contraction at higher frequencies.

Hennemann and his colleagues (1965) investigated the excitability of motoneurones and the order of their recruitment during movement. The size of the cell body of a motoneurone is related to the number of muscle fibres that it innervates. Large motoneurones have larger cell bodies, large diameter axons (and high conductance velocities) and a lower input resistance to an applied input current than do small neurones. For a similar input current, small motoneurones reach their threshold for firing sooner than large motoneurones. Hennemann showed that the excitability or firing pattern of a motoneurone was directly correlated with its size and that, in any given movement, motoneurones were recruited in an orderly manner according to their size.

Later, in 1973, Milner-Brown and his colleagues showed, in humans, that slower-contracting motor units are recruited first in both reflex and voluntary movements involving low tensions and that the larger, faster, motor units are activated 'only by rapid vigorous and briefly sustained contractions' with bursts of rapid firing. Patterns of firing and of recruitment of voluntary muscle force can be increased both by increasing the firing frequency of motoneurones and by recruiting additional motor units.

Only in very fast (ballistic) movements, where speed is of the essence, does the faster conduction speed of the large motoneurones play a part; the slow motor units, because of the slower conduction times of their axons, may fire after the faster motor units.

Normal frequencies of firing of motoneurones in human muscles rarely exceed 40 Hz and are rarely less than 6–8 Hz. Under most conditions motor units fire asychronously; they only fire sychronously during powerful contractions and during fatigue.

Influence of Motoneurone

The change of muscle properties in response to a change of neural input was first demonstrated by Buller and his colleagues in 1960. They sutured the nerve that normally supplied the slow-contracting muscle of the cat into the fast-contracting flexor digitorum longus (FDL), and soleus was innervated by suturing the nerve from FDL. This experiment showed that not only were the contractile properties of the two muscles exchanged but that there were also extensive sequential changes in their metabolic and histological properties.

The close association of the activity pattern of the motoneurone and the contractile properties of the motor unit was underlined when it was shown, using chronic stimulation at 10 Hz, that it was possible to preserve the contractile characteristics of the soleus muscle of the rabbit following tenotomy (Vrbová, 1966).

The slow soleus would normally have become fast-contracting following section of its tendon and the spinal chord. However, when the muscle was stimulated chronically at 5–10Hz for 8 hours each day, its contractile properties remained slow. If higher frequencies of stimulation were used i.e. 20–40 Hz, the silenced soleus muscle became fast contracting (Vrbová, 1966; Salmons and Vrbová, 1969). This matching of the pattern of activity of motoneurones to the properties of the muscle fibres is fundamental.

Effect of Immobilization

The force developed by a muscle is dependent upon the number of cross bridges which can be engaged between actin and myosin filaments, and this, in turn, depends on the overlap of these filaments in the sarcomeres. The number of sarcomeres in series determines the distance through which a muscle can shorten, and regulation of the sarcomere number is considered to be an adaptation to changes in the functional length of muscle. If a muscle is immobilized in a shortened position there is a reduction in the number of sarcomeres and, conversely, if the muscle is immobilized in a lengthened position there is an increase in the number of sarcomeres

Afferent Input to the Central Nervous System

The nervous system receives information from a wide variety of receptors. There are receptors that respond to light, to sound, to mechanical stimuli, or to heat and to cold; some stimuli are perceived as pain; some chemical influences are perceived as tastes by the taste buds in the tongue. Sensory nerve fibres are also called *afferent* nerve fibres because they transmit information from external sources into the central nervous system. The ability to react to external stimuli depends on inputs of information from external sources into the central nervous system.

Sensory Pathways

The central nervous system not only receives information from sensory receptors but also acts upon them to modify their responses. Afferent neurones convey information from receptors at their peripheral endings to the CNS. Such neurones are sometimes called primary or first-order neurones because they are the first cells entering the CNS in the synaptically-linked chains of neurones that handle the incoming information.

All information coming into the CNS is subjected to control mechanisms at synaptic junctions either by other afferent neurones or by descending pathways from higher regions such as the reticular formation and the cerebral cortex. These inhibitory controls are exerted at two main sites:

1 The axon terminals of the afferent nerves; and
2 The interneurones that are activated directly by the afferent neurones.

Motoneurones that innervate a particular muscle form a *motoneurone pool*, α and γ motoneurones are mixed together in this pool, which is located in the ventral horn of one of several segments of the spinal chord. All motoneurones receive afferent fibres from all of the muscle spindles in the innervated muscle. The group Ia and group II afferent fibres make monosynaptic and polysynaptic excitatory connections on the motoneurones in the spinal chord.

The signals are either carried in ascending pathways to the brainstem and thalamus and then relayed to a specific area of the cerebral cortex, or the information is relayed from the interneurones along non-specific ascending pathways into the brain reticular formation and regions of the thalamus and cortex that are not highly discriminative.

Transmission of Impulses from Receptors

A great deal of research has been undertaken on the ways in which sensory receptors generate electrical signals. Mathews, in his book published in 1972, reviewed his outstanding work on muscle stretch receptors and very detailed information is now available on the visual field and on the mechanism of hearing. The skin is equipped with three categories of cutaneous receptor: mechanoceptors or pressure receptors, thermoceptors for sensing hot and cold, and nociceptors signalling damage to the skin.

Afferent neurones differ from motoneurones in that they have no dendrites and only one process or axon. On leaving the cell body, the axon divides into two branches: one, the peripheral process, which may end in a receptor and the other, the central process, enters the CNS and makes synaptic contact with its target neurones. In response to an adequate stimulus, the receptor generates a receptor potential that reflects the intensity, duration and location of the stimulus. A stimulus that is too weak to initiate nerve impulses is said to be *subthreshold*.

Adequate stimuli generate receptor potentials which result in trains of action potentials that are propagated along the afferent nerves fibres some synapsing on motoneurones and some synapsing in the medulla. These stimuli have the same all-or-none nature of action potentials as described earlier for motoneurones. The greater the intensity of the stimulus the higher the frequency of action potentials; and the more widespread the stimulus the greater the number of receptors that are stimulated. Location of the input signal is determined by the size of each afferent nerve's receptor site and the amount of overlap of nearby receptor fields.

In a few cases, e.g. the Pacinian, Meissner and Ruffini corpuscles (pressure receptors present in the skin), a single afferent neurone ends in one receptor. More commonly, the afferent neurone divides into many fine branches, each terminating in a receptor, all of which are preferentially sensitive to the same type of stimulus or input. A single afferent neurone and all of its receptor endings make up a sensory unit, a concept similar to the motor unit described above. Sensory receptors act as transducers and the input stimulus is transformed into an electrical signal.

Adaptation

A stimulus that is applied and maintained results in different patterns of impulses according to the particular receptor that is being stimulated. In some receptors, there is an initial burst of impulses on stimulation and then the discharge rate falls greatly or may cease altogether. This process is called *adaptation* and is a decline in the intensity of response during sustained stimulation at constant intensity. Other receptors show no adaptation and the pattern of impulses accurately reflects the duration and intensity of the input stimulus. Adaptation of the subject to the sensory effects of electrical stimulation is important and is sometimes overlooked in evaluating tolerance to superimposed electrical stimulation (see sections on *Pain* and *Low Frequency Stimulation*).

Classification of Afferent Nerve Fibres

Sensory nerves, like motor nerves, may be myelinated and have been classified according to their function and the receptors that they innervate. Two methods of classification have been used (see Table 4.1). LLoyd (1948) proposed a system of classification, I–IV for muscle afferents, based on fibre diameter which is inversely related to conduction velocities. The largest and fastest conducting sensory nerves are group I afferents (12–21 μm in diameter) and have the lowest threshold of any sensory nerves to electrical stimulation. Their terminals are found in the central parts of both bag and chain fibres (see Figure 4.9) and form the primary endings. They correspond to α motoneurones having conduction velocities that range from 50–70 m/s. Group Ib afferents are slightly smaller and come from Golgi tendon organs. The smaller Group II (6–12 μm in diameter) afferents come from terminals found in less central positions of the muscle spindles where they form secondary endings (see Figure 4.9). The other afferent nerves share Erlanger's A, B, and C classification based on the conduction velocities for the motor nerves. The A group have a wide spectrum of fibre diameter (1–20 μm). Erlanger and Gasser (1937) were the first to realise that the compound action potential of a peripheral nerve in a frog shows several distinct peaks. For convenience, these were divided according to their conduction velocity; peak A is subdivided into α, β, γ and δ. Each peak contains nerve fibres with particular functions. The Aα and γ peaks include efferent nerve fibres that supply the extrafusal and intrafusal muscle fibres.

Figure 4.9   Diagrammatic representation of a muscle spindle. The two types of afferent sensory ending (group Ia and group II) are shown on the upper chain, and bag fibres and the efferent endings on the lower fibres.

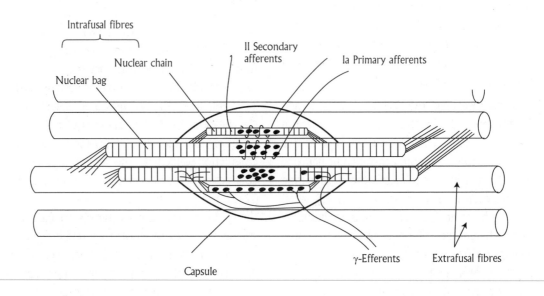

Sensory Receptors in Skeletal Muscle

Skeletal muscle contains the following sensory receptors: free nerve endings, Golgi tendon organs, Pacinian corpuscles and muscle spindles. Receptors in skeletal muscles are sophisticated, and their response to stretch is moderated by the central nervous system. (For a detailed review of muscle receptors see Mathews, 1972.)

Free nerve endings are found in association with every structure in muscle; they are the endings of all non-myelinated afferent fibres and the smallest myelinated nerve endings' type Aδ fibres. Types of stimuli that excite these endings are pressure, pain, increase in osmolarity, tetanus and infusion of potassium ions. All conditions that might be expected to exist in exercising or stimulated muscle.

Golgi tendon organs are mechanoreceptors found at the points of attachment of muscle fibres to tendinous tissue. They are encapsulated structures composed of collagen bundles innervated by large, myelinated (8–12 μm diameter) Ib afferent fibres. Golgi tendon organs were thought originally to be high-threshold stretch receptors. It is now accepted that they have low threshold and a dynamic sensitivity which signals small and rapid changes in contractile forces in the muscle. Their widespread distribution at the musculotendinous junction enables monitoring of contractions of every portion of muscle. In addition to ascending pathways, activation of Ib axons from the tendon organs produces inhibition of homonymous and synergic motoneurones and excitation of antagonist motoneurones. Pacinian corpuscles are usually found in association with Golgi tendon organs and are supplied by group II (3 μm diameter) myelinated fibres.

Muscle spindles are highly complicated receptors and are found in greatest number in skeletal muscles which undergo small length variation requiring precision movement. Figure 4.9 shows schematic diagram of a spindle. The spindles are structures of about 10 mm in length which lie parallel to the extrafusal muscle fibres. They are attached at either end to extrafusal fibres or to tendinous insertions and consist of a bundle of specialized muscle fibres or intrafusal fibres. They have a rich nerve supply, the role of which is not yet fully established. The central part of the spindle is contained within a thick connective tissue capsule. There are two types of intrafusal muscle fibres in the spindle: two or three bag fibres, and up to eight chain fibres. Bag fibres can be further subdivided into bag_1 and bag_2 fibres.

The large, Ia afferent fibres (12–20 μm diameter) have primary spiral endings on all of the muscle fibres in a spindle. These endings are on the most central region of each fibre. On either side of them, there may be up to five secondary spiral endings of the group II afferent neurones, lying mainly on the bag_2 and chain fibres. The primary and secondary afferent endings differ in their response to stretch and to vibration.

The primary endings respond with a rapid discharge during actual extension, have a slower rate of discharge during static stretch, and do not fire during the release of stretch. The secondary endings fire during static stretch. The primary endings are more highly sensitive to vibration than the secondary endings.

The motor supply to the spindles is provided mainly by small motor nerves (2–8 μm in diameter) fusimotor or γ fibres which are found at the poles of the spindles within the capsule. There are two main classes of γ efferent motor fibres. One group, $γ_d$, innervate the dynamic bag fibres, whereas $γ_s$ innervate ends on static bag_2 fibres and chain fibres. Stimulation of the fusimotor nerves elicits no increase in muscle tension but produces an increase in sensory Aβ discharge. More recently it has been recognized that some of the motor supply to the spindles comes from branches of the motoneurone supplying the extrafusal muscles.

The primary endings are very sensitive to stretch and are thought to be the mechanical response of the bag_1 fibre, and these endings are thought to be length and velocity sensitive.

Nociceptive Systems and Pain

The pain receptors are free nerve endings without specialized accessory structures. Information about noxious or painful stimuli is passed to the spinal chord by two distinct sets of fibres. The myelinated Aδ axons (1–4 μm in diameter) conduct at 6–24 m/s. They are stimulated by sharp, pricking, well localized pain, respond to noxious stimuli such as burning and cutting, and are mechanothermal receptors. The nonmyelinated C axons at 0.1–1 μm in diameter conduct more slowly (at 0.5–2 m/s) and provide the second wave of pain, which is associated with a burning or aching sensation and is poorly localized.

These afferent fibres form synapses with second order cells in the dorsal horn, sending their axons to the contralateral side and ascending in the spinothalamic tracts to the thalamus. The subject of pain modulation has received considerable attention and will be addressed in detail in Chapter 5. Many experiments have shown that no noxious stimulus can fail to activate other receptors responding to touch, pressure, displacement, stretch, and cooling and much interest in the treatment of pain by stimulation of the afferent system is based on these findings.

References

Adrian, ED, Bronk, DW (1929) The discharge of impulses in motor nerve fibres II, the frequency of discharge in reflex and voluntary contractions. *Journal of Physiology* **67**: 119–151.

Bárány, M (1967) ATPase activity of myosin correlated with speed of muscle shortening. *Journal of Genetics and Physiology* **50**: 197–218.

Barnard, RJ, Edgerton, VR, Furukawa, T and Peter, JB (1971) Histochemical, biochemical and contractile properties of red, white and intermediate fibres. *Am J Physiol* 220: 410–414.

Basmajian, JV, De Luca, CJ (1985) *Muscles alive. Their functions revealed by electromyography*, 5th edn, Williams & Williams, Baltimore.

Bernstein, J (1902) Untersuchungen zur Thermodynamik der bioelktrishen Strome. *PflügersArch* 92: 521–562.

Brown, MD, Cotter, MA, Hudlická, O, Vrbová, G (1976) The effects of different patterns of muscle activity on capillary density, mechanical properties and structure of slow and fast rabbit muscles. *Pflügers Arch* 361: 241–250.

Buchtal, F, Rosenfaalck, A (1966) Evoked action potentials and conduction velocity in human sensory nerves. *Brain Research* 3: 1.

Buller, AJ, Eccles, JC, Eccles, RW (1960a) Differentiation of fast and slow muscles in the cat hind limb. *Journal of Physiology* 150: 399–416.

Buller, AJ, Eccles, JC, Eccles, RW (1960b) Interactions between motoneurones and muscles in respect of the characterisitc speeds of their responses. *Journal of Physiology* 150: 417–439.

Burke, RE, Levine, DN, Tsiaris, P, Zajac, FE (1973) Physiological types and histochemical profiles in motor units of the cat gastrocnemius. *Journal of Physiology (Lond)* 234: 723–748.

Cotter, M, Hudlická, O (1977) Effects of chronic stimulation on muscles in ageing rats. *Journal of Physiology (Lond)* 266: 102P–103P.

Cotter, M, Phillips, P (1986) Rapid to slow fibre type transformation in response to chronic stimulation of immobilised muscles of the rabbit. *Experimental Neurology* 93: 531–545.

Denny Brown, D (1929) The histological features of striped muscle in relation to its functional activity. *Proceedings of the Royal Society (Series B)* 104: 371–411.

Eccles, JC, Eccles, RN, Lundberg, A (1958) The action potentials of the alpha neurones supplying fast and slow muscles. *J Physiol* 142: 275–291.

Edström, L, Krugelberg, E (1968) Histochemical composition, distribution of units and fatigueablity of single motor units. *J Neurol, Neurosurg, Psychiat* 31: 424–433.

Edström, L, Grimby, L (1986) Effect of exercise on the motor unit. *Muscle and Nerve* 9: 104–126.

Enoka, RM (1988) Muscle strength and its development: new perspectives. *Sports Medicine* 6: 146–168.

Erlanger, J, Gassner, HS (1937) *Electrical signs of nervous activity*. University of Pennsylvania Press.

Erlanger, J, Gassner, HS *Human Neurophysiology*, Oliver Holmes, 2nd edition, Chapman & Hall, London.

Garnett, RAF, O'Donnavan, MJ, Stephens, JA *et al.* (1979) Motor unit organisation of human gastrocnemius. *Journal of Physiology* 287: 33–43.

Garnett, RAF, Stephens, JA (1981) Changes in the recruitment threshold of motor units produced by cutaneous stimulation in man. *Journal of Physiology* 311: 463–473.

Hennemann, E, Olson, C (1965) Relations between structure and function in the design of skeletal muscles. *Journal of Neurophysiology* 28: 581–598.

Hodgkin, AL, Keynes, RD (1955) Active transport of cations in giant axons from Sepia and Lologo. *Journal of Physiology* 128: 28–60.

Hodgkin, AL, Huxley, AF (1952a) Currents carried by sodium and potassium ion through the membrane of the giant axon of Loligo. *Journal of Physiology* 116: 449–472.

Huxley, AF (1957) Muscle structure and theories of contraction. *Progress in Biophysics* 7: 255–318.

Huxley, AF, Simmons, RM (1971) Proposed mechanism of force generation in striated muscle. *Nature* 233: 533–538.

Jami, L (1992) Golgi tendon organs in mammalian skeletal muscle: Functional properties and central actions. *Physiology Review* 72: 623–666.

Jones, DA, Rutherford, OM, Parker, DF (1989) Physiological changes in skeletal muscle as a result of strength training. *Quarterly Journal of Experimental Physiology* 74: 233–256.

Katz, B (1966) *Nerve, Muscle and Synapse*. McGraw Hill, New York.

Lieber, RL (1992) *Skeletal Muscle Structure and Function*. Williams & Wilkins, Baltimore, Maryland, USA.

Lloyd, DPC, Chang, HT (1948) Afferent nerves in muscle nerves. *J ournal of Neurophysiology* 11: 488–518.

Low, J, Reed, A (1995) *Electrotherapy Explained*, 2nd edition, Butterworth-Heinemann Ltd, Oxford.

Martin, TP, Bodine-Fowler, S, Roy, RR, Eldred, E, Edgerton, VR (1988) Metabolic and fibre size properties of cat tibialis anterior motor units. *American Journal of Physiology* 255: C43–C50.

Mathews, PBC (1972) *Mammalian Muscle Receptors and their Central Actions*. Edward Arnold, London.

Milner-Brown, HS, Stein, RB, Yemm, R (1973) The orderly recruitment of human motor units under voluntary isometric contractions. *Journal of Physiology* 230: 371–390.

Nicholls, JG, Martin, AR, Wallace, BG (1992) *From Neuron to Brain a Cellular and Molecular Approach to the Function of the Nervous System*. International student series, 3rd edition. Sinauer Associates Inc., Sunderland, Massachusetts, USA.

Pette, D, Vrbová, G (1992) Adaptation of mammalian skeletal muscle fibers to chronic electrical stimulation. *Rev Physiol Biochem* 120: 116–202

Ranvier, L (1874) De quelques faits relatifs a l'histologie et á la physiologie des muscles striés. *Archives of Physiology and Normal Pathology* 6: 1–15.

Rothwell, J (1994) *Control of Human Voluntary Movement*, 2nd edition, Chapman & Hall, London.

Salmons, S, Vrbová, V (1969) The influence of activity on some contractile characteristics of mammalian fast and slow muscles. *Journal of Physiology* 201: 535–549.

Singer, B (1987) Functional electrical stimulation of the extremities in the Neurological patient: a review. *Australian Journal of Physiotherapy* 33: No. 1, 33–42.

Sherrington, CS (1906) *The Integrative Action of the Nervous System*, 1961 ed., Yale University Press, New Haven, USA.

Trimble, MH, Enoka, RM (1991) Mechanisms underlying the training effects associated with neuromuscular electrical stimulation. *Physical Therapy* 71: No. 4, 273–282.

Vrbová, G (1966) Factors determining the speed of contraction of striated muscle. *Journal of Physiology* 185: 17P–18P.

Winter, DA (1990) *Biomechanics and Motor Control of Human Movement*, 2nd ed, John Wiley & Sons, New York.

5

Physiology of Pain

LESLIE WOOD

Introduction
•
Peripheral Aspects of Pain
•
Central Aspects of Pain
•
Referred Pain
•
Phantom Limb Pain

Introduction

Pain is the combination of subjective sensations that accompany the activation of nociceptors. These sensations are variable in quality and can have serious effects on the physical and emotional well-being of the subject; pain sensations can range from mild irritation to severe, intractable pain that can be beyond endurance. Despite this, pain is a necessary sensation for normal functioning of the body; it serves a protective function by providing information concerning the location and strength of noxious and potentially tissue-damaging stimuli.

The physiology of pain, and the potential for reducing the pain sensations has only fairly recently been investigated in any great depth. Related to this is the importance of the psychology of pain. The influence of higher brain centres on the perception of pain can be an important tool in pain relief.

Peripheral Aspects of Pain

The types of sensory receptors responsible for the detection of painful stimuli – the *nociceptors* – are mostly found to be *free nerve endings*. These are nerve endings which possess no specialized accessory structures, and are found in almost all types of tissue in the body.

The nociceptors give rise to two types of afferent nerve fibre:

1 *Small diameter myelinated fibres* – group III afferents, which conduct impulses at 5–30 m/s, and are usually associated with sharp, pricking pain sensations – so-called *acute* or *fast pain*. These pain sensations have a short latency and are well localized to the specific areas of the body where the stimulus has arisen. The duration of these sensations is relatively short and the pain has less emotional involvement.

2 *Small diameter unmyelinated fibres* – group IV afferents, which have a much slower conduction velocity (about 0.5–2 m/s). These fibres are usually associated with longer lasting, dull throbbing or burning-type pain sensations – so-called *chronic* or *slow pain*. These pain sensations have a much slower onset following the painful stimulus, and are more diffuse. Pain sensations associated with group IV activation are longer lasting and may be difficult to endure, promoting greater emotional associations, and can be accompanied by autonomic responses such as sweating, increased heart rate and blood pressure, and nausea.

Both types of nociceptor are *polymodal* receptors, in that they can respond to a variety of different stimuli – mechanical, thermal and chemical. These can be light and heavy pressure, extremes of temperature, or chemical factors. All of these are stimuli that are potentially damaging to the tissues. The nociceptors are usually inactive (silent) in uninjured tissue; indeed, some nociceptors may never be activated throughout a person's life. However, following tissue injury the nociceptors increase their activity and become more sensitive to stimulation.

Chemical mediators of pain are released by damaged tissue and will activate the nociceptors. These include bradykinin, substance P, histamine, prostaglandins and 5-hydroxytryptamine (5-HT). Such chemical mediators are also released in pathological situations such as inflammation, arthritis, coronary occlusion and ulceration.

These chemical mediators are responsible for the longer-lasting aspects of the pain once the initial physical stimulus has ceased.

A short, noxious stimulus to the skin, joints or muscles, such as might be produced if a thumb is struck with a hammer, results in a 'double' pain response. There is an initial fast component due to activation of the group III afferents by the mechanical stimulus, followed by a slower response due to activation of group IV afferents by the release of chemical mediators from the damaged tissue. The pain sensations accompanying striking of the thumb with a hammer are therefore an initial sharp pain, followed by a longer-lasting dull, throbbing pain.

Central Aspects of Pain

Both group III and group IV afferent fibres project to the spinal cord where they synapse (both directly and via interneurones) with neurones in the dorsal horn of the grey matter. These neurones – *transmission cells* (or *T cells*) – are either involved in local spinal reflexes, or project to higher centres of the nervous system via the spinothalamic tracts (see later). The T cells are therefore responsible for relaying peripheral information regarding pain sensation to the higher centres. The excitability of these spinal interneurones can be elevated for a considerable time (up to several hours) following activation of group IV afferents.

As well as receiving excitatory input from the

primary afferent nociceptive fibres, the T cells are also subject to an inhibitory input from inter-neurones arising in the *substantia gelatinosa* of the spinal cord dorsal horn grey matter. These substantia gelatinosa interneurones (SG cells), in turn, are excited by input from large diameter, low threshold, mechanosensitive afferents. The transmission cells therefore receive excitatory inputs from nociceptive afferents, and inhibitory inputs from large diameter mechanosensitive afferents – via SG cells (Figure 5.1). The overall balance of the levels of excitatory and inhibitory influences on the transmission cells is of great importance in determining whether or not pain sensation is relayed to higher cognitive centres of the brain. Therefore, activation of low threshold mechano-receptors, whether by electrical or mechanical means, can inhibit the transmission of pain signals through the T cell by altering the balance of excitatory and inhibitory inputs to the cell (Figure 5.1).

This modulation of pain transmission by altering afferent input to the spinal cord is known as the *gate-control theory,* which was established by Melzack and Wall in 1965. In this theory, the activation of large diameter, myelinated axons in the periphery increases the amount of inhibition

impinging on the T cells in the spinal cord via the cells of the substantia gelatinosa. Even though a certain level of excitatory input to the T cells is still present via the nociceptive afferents, this is effectively abolished by the higher level of inhibition from the SG cells (Figure 5.2). The inhibitory input caused by stimulation of the large diameter, mechanosensitive afferents is said to 'close the gate' to pain transmission through the T cells in the spinal cord.

This theory has important implications for the management of pain in physiotherapy. Any technique that involves the activation of large diameter mechanosensitive afferents has the potential to modulate pain transmission in the spinal cord. Techniques such as massage, joint manipulation, traction and compression, thermal stimulation and electrotherapy all have the capability to produce sensory inputs from low threshold afferents, which can ultimately inhibit pain transmission in the spinal cord by 'closing the gate' i.e. inhibiting T cell excitability via the SG cells.

The ascending pathways responsible for relaying pain sensation to higher brain centres form part of the *anterolateral* system in the spinal cord. The anterolateral system conveys information

---

Figure 5.1 Peripheral influences on transmission of information through the T cells of the dorsal horn of the spinal cord grey matter. Nociceptive afferents stimulate the T cell, thereby transmitting nociceptive information to higher centres. Excitation of large diameter mechanosensitive afferents stimulates cells of the substantia gelatinosa (SG) that inhibit this transmission.

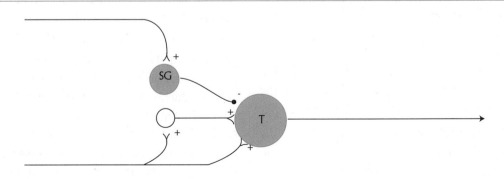

Figure 5.2 Balance of excitatory and inhibitory influences on the T cell determines the transmission of pain to higher centres. In this case, the larger amount of inhibitory activity, produced by activation of large diameter afferents (large arrow), overrides the amount of excitatory activity produced by activation of nociceptors (small arrow).

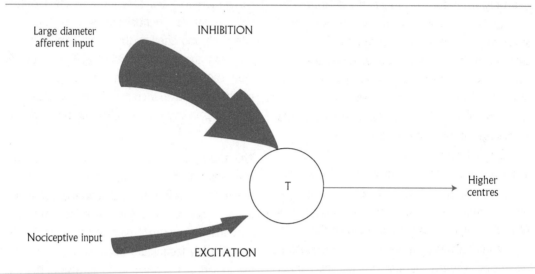

concerning pain and temperature sensation and some information about crude touch to the higher centres. This system can be subdivided into three main pathways: the *spinothalamic*, *spinoreticular* and *spinotectal* pathways.

Axons in the anterolateral system cross the midline at the level of the spinal cord, and this can occur over several spinal segments. The fibres travelling in the anterolateral system are always second-order axons that have their cell bodies in the marginal zone or substantia gelatinosa of the dorsal horn of the spinal cord grey matter. The primary afferents therefore make synaptic connections with these second-order neurones in these dorsal horn nuclei. Some of these second-order axons will ascend ipsilaterally for a few spinal segments before crossing the midline, while others will cross immediately. Anterolateral fibres terminate throughout the whole of the brainstem as well as in the thalamus (Figure 5.3).

The spinothalamic tract is concerned with the relay of information concerning pain to the higher centres. It is mostly concerned with 'fast' pain mediated by group III and IV fibres, whereas the spinoreticular tract is more concerned with 'slow' pain mediated by unmyelinated group IV fibres. The spinoreticular tract also relays information to the *periaqueductal grey matter* – an area of the brain associated with pain modulation.

Transcutaneous electrical nerve stimulation (*TENS*) can be used to directly stimulate these afferents in an appropriate area and at an appropriate voltage which will influence pain transmission in the relevant spinal segments. Both the therapist and the patient can therefore have control over pain modulation and can adjust the levels of this at any time.

The inhibitory interneurones in the substantia gelatinosa of the spinal cord can also be influenced by descending inputs from higher brain centres. Stimulation of the grey matter which surrounds the cerebral aqueduct (*periaqueductal grey matter* – *PAGM*) and of the *raphe nucleus* in the medulla can produce analgesia by inhibiting pain transmission in the spinal cord.

Figure 5.3   Anatomical organization of the anterolateral system. This is a three-neurone pathway. The primary nociceptive afferents (I) terminate in the dorsal horn of the spinal cord grey matter where they synapse with the second-order neurones (II) which ascend in the anterolateral tracts. The second-order neurones terminate in nuclei in the thalamus where they synapse with the third-order neurone (III) which ascends to the cortex.

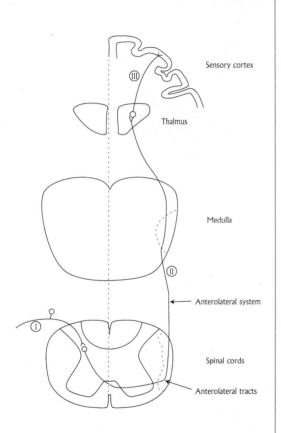

Sensory cortex

(III)

Thalmus

Medulla

(II)

Anterolateral system

(I)

Spinal cords

Anterolateral tracts

interneurones of the substantia gelatinosa by releasing monoaminergic neurotransmitters such as 5-hydroxytryptamine and noradrenaline. The action of opiates on the cells of the periaqueductal grey matter and the raphe nucleus is thought to be via suppression of the action of the inhibitory neurotransmitter GABA (gamma-amino butyric acid) released by an interneurone acting on the cells. The analgesic effects of opiates are therefore brought about by a removal of normal inhibition of the descending inputs to the spinal cord.

Higher cognitive functions of the brain such as emotions can also influence pain transmission. Fear, stress and excitement can reduce, or even abolish, the feelings of pain associated with injury. A well-known example of this is the so-called 'battlefield analgesia', where a soldier may have sustained a severe injury to a part of the body but is unaware of it until some time later, usually after reaching safety. Similar reduced responses to pain are observed in many sports, with players managing to continue while injured. This suggests that there is modulation of pain transmission brought about by the influences of higher centres such as the limbic system, probably mediated by the PAGM and raphe nucleus (see Figure 5.3). This also has important therapeutic implications at a psychological level, since the fact that a patient may simply be receiving attention from a therapist, regardless of the techniques being employed, may be sufficient to induce an emotional response which may modulate the pain they are experiencing.

These structures possess receptors for opiates, and can be activated by drugs such as morphine. Endogenous opiates such as the enkephalins and endorphins also activate these structures to produce analgesia through descending influences on the inhibitory interneurones in the substantia gelatinosa (Figure 5.4).

These descending inputs to the spinal cord are thought to modulate activity in the inhibitory

Figure 5.4 Descending influences on SG cell excitability. The peri-aqueductal grey matter and the raphe nucleus are normally inhibited by the action of inhibitory GABA-ergic interneurones. Opiates interfere with this inhibition, releasing the excitatory influence of these structures on the SG cells (mediated by 5-hydroxytryptamine). This therefore suppresses pain transmission in the spinal cord.

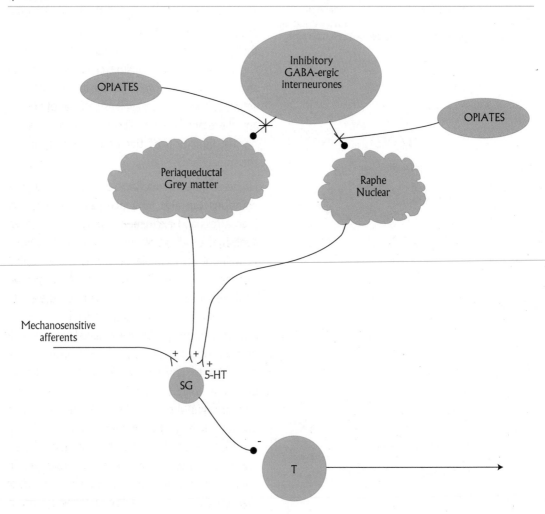

Referred Pain

Pain which arises from deep structures in the body — *visceral pain* — is often felt by the subject in locations that are far removed from the site of origin. Such translocation of pain sensation is known as *referred pain*. An example of this is the pain associated with anginal episodes. Here,

the organ that is affected is the heart, but the pain is often described as arising in the upper chest, left shoulder and arm. Similar patterns of referred pain are seen for pain arising in other structures, such as the diaphragm and appendix.

The explanation for the pattern of referred pain lies in the pattern of convergence of afferent nerve fibres in the dorsal horn of the spinal cord. Dorsal horn neurones, including those which act as transmission cells, receive input from several sources that are innervated by the same spinal segments (TI–T4 in the case of the heart and left arm). These may include nociceptive input both from cutaneous areas and visceral areas (Figure 5.5).

As previously discussed, these transmission cells pass this nociceptive information to higher centres where it is perceived as pain sensation. However, the higher centres cannot distinguish the source of this information as being either cutaneous or visceral in origin since they only receive input from single transmission cells. Peripheral input from cutaneous receptors normally predominates, and this may account for the pain sensation being incorrectly ascribed to the skin rather than the visceral organ.

It is important for the physiotherapist to be aware of the possible patterns of referred pain, since the patient might describe pain as arising in a structure which has no underlying lesion, misleading the therapist as to the real source of complaint.

Phantom Limb Pain

When a limb has been amputated or the sensory nerves from a limb have been destroyed, the sensation of the limb still being present can exist in some cases (phantom limb) and, sometimes, pain referred to the missing limb can be perceived. Pain associated with a missing limb is known as *phantom limb pain*.

Phantom limb pain is often described as burning, electric or cramping sensations, and may persist for many years after the loss of the limb.

The source of this phantom limb pain may be the severed ends of the peripheral nerves that were cut during the amputation or injury. This may set up abnormal patterns of discharge in the peripheral nerve fibres, particularly nociceptors, which are then relayed to higher centres and perceived as pain sensations arising in the areas these nerves formerly supplied. Additionally, there may be altered activity in the neurones of the dorsal horn associated with pain transmission. This

Figure 5.5 Convergence of nociceptors from different structures onto the same transmission cell. Input from cardiac nociceptors (arrow) is interpreted by higher centres as input from cutaneous nociceptors which impinge on the same transmission cell.

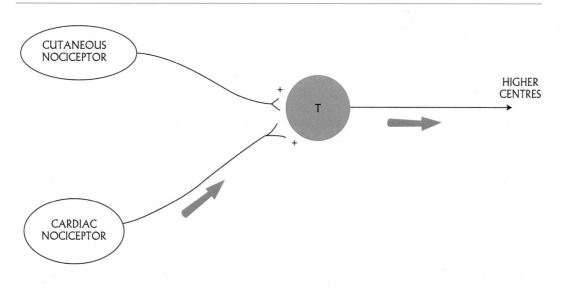

altered activity may arise as a result of afferent degeneration inducing post-synaptic changes in the dorsal horn neurones.

Recent research has suggested a further cause of phantom limb pain. This proposes that phantom limbs and the sensations associated with them are a consequence of activity in neural networks in higher centres of the brain. These neural networks form a so-called *neuromatrix*, the structure and functioning of which may be genetically determined, and which is susceptible to inputs from peripheral structures. This neuromatrix is not localized, but is widespread throughout the brain. It provides a neural framework which underpins the subject's experience of their own body as a physical entity which 'belongs' to them. Sensory inputs from all areas of the body can manipulate and modify the activity of the neuromatrix. It has been suggested that phantom limb pain arises as a result of abnormal or absent modulating input to this neuromatrix and missing channels of output from the neuromatrix to the muscles.

Bibliography

Kandel, ER, Schwartz, JH, Jessel, TM (1991) *Principles of Neural Science*, 3rd edition. Appleton and Lange.

Melzack, R (1990) Phantom limbs and the concept of a neuromatrix. *Trends in Neuroscience* 13: 88–92.

Melzack, R, Wall, P (1989) *The Challenge of Pain*, 2nd edition. Penguin Books.

Melzack, R, Wall, P (eds) (1989) Textbook of Pain.

B

Scientific Basis of Therapy

6

Thermal Effects

KENNETH COLLINS

Introduction
•
Heat and Temperature
•
Physical Effects of Heat
•
Heat Transfer
•
Thermal Homeostasis
•
Physiological Effects of Heat
•
Physiological Effects of Cold

Introduction

For centuries, early philosophers have speculated on the nature of heat and cold. Opinions have been divided as to whether heat was a substance or an effect of the motion of particles, but in the eighteenth century, physicists and physical chemists came to the conclusion that what gave our senses the impression of heat or cold was the speed of motion of the constituent molecules within the body or object. The accurate investigation of the relationship between the work done in driving an apparatus designed to churn water, and the heat developed while doing so, was taken up by Dr JP Joule of Manchester in the year 1840. He showed quite clearly that the amount of heat produced by friction depended on the amount of work done. Subsequently, his work also contributed to the theory of the correlation of forces, and in 1847 he stated the law of the Conservation of Energy (the basis of the 1st Law of Thermodynamics).

It became the accepted view that heat can be regarded as a form of energy which is interchangeable with other forms of energy such as electrical or mechanical energy. The theory supposed that when a body is heated, the rise in temperature is due to the increased energy of motion of molecules in that body. The theory went further, and explained the transmission of radiant energy from one body to another, as from the sun to an individual on earth. Evidence was found in favour of the supposition that light is an electromagnetic wave, and exactly the same evidence was adduced with regard to radiant energy. Apart from the fact that radiant heat waves (e.g. infrared radiations) have a longer wavelength than light waves, their physical characteristics are the same. It was therefore suggested that molecules of a hot body are in a state of rapid vibration, or are the centre of rapid periodic disturbances, producing electromagnetic waves, and that these waves travel between the hot body to the receiving body causing similar motion in the molecules. The sense of heat may thus be excited in an organism by waves of radiant heat energy which start from a hot object just as the sense of sight is excited by waves of light which start from a luminous object.

Heat and Temperature

The fact that when various forms of energy are converted into heat there is always a constant ratio between the amount of energy that disappears and the amount of heat produced, suggests that in all these processes energy is neither created nor destroyed. This principle is a partial expression of the *1st Law of Thermodynamics*: 'in all processes occurring in an isolated system, the energy of the system remains constant'. Electrical, chemical, magnetic and other forms of energy can be converted into heat energy with 100% efficiency, but it is not possible to achieve the reverse and transform all heat energy stored in the microstructure of matter to some other energy form. Again, if one form of energy is converted to another, e.g. chemical to mechanical, the process is not 100% efficient and some of the energy is always converted to heat. The

tendency eventually to randomize molecular motion into heat energy suggests that heat is a primordial component in the structure of matter.

The concepts of *heat* and *temperature* are rigorously differentiated in physics and the distinction needs to be similarly maintained in the theory of electrotherapy. If we suppose that the same quantity of heat (Q) is distributed over a large and a small amount of the same material, the larger amount of material will have a lower temperature (T_1) than the smaller (T_2). Thus, while the quantity of heat is a form of energy, the temperature of an object is a measure of the *average kinetic energy* of the constituent molecules. Since it is related to the 'average' movement of molecules, the concept of temperature can be applied only to bodies consisting of a large number of molecules. Furthermore the simple relationship no longer applies at very low temperatures.

The only term for temperature that allows consistent expression of all states of matter, solid, liquid and gas, in accord with the laws of thermodynamics, is the thermodynamic temperature, the base unit of which is the *kelvin* (K). In the system introduced by Lord Kelvin in 1848, the linear scale starts at the absolute zero of temperature (0 degrees K). The thermodynamic *Celsius* scale is subdivided into the same intervals as the Kelvin scale but has a zero point displaced by 273.15. The Celsius scale is divided into 100 unit intervals between two fixed points, the condensing point of steam (100°C = 373.15K) and the melting point of ice (0°C = 273.15K). Absolute zero on the Celsius scale is −273.15°C. The *Fahrenheit* (F) scale does not conform to the International System of Units (SI) but continues to be used in many regions of the world particularly in meteorological data (0°C = 32°F; 100°C = 212°F).

Heat Units

Energy, work and the *amount of heat* are physical quantities with the same dimensions and ideally should be measured by a common unit. Traditional units such as the calorie are deeply rooted in technical as well as in dietary usage, but in accord with SI strategy, the calorie is a 'non-coherent' unit. To conform with the SI, a quantity of heat should be expressed in *joules* (J). Heat exchanges are usually considered in terms of *power* (energy per unit time) e.g. joules per second (= 1 watt or W). The watt is probably more familiar in everyday use as a measure of power consumption of electrical appliances e.g in kilowatt hours (kWh), which is actually energy per unit time × time. Table 6.1 derives the relationship between the physical expressions of *force*, *energy* and *power*.

The amount of heat energy required to raise a unit mass of material by 1°C is known as the *specific heat* of the material. The specific heat of water is 4.185 J/g/°C. Far less heat is needed to raise the temperature of a gas (e.g. specific heat of air = 1.01 J/g/°C). The human body contains approximately 60% water and not surprisingly has a relatively high specific heat (3.56 J/g/°C). The specific heats of skin, muscle, fat and bone are respectively 3.77, 3.75, 2.3 and 1.59 J/g/°C. It is thus readily calculated that if the mean body temperature of a 65 kg person is increased by 1°C over a period of 1 h, then an extra 231 kJ of heat has been stored in the body.

Table 6.1
Derivation of Coherent Heat Units

Physical quantity	Definition	SI unit	Dimension
Force	mass × acceleration	newton (N) (kg × metre.sec^{-2})	$M L T^{-2}$
Energy	force × distance	joule (J) (newton × metre)	$M L^2 T^{-2}$
Power	energy/unit time	watt (W) (joule.sec^{-1})	$M L^2 T^{-3}$

M = mass
L = distance
T = time
Non-coherent units:
1 calorie = 4.185 joules
1 kcal/hour = 1.16 watts

Physical Effects of Heat

When heat is added to matter, a number of physical phenomena result from increasing the kinetic energy of its microstructure. These may be summarized as follows:

1. Rise in temperature: The average kinetic energy of constituent molecules increases.
2. Expansion of the material: Increased kinetic energy produces a greater vibration of molecules which move further apart and expand the material. Gases will expand more than liquids and liquids more than solids. If, for example, a gas is enclosed so that expansion cannot take place, a rise in gas pressure will occur instead.
3. Change in physical state: Changing a substance from one physical state (phase) to another requires a specific amount of heat energy i.e. latent heat. The latent heat of fusion is the energy required for, or released by, 1 gram of ice at 0°C in order to convert it to 1 gram of water at 0°C (336 joules), and the latent heat of vaporization is the energy needed to convert 1 gram of water at 100°C to 1 gram of steam at 100°C (2268 joules).
4. Acceleration of chemical reactions: Van't Hoff's Law states that 'any chemical reaction

capable of being accelerated, is accelerated by a rise in temperature. The ratio of the reaction rate constants for a reaction occurring at two temperatures 10°C apart is the Q_{10} of the reaction'.

5   Production of an electrical potential difference: if the junction of two dissimilar metals, e.g. copper and antimony, is heated, an e.m.f. (electromotive force or electrical potential difference) is produced between their free ends (the Seebeck, or thermocouple effect). Conversely, an e.m.f. applied to the junction of two metals can cause a rise in temperature at the junction (Peltier effect).

6   Production of electromagnetic waves: When energy is added to an atom, e.g. by heating, an electron may move out into a higher-energy electron shell. When the electron returns to its normal level, energy is released as a pulse of electromagnetic energy (a photon).

7   Thermionic emission: Heating of some materials, e.g. tungsten, may cause such molecular agitation that some electrons leave their atoms and may break free of the metal. This leaves a positive charge which tends to attract electrons back. A point is reached where the rate of loss of electrons equals the rate of return, and a cloud of electrons then exists as a space charge around the metal. This process is known as thermionic emission.

8   Reduction in viscosity of fluids: Dynamic viscosity is the property of a fluid (liquid or gas) of offering resistance (internal friction) to the non-accelerated displacement of two adjacent layers. The molecules in a viscous fluid are quite strongly attracted to one another. Heating increases the kinetic movement of these molecules, reducing their cohesive mutual attraction and making the fluid less viscous.

Heat Transfer

Processes involving the movement of heat energy from one point to another are governed by the Laws of Thermodynamics. Previously, mention has been made of the 1st Law which deals with the conservation and interchange of different forms of energy. The *2nd Law of Thermodynamics* states that 'heat cannot by itself, i.e. without performance of work by some external agency, pass from a colder to a warmer body'. These general laws establish the principles that govern heat exchanges (gain or loss) within the body and between the body and its environment. In electrotherapy we are concerned with the transfer of heat energy between the external environment and the body surface, and between the component tissues and fluids of the body itself as well as with the therapeutic effects of heat.

Conduction

Conduction is the mechanism of energy exchange between regions of different temperature, from hotter to colder, which is accomplished by direct molecular collision. The energy thus transferred causes an increased vibration of molecules which is transmitted to adjacent molecules. A simple example of this process is the metal bar heated at one end which, by heat conduction, eventually becomes hot at its other end. The application of a cold pack to the skin surface induces skin cooling by heat conduction from the warm skin, and *vice versa* for a hot pack. The rate of heat transfer depends on the difference in temperature between the regions in contact, the surface area of contact at the boundary, and the thermal conductivity of the materials in contact. Thermal conductivity is a specific property of the material itself, e.g. metals are better conductors than wood, water a better conductor than air.

Convection

Convection is the heat transfer mechanism that occurs in a fluid due to gross movements of molecules within the mass of fluid. If a part of a fluid is heated, the kinetic energy of the molecules in that part is increased, the molecules move further apart, and the fluid becomes less dense. In consequence, that part of the fluid rises and displaces the more dense fluid above, which in turn descends to take its place. The immediate process of energy transfer from one fluid particle to another remains one of conduction, but the energy is transported from one point in space to another primarily by convective displacement of the fluid itself. Pure conduction is rarely observed in a fluid, due to the ease with which even small temperature differences initiate free convection currents.

Thermal Radiation

Heat may be transmitted by electromagnetic radiation emitted from the surface of a body whose surface temperature is above absolute zero. The heating of certain atoms causes an electron to move to a higher-energy electron shell. As it returns to its normal shell, the energy is released as a pulse of electromagnetic energy. This radiation occurs primarily in the infrared band from wavelengths of about 10^{-5} cm to 10^{-2} cm (0.1–100 μm, or 10^3–10^6 Å). A thermal radiation incident upon a surface can be:

1 reflected back from that surface;
2 transmitted through it;
3 absorbed.

In many everyday circumstances, objects are radiating and absorbing the same amount of infrared energy, thus maintaining a constant temperature. The amount of radiation from an object is proportional to the fourth power of the temperature (in kelvin). The rate of emission from a surface also depends on the nature of the surface, being greatest for a black body. A perfect black body absorbs all the radiation, while other surfaces absorb some and reflect the remainder.

Evaporation

Thermal energy is required to transform a liquid into vapour and the rate at which this proceeds is determined by the rate at which the vapour diffuses away from the surface. The rate depends on the power supplied and the vapour pressure of the air above the liquid. Evaporation follows laws very similar to those governing convection. When water vaporizes from the body surface (e.g. during sweating) the latent heat required is extracted from the surface tissue, thereby cooling it. The converse process, condensation, entails latent heat gain at the surface as vapour is changed into liquid.

Body Heat Transfer

In thermoregulation, heat is exchanged by conductive, convective, radiative and evaporative transfer processes between the body surface and the environment so that the body's core temperature remains constant and equilibrium is maintained between internal (metabolic) heat production and heat loss (or gain) at the skin surface.

Heat transfer within tissues takes place primarily by *conduction* and *convection*. The temperature distribution will depend on the amount of energy converted into heat at a given tissue depth, and thermal properties of the tissue (e.g. specific heat, thermal conductivity). Physiological factors are important in determining tissue temperature, e.g. when raised tissue temperature produces an increased local blood flow, cooler blood re-perfusing the heated tissue will selectively tend to cool the tissue. The technique of application of a treatment modality will also clearly modify the tissue temperature through variations in time and intensity, etc. When deep-treatment is applied (e.g. short-wave dia-thermy, microwave, ultrasound) conversion of the energy into heat occurs as it penetrates into the tissues. Heating modalities may be subdivided according to their primary mode of heat transfer during selective heating of superficial or deep tissues (Table 6.2).

In thermotherapy, the important properties concerned with heat conduction in tissues are thermal conductivity, tissue density and specific heat. Convection involves these properties also, but in addition, fluid viscosity becomes import-ant. Understanding of the interaction of electromagnetic waves within biological media requires knowledge of the dielectric properties of tissues with different water content (Guy, 1990).

Table 6.2
Heating modalities and their primary mode of heat transfer (after Lehman, JF, De Lateur, BJ, 1990)

Primary mode of heat transfer	Modality	
Conduction	Hot packs Paraffin bath	⎫
Convection	Fluidotherapy Hydrotherapy Moist air	⎬ Superficial heat
'Conversion'	Radiant heat Laser	⎭
	Microwave Shortwave Ultrasound	⎬ Deep heat

Thermal Homoeostasis

In health, humans maintain internal and external heat exchanges and preserve a constant body temperature by means of a highly efficient ther-moregulatory system. This process of homo-eothermy is defined as 'a pattern of temperature regulation in which cyclic variations in deep body (core) temperature is maintained within arbitrary limits of $\pm$ 2°C despite much larger variations in ambient temperature' (I.U.P.S., 1987). Thus, with a normal body temperature of about 37°C, hyperthermia may be regarded as a core tempera-ture in excess of 39°C and hypothermia below 35°C. At rest, and in a neutral environment, core temperature can be kept within a much more narrow band of control ($\pm$ 0.3°C) in accord with the body's intrinsic diurnal temperature rhythm. Claude Bernard's concept of thermal homoeostasis depicting a virtual straight-line constancy is shown to be not so precise, since spontaneous rhythmic variations in body tem-perature occur with diurnal, monthly (e.g. ovulatory) and seasonal temperature cycles.

Body Temperature

The body is usually considered to consist of two thermal compartments, the core or central com-partment, and the shell or superficial layer. The core temperature is controlled at a constant level by physiological mechanisms. The shell, at the interface between the body and the environ-ment, is subject to much greater variations in temperature. Though the core temperature is kept within a narrow range around 37°C, it must not be regarded as a simple fixed entity, for there are significant temperature gradients within the anatomical core. Organs such as the liver and active skeletal muscles, for example, have a higher rate of metabolic heat production than other tissues and therefore maintain a higher temperature. Similarly, there are temperature gradients within the vascular compartment perfusing both the core and the shell.

The diurnal (circadian) core temperature rhythm is one of the most stable of biological rhythms, with a well-marked intrinsic component (Figure 6.1). Body temperature is lowest in the early morning and highest in the evening, though in a small minority of people the phase is reversed. The diurnal range of variation is usually about 0.5–1.5°C in adults, depending on other external factors such as the effects of meals, activity, sleep and ambient temperature (which can sometimes influence the oral temperature). Different intrinsic biological rhythms are often in phase with each other. There is evidence that desynchronization of different rhythms is deleterious to function, e.g. desynchronization of the sleep-wake cycle and the core temperature cycle by continuous light exposure can bring about impairment of thermo-regulatory function (Moore-Ede and Sulzman, 1981).

Across approximately 1 cm of the body shell, from the skin surface to the superficial layer of muscle, there is a temperature gradient that varies according to the temperature of the core and the external environment. The gradient is not uniform, but changes with the thermal conductivity of the tissue layers and the rate of blood flow in the different regions (Figure 6.2). Skin temperatures differ widely over the body surface, especially in hot or cold conditions. When an individual is in a comfortable environment of, say, 24°C, the skin of the toes may be 27°C, the upper arms and legs 31°C, the forehead 34°C, while the core is maintained at 37°C.

Body Temperature Measurement

Core temperature is measured conventionally by a mercury-in-glass thermometer placed in the mouth. The instruments for clinical use comply with the British and EC Standards (BS 691, 1987).

Figure 6.1   Diurnal variation in body temperature showing the influence of ambient (room) temperature on the oral temperature when ambient temperature, meals and physical activity are kept constant. [E = intrinsic temperature rhythm].

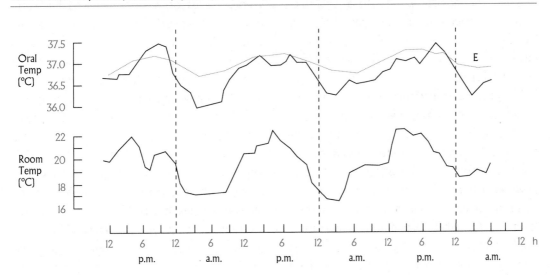

Figure 6.2   Temperature gradients in the forearm between the skin surface and deep tissues in A comfortably warm conditions and B cold conditions.

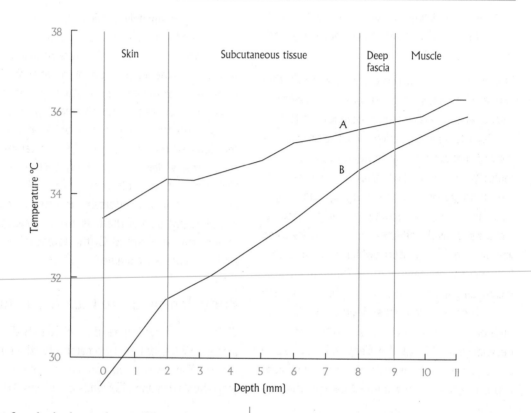

The Standards also apply to subnormal temperature, ovulation and dual scale (Fahrenheit and Celsius) thermometers. Electronic thermometers are widely used, but apart from the increase in range of measurement they are no quicker or more accurate than the mercury thermometer. Errors in taking oral temperature arise with any thermometer if there is mouth breathing or talking during measurement, or if hot or cold drinks have been taken just previously, or if the tissues of the mouth are affected by a hot or cold external environments. The rectal temperature is a slowly-equilibrating but often more reliable measurement of core temperature and on average about 0.5°C higher than mouth temperature. Cold blood from chilled legs or warmed blood from active leg muscles can affect the rectal temperature. The reading will depend on the position of the probe in relation to the rectal venous plexus of vessels influenced by blood from the lower limbs. The temperature of the urine is also a reliable measure of core temperature, provided that it is possible to void a stream of 50–100 ml or more. For accurate and fast recording, measurement can be made in the ear canal (near but not touching the tympanic membrane) by thermistor or thermocouple, but unless this is done in a warm environment and with lagging placed over the ear, errors are introduced because of heat conduction from the ear canal to the colder pinna. It is possible to overcome this problem by employing a zero-gradient self-correcting electronic thermometer (Keatinge and Sloane, 1975). Oesophageal temperature also provides an accurate measurement of core temperature, but placement of the thermistor probe is important in order to avoid cooling from the trachea and warming from the stomach. Telemetric monitoring is sometimes appropriate for measuring intestinal temperature by a temperature sensitive pill that is easily swallowed. Internal temperature is thus continuously transmitted to an external receiver.

Average values for skin temperature can be obtained by applying a number of separate thermistors or thermocouples over the skin surface and applying weighting factors for the different areas of skin represented. Contact temperatures of this nature are, however, prone to errors, notably from changes in skin temperature produced by the probe and tape, the effect of pressure on the skin, sweating, and heat transfer from the detector to the air. Regional variations can be visualized and an integrated mean skin temperature computed by infrared thermography.

Temperatures in the shell and in deeper tissues of the body can be determined locally by inserting thermocouples or thermistors into the tissues. Thermocouples can be made very small and probes inserted in 29-gauge needles. Techniques for constructing probes of the order of 10 μm diameter have been described. This is an invasive procedure, but non-invasive thermometry has become possible by thermal tomography, a technique that is particularly relevant for monitoring hyperthermia treatments. Most existing systems have, however, inherent inaccuracies in their temperature sensitivity and spatial discrimination that require care in interpretation.

Thermal Balance

Whilst core temperature remains constant, there is an equilibrium between internal heat production and external heat loss. This is expressed in the form of a Heat Balance Equation:

$$M \pm w = \pm K \pm C \pm R - E \pm S$$

where:

- M is the rate of metabolic heat production;
- w the external work performed by or on the body;
- K, C and R the loss or gain of heat by conduction, convection and radiation;
- E the evaporative heat loss from the skin and respiratory tract; and
- S the rate of change of body heat storage (= 0 at thermal equilibrium).

Metabolic heat production (M) can be derived from the measurement of total body oxygen consumption. Basal metabolic rate during complete physical and mental rest is about 45 W/m^2 (i.e. watts per square metre of body surface) for an adult male of 30 years and 41 W/m^2 for a female of the same age. Maximum values of heat production occur during severe physical work and may be as high as 900 W/m^2 for brief periods. Heat production can increase at rest in cold conditions by involuntary muscle contractions that produce shivering. A small increase in M follows eating a meal, the thermogenic response to food.

Heat loss or gain by conduction (K) depends on the temperature difference between the body and the surrounding medium, on the thermal conductivities, and the area of contact. Little heat is normally lost by conduction to the air since air is a poor heat conductor. The amount of subcutaneous fat is an important factor determining tissue cooling by providing tissue insulation (the reciprocal of conductance) and it is especially important for preventing conductive heat loss in cold water immersion.

Normally, the surface temperature of a person is

higher than that of the surrounding air so that heated air close to the body moves upwards by natural convection as colder air takes its place. The value of *convective heat exchange* (C) depends on the nature of the surrounding fluid and the existing characteristics of its flow.

Radiant heat transfer (R) depends on the nature of the radiating surfaces, their temperature and the geometrical relationship between them. Extending the arms and legs effectively increases the surface area over which convective and radiant heat exchange can take place.

At rest in a comfortable ambient temperature, an individual loses weight by evaporation of water diffusing through the skin and from the respiratory tract. This is described as insensible water loss, normally about 30 g per hour, which produces a heat loss of about $10 \, W/m^2$. Sweating (sensible water loss) contributes a much greater potential *evaporative heat loss* (E). Complete evaporation of 1 litre of sweat from the body surface in 1 hour will dissipate about $400 \, W/m^2$.

The specific heat of the human body is $3.5 \, kJ/kg$. If a person of 65 kg increases mean core temperature by 1°C over a period of 1 hour, the *rate of heat storage* (S) becomes 230 kJ per hour, or 64 W S can be positive or negative, but in determining heat storage the difficulty is to assess the change in mean body temperature. The change in mean core temperature is not sufficient because different weightings are contributed by the core and shell. During cold exposure for example, the volume of the core of the body is effectively reduced, thereby altering the skin–core weighting coefficients. Various formulae have been suggested, e.g. 0.90 core temperature + 0.10 skin temperature in hot conditions; and 0.67 core temperature + 0.33 skin temperature in cold conditions.

In recent years, thermotherapy has developed numerical methods for quantitatively analyzing the complex interactions between diathermy energy and the tissues by computer modelling (Emery and Sekins, 1990). It has particular applications in hyperthermia treatment of malignancies where there are critical thresholds for cell viability. Thermal modelling by computer has similarly led to increased understanding of safe exposure times and the processes of heat exchange in whole-body exposures to hot and cold temperatures (Wissler, 1988).

Control of Body Temperature

Thermoregulation is integrated by a controlling system in the central nervous system that responds to the heat content of tissues signalled by thermoreceptors. These receptors are sensitive to heat and cold thermal information arising in the skin, deep tissues and the central nervous system itself. They provide feedback signals to central nervous structures situated mainly in the hypothalamus of the brain in a servo- or loop-system (Figure 6.3). The temperature of the blood perfusing the hypothalamus is a major physiological drive to thermoregulation, in addition to the neural inputs from thermoreceptors. The hypothalamus thus monitors ambient thermal load or deficit in the heat balance of the body and initiates appropriate physiological responses (vasodilatation and sweating in hot conditions, vasoconstriction and shivering in cold) that prevent any deviation of core temperature. Apart from these involuntary responses, thermal information is also transmitted by afferent nerves to other regions of the brain controlling endocrine functions, and to the cerebral cortex signalling thermal sensations and inducing behavioural thermoregulation.

Figure 6.3   Schematic diagram of the human thermoregulatory control system.

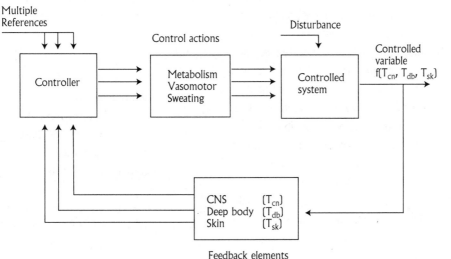

An essential role in processing thermal signals is ascribed to the pre-optic region of the anterior hypothalamus and a region in the posterior hypothalamus, described respectively as the 'heat loss' and 'heat gain' centres, since they are considered to exert the primary control on vasodilatation / sweating in heat and vasoconstriction / shivering in cold. The integration of incoming and outgoing information, and the 'set-point' or 'gain' at which the hypothalamic centres operate is the basis on which present views of thermoregulatory control are constructed (Hensel, 1981; Collins, 1992).

Physiological Effects of Heat

Heating the tissues brings about the physical effects of heat on matter already described (see p. 95). Heat generated within any specific tissue is not confined to that tissue, but is distributed within adjacent parts according to the laws of heat

flow and by changes in local blood flow. In biological systems, the reactions are considerably more complicated than in non-biological material however. Other thermal changes are produced by local, general or remote effects involving different physiological processes. Nevertheless, the same physical principles apply initially as for all materials, and heat distribution will depend on factors such as:

1   Size of heated area;
2   Depth of absorption of specific radiation;
3   Duration of heating;
4   Intensity of irradiation;
5   Method of application.

Local Effects

CELL METABOLISM

Chemical reactions involved in metabolic activity are increased by a rise in temperature (Van't Hoff's Law). Metabolic rate may increase by about 13%

for each 1°C rise in tissue temperature, the increase in metabolism being greatest in the region where most heat is generated. As a result, there is an elevated tissue demand for oxygen and nutrients and enhanced output of metabolic waste products. Accelerated cellular metabolism can produce many beneficial therapeutic effects to treat injury or infection. However, components of enzyme systems, such as proteins, are heat sensitive and increasingly destroyed by raising temperature beyond a threshold value. Rising tissue temperature first produces an increase in enzyme activity to a peak value, followed by a decline, and then finally abolition of enzyme activity. As an example, a specific destructive enzyme such as collagenase (found to have an important role in rheumatoid arthritis) brings about an increase in collagenolysis at 36°C when compared with that at 30°C in tissue experiments (Harris and McCroskery, 1974). Clinically, it has been demonstrated that normal knee joints have a temperature of 30.5–33°C, whereas joints with active synovitis have temperatures between 34–37.6°C. It might be anticipated that had the joint temperature been raised to say the range 40–45°C, the destructive collagenase may be inactivated. The problem is, of course, that *in vivo*, other enzyme systems with lower thresholds may also be destroyed. At temperatures about 45°C, so much protein damage occurs that there is destruction of cells and tissues. At 45°C, skin burns occur if contact is maintained for long enough. It is found that 'heat-shock proteins' accumulate in cells and tissues exposed to high temperatures, the function of which, though not yet clearly agreed, is thought to confer a degree of protection to cells upon subsequent heat exposure. Temperature has an all-pervasive influence on cellular function, and heat damage can occur at multiple sites. Cell membranes are particularly sensitive, the lipoprotein structure of membranes may become more fluid with increasing temperature and cause breakdown in permeability (Bowler, 1987).

BLOOD FLOW

When the skin is heated, the surface reddens (erythema) and blood vessels become vasodilated leading to increased blood flow. A good blood supply is essential for healing and, if there is infection, the increased number of white cells and fluid exudate available assist in destroying bacteria. The vasodilatation is caused by several mechanisms. Firstly, temperature elevation has a direct effect on the state of dilatation of arterioles and venules by acting on the smooth muscle of the vessels. If any local tissue damage occurs during heating, further dilatation may be produced by the release of histamine-like and tissue dilator substances such as bradykinin. Vasodilatation may also be produced in the skin by a local axon reflex in which stimulation of sensory cutaneous nerve endings produce antidromic nerve impulses in branches of the sensory nerves arborizing around skin blood vessels. Increased skin blood flow occurs in areas remote from the heated tissue due to long spinal nervous reflexes (Kerslake and Cooper, 1950).

Veins commonly run close to arteries allowing ready exchange of heat between vessels. By a counter-current exchange, heat flows from the arterial blood to the cooler venous blood, thus returning some of the heat to the core. Its effect is to reduce body convective heat transfer by the blood but, in a warm environment, its effect is considerably diminished because of dilatation in the large superficial veins. Much of the variation in skin blood flow, however, is due to the presence of arteriovenous anastomoses deep to the skin capillaries. When these vessels open, the fall in temperature along the artery is reduced, thus raising skin temperature and increasing heat loss.

Increased blood flow in deeper organs and tissues has been shown to occur as the consequence of heating, but it is usually less marked than in the skin. Part of the overall circulatory response in thermoregulation involves a redistribution of circulating blood in favour of the skin blood vessels for the purpose of heat exchange and at the expense of blood supply to the core. There is consequently a complex blood flow response in deeper tissues, involving direct vasodilatation due to heat, increased blood flow due to increased metabolic activity, e.g. in skeletal muscle, and a reduced blood flow because of a relative vasoconstriction brought about by thermoregulation.

OTHER TISSUE EFFECTS

The properties of specific tissues may be changed by heating. For example, tendon extensibility can be increased by raising the temperature with the result that a stretch producing a given elongation will alter the strength of the tissue less when heat is applied. Joint temperature influences the resistance to movement, with low temperature increasing and higher temperature reducing the resistance. These changes in joint movement can be in part attributed to changes in viscosity of the synovial fluid. It is commonly observed that muscle spasms, secondary to underlying pathology, can often be relieved through the use of heat. On the basis of studies on the effect of temperature on muscle spindles, it has been postulated that there is a selective cessation of firing from secondary spindle afferent endings which may result in reduced muscle tone (Lehmann and De Lateur, 1990). Heat is often used to relieve pain in a variety of musculoskeletal disorders, though the mechanism is uncertain. In some cases, pain may be relieved by reducing secondary muscle spasm, or pain alleged to be related to ischaemia can be reduced by heat-induced vasodilatation. Heat has also been applied as a 'counter irritant', e.g. the thermal stimulus may affect pain sensation in accord with the 'gate theory' of Melzack and Wall (1965) (see Chapter 5, p. 85), as one explanation of the phenomenon.

Systemic Effects

Local heating causes a *rise in temperature of tissues* and *reflex vasodilatation* in remote areas of the body, but if heating is extensive and prolonged, a general rise in core temperature can ensue. Blood heated by the local tissues carries heat throughout the circulation. The hypothalamic centres are thus stimulated both by reflex mechanisms arising from peripheral thermoreceptors and from the direct blood-borne heat stimulus.

The immediate systemic response is a *generalized skin vasodilatation* which serves to transport heat by conduction and convection from the core to the shell. There is a concomitant reduction in splanchnic blood flow resulting in reduced hepatic clearance rate and reduction in urine flow. If the heat stress is great, the skin temperature rises and approaches 35°C over the whole of the body. At, or near this point, the body temperature becomes stabilized by the stimulation of sweat glands which secrete hypotonic sweat onto the body surface so that increased evaporative cooling may take place. High radiant temperatures can be tolerated for many minutes if the environment is dry (as in a sauna). An increase in ambient humidity makes these conditions immediately unbearable. This is because the vapour pressure gradient between the skin and air is reduced, allowing sweat to run off the body instead of dissipating heat by evaporation.

Heat illness may occur with sudden increases in heat stress, most readily in those who are not adapted (acclimatized) to heat. Generalized skin vasodilatation may cause swelling of the feet and ankles (heat oedema) or syncope during postural change or prolonged standing. Prickly heat, a papulovesicular rash accompanied by a dermal prickling sensation when sweating is provoked, occurs in some people when areas of the skin are continuously wetted by sweat. More serious heat illnesses such as water-deficiency or salt-deficiency heat exhaustion are due to imbalance of body water and salt respectively with excessive sweating and lead to collapse. Left untreated, they may result in potentially fatal heat stroke when core temperature reaches high levels of 41°C and above and the central heat regulatory mechanisms fail (Khogali and Hales, 1983).

Physiological Effects of Cold

The application of cold to tissues (cryotherapy) involves the tranference of heat energy away from the tissues and is therefore considered only in a 'negative sense' to be a part of electrotherapy. It is included usually because of its value in physical therapy. Some effects are similar to those of heating and some are not; the common indications are in treatment of muscle spasm, pain from injury and reduction in bleeding and swelling. The effects of cold can be examined at both the local level and for the overall systemic effect. As with heat gain, the rate of removal of heat from tissues depends on area, depth, duration, intensity and method of cooling.

Local Effects

CELL METABOLISM

It is generally, but not universally, true that chemical and biological processes slow down with decreasing temperature. Since most enzyme systems operate at an optimum temperature, lowering the temperature results in a slow inactivation of chemical processes. Cell viability is critically-dependent on membrane transport systems involving active biochemical pumps and passive leaks in membranes, which maintain intracellular ionic composition. The failure of pumps at low temperatures relative to leaks brings about a gain in Na^+, Ca^{++} and loss of K^+ at reduced temperature in the cells of many species, i.e. membranes lose their selective permeability in cold conditions. Freezing damage to cells occurs when local temperature drops to zero. Viscosity increases, ice crystallizes and the remaining solution in the cells is reduced in volume as water leaks into the interstitial space. A characteristic feature of cold injury is the vascular damage which occurs with intravascular aggregation of platelets and red blood cells and the formation of occlusion masses in the vessels.

BLOOD FLOW

Cooling the skin causes an immediate vasoconstriction which acts to diminish body heat loss. Thermoreceptors in the skin are stimulated and produce an autonomic reflex vasoconstriction over the body surface. In addition, there is a direct constrictor effect of cold on the smooth muscle of arterioles and venules. Counter-current heat exchange helps to reduce heat transfer to the periphery. This is most effective in the limbs because of the relatively long parallel pathways between the deep arteries and veins. In this way, body core temperature is prevented from falling rapidly. Arteriovenous anastomoses that open to allow more blood flow to the skin in hot conditions are constricted in the cold.

Although immersion of the hands in water at 0–12°C at first causes the expected vasoconstriction, this is followed after a delay of 5 min or more by a marked vasodilatation. This is then interrupted by another burst of vasoconstriction and subsequent waves of increased and decreased local blood flow. This phenomenon is known as cold-induced vasodilatation (CIVD) and demonstrates a hunting reaction of the vessels that can be measured simply by thermocouple readings on the cooled skin (Figure 6.4). At first, CIVD was thought to be caused by a local neurogenic axon reflex and/or the local release of vasodilator hormones into the tissues. Later work on isolated strips of vascular tissue revealed that CIVD is most likely to be due to the direct effect of low temperature causing paralysis of smooth muscle contraction in blood vessels (Keatinge, 1978). The reaction may provide protection to tissues from damage caused by prolonged cooling and relative ischaemia.

Muscle blood flow is not much influenced by thermal reflexes but is determined largely by local muscle metabolic rate. During exercise there is a large increase in muscle blood flow due to metabolite accumulation, and stress release of adrenaline also causes substantial vasodilatation in muscle vessels. A striking feature of attempts at muscle cooling in cryotherapy is the prolonged period taken to reach maximum cooling. Muscles are generally shielded from temperature changes at the skin surface by the insulative layer of subcutaneous fat.

OTHER TISSUE EFFECTS

There is a marked difference in the appearance of the *skin erythema* due to CIVD as compared with skin heating. In CIVD the skin has a brighter red colour due to the presence of more oxyhaemoglobin and less reduced-haemoglobin in blood. It is apparent in the skin of babies who appear bright pink instead of pale when they are hypothermic or suffering from cold injury. The reason for this is that at low temperatures there is a shift in the

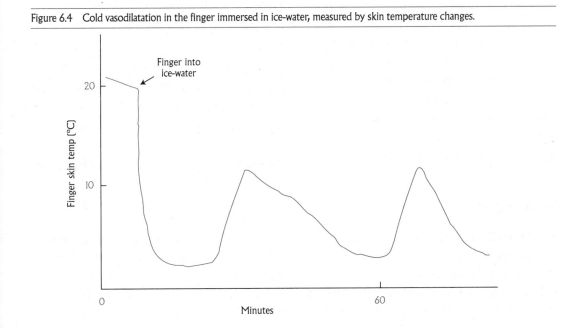

Figure 6.4 Cold vasodilatation in the finger immersed in ice-water, measured by skin temperature changes.

oxygen dissociation curve and blood tends to hold on to its oxygen with oxyhaemoglobin dissociating less readily. One result of this is that although cooling is immediately useful for haemostasis, cryotherapy probably does not benefit healing.

Cold applied to the skin stimulates *cold* and *pain sensation*. If the cold is sufficiently intense, both sensations are suppressed because of inhibition of nerve conduction. Not all nerve fibres are equally affected: the smaller diameter non-myelinated group IV C fibres are least affected as also are small myelinated pre-ganglionic autonomic fibres (essential for vasomotor function). Small, thinly myelinated Aδ fibres subserving pain and temperature sensations are most susceptible to cold.

Muscle strength is diminished by cooling, probably because of increased fluid viscosity and reduced metabolism, but there is evidence that strength may increase over its initial value approximately 1 hour after cooling has ceased. Cold is often used to reduce muscle spasticity and spasm. Reduced nerve conduction velocity may be involved, but because of the rapid effect produced by skin cooling (30 s after application of ice) other explanations have been sought. It is postulated that reflexes from the cold skin may inhibit the dominant excitatory stimuli which operate in the region of the anterior horn neurones of the spinal cord causing spasticity and spasm (Lehmann and De Lateur, 1990).

Systemic Effects

A *generalized vasoconstriction* develops over the skin surface when a cold stimulus is applied. The effect on heat transfer may be judged from calculations showing that 60 W/m^2 can be transferred across the shell of the body when peripheral blood vessels are fully dilated, compared to 10 W/m^2 in the vasoconstricted state. Skin vasoconstriction and increased blood viscosity raises peripheral resistance and produces an increase in arterial blood pressure.

As skin temperature decreases, the drive to *internal heat production* grows. This is brought about by an involuntary increase in muscle tone (pre-shivering tone) that eventually develops into shivering. Voluntary movement and muscular exercise tend to inhibit shivering, mostly by helping to raise body temperature and reduce the central nervous drive. Behavioural responses such as adopting a contracted posture with arms and legs drawn up to the body can reduce the surface area exposed for heat loss by up to 50%. Many animals possess another mechanism for thermogenesis in the cold that involves the biochemical uncoupling of metabolic pathways within the mitochondria of cells of brown fat tissue. The human neonate relies strongly on this process of non-shivering thermogenesis to balance body heat loss, but there is usually little evidence of this tissue in the adult as brown fat disappears during development.

Severe local cooling of the limbs can induce *non-freezing cold injury* in the extremities. Cooling for short periods below 12°C may cause sensory and motor paralysis of local nerves. Trench foot is due to prolonged cooling of the feet in mud or water resulting in damage to nerve and muscle with subsequent long-term diminution of function when normal body temperature and blood flow is restored. Hypothermia is a condition of low core temperature defined as a deep body temperature below 35°C (Collins, 1983). It is potentially life-threatening and often develops insidiously without the subject being aware of the threat. As body temperature falls below 35°C there are increasing disturbances of brain and cardiac function. Consciousness is lost at a body temperature between 33° and 26°C with considerable variability between individuals.

References

Bowler, K (1987) Cellular heat injury: are membranes involved? In Bowler, K, Fuller, BJ (eds) *Temperature and Animal Cells.* pp. 157–185. The Company of Biologists Ltd, Cambridge.

BS 691 (1987) *Specification for solid stem clinical maximum thermometers (mercury in glass).* British Standards Institution, London.

Collins, KJ (1983) *Hypothermia the Facts.* Oxford Univ Press, Oxford.

Collins, KJ (1992) Regulation of body temperature. In Tinker, J, Zapol, WM (eds) *Care of the Critically Ill Patient, 2nd Edn.* pp. 155–173. Springer-Verlag, London.

Emery, AF, Sekins, KM (1990) Computer modeling of thermotherapy. In Lehman, JF, (ed) *Therapeutic Heat and Cold, 4th Edn.* pp. 113–149. Baltimore: Williams & Wilkins.

Guy, AW (1990) Biophysics of high-frequency currents and electromagnetic radiation. In Lehmann, JF (ed) *Therapeutic Heat and Cold, 4th Edn.* pp. 179–236. Baltimore: Williams & Wilkins.

Harris, ED, Jr, McCroskery, PA (1974) The influence of temperature and fibril stability on degradation of cartilage collagen by rheumatoid synovial collagenase. *N Engl J Med,* **290**: 1–6.

Hensel, H (1981) *Thermoreception and Temperature Regulation.* Monogr of the Physiol Soc No 38. London: Academic Press.

International Union of Physiological Sciences (1987) Commission for Thermal Physiology. A glossary of terms for thermal physiology. *Pflug Arch,* **410**: 567–587.

Keatinge, WR (1978) *Survival in Cold Water.* pp. 39–50. Oxford: Blackwell.

Keatinge, WR, Sloane, REG (1975) Deep body temperatures from aural canal with servo-controlled heating to outer ear. *J appl Physiol,* **38**: 919–921.

Kerslake, D McK, Cooper, KE (1950) Vasodilatation in the hand in response to heating the skin elsewhere. *Clin Sci,* **9**: 31–47.

Khogali, M, Hales, JRS (1983) *Heat Stroke and Temperature Regulation,* London: Academic Press.

Lehmann, JF, De Lateur, BJ (1990) Therapeutic heat. In *Lehmann, JF (ed) Therapeutic Heat and Cold, 4th Edn,* p. 444. Baltimore: Williams & Wilkins.

Lehmann, JF, De Lateur, BJ (1990) Cryotherapy. In Lehmann, JF (ed) *Therapeutic Heat and Cold, 4th Edn,* pp. 590–632. Baltimore: Williams & Wilkins.

Melzack, R, Wall, PD (1965) Pain mechanisms: a new theory. *Science,* **150**: 971–979.

Moore-Ede, MC, Sulzman, FM (1981) Internal temporal order. In Aschoff, J (ed) *Handbook of Behavior Neurobiology,* pp. 215–241. New York: Plenum.

Wissler, EH (1988) A review of human thermal models. In Mekjavic, IB, Banister, EW, Morrison, JB (eds) *Environmental Ergonomics,* pp. 267–285. London: Taylor & Francis.

7

Low Energy Treatments: Nonthermal or Microthermal?

SHEILA KITCHEN AND MARY DYSON

Introduction
•
Interactive Targets
•
The Effect of Dosage Parameters
•
Conclusion

Introduction

Chapter 6 outlined the thermal changes which can arise both locally and generally in the human subject following the use of electrophysical agents such as infrared irradiation and shortwave diathermy. Heating is not, however, the only way in which physiological changes can be brought about in body tissues by electrophysical agents. Other effects include the use of low-frequency currents to produce stimulation of muscle or nervous tissue and the use of the predominantly nonthermal effects of high-frequency agents to facilitate tissue repair and/or reduce pain. Chapter 8 addresses the former aspects whilst this chapter addresses the latter.

The term 'nonthermal' is frequently used in clinical practice to mean a treatment which does not result in the patient being conscious of any thermal sensations. It must be remembered, however, that almost all forms of energy can degrade ultimately into heat energy. 'Nonthermal' treatments may, therefore, still involve the production of low levels of heat which it may be possible for the tissues to convert to chemical changes within the cell. In addition to any such microthermal changes, some agents are known to produce specific effects which do not depend on heat for their occurrence. All of these will be discussed in this chapter.

Although there is clear evidence of the nonthermal effects of agents such as ultraviolet irradiation, x-rays and gamma rays, there is currently much controversy surrounding the possible existence of such effects due to the use of low-intensity, non-ionizing radiations and mechanical waves in physiotherapy practice. Arguments for and against their existence arose early in the development and evaluation of a number of agents (including ultrasound and pulsed short-wave diathermy) and the controversies have continued into recent times. For example, Frizzell and Dunn (1990) believe there to be no evidence to support the idea that biological effects are produced through the use of low-energy ultrasound; Barker and Freestone (1985) and Barker (1993) have similar reservations with respect to pulsed short-wave diathermy; and the American Drug Administration Board have yet to be convinced of the efficacy of low-level laser therapy. It has been suggested that almost all effects are mediated through thermal changes, albeit at microthermal levels, whilst others have indicated that additional mechanisms might be active.

A variety of suggestions has been made about the ways in which notionally nonthermal effects may occur. Many of those postulated are based on the suggestion that electrophysical agents can influence the mechanisms which lead to cell communication. Tsong (1989) suggests that cells communicate both *directly* through chemical means and *indirectly* through the influence of electrical, physical and acoustic signals, and it is thought that electrophysical agents may produce physiological changes through these mechanisms.

Interactive Targets

'Interactive targets' are cellular components that may be receptive to interventions. These interactive targets include the cell itself, its membrane, and intracellular structures such as intracellular membranes, microtubules, mitochondria, chromophores, cell-associated ions and the nucleus.

Cell Membrane

The cell was described in terms of its electrical structure and function in Chapter 2, and it will be recalled that the cell membrane consists of a bilayered, phospholipid structure which surrounds the central core of the cell, and is studded with transmembranous proteins (Figure 7.2). These proteins have a number of functions: they strengthen the membrane, they transport substances such as proteins, sugars, fats and ions across the membrane, and they form specialist receptors sites for proteins (such as hormones and neurotransmitters) and enzymes. In addition, the cell membrane is electrically charged, possessing a negative charge on its internal surface and a positive charge on its external surface. The resulting potential difference of approximately -70 mV is maintained through the passive and active movement of ions across the cell membrane.

A number of electrophysical agents are thought to effect changes at the level of the cell membrane. For example, Adey, in 1988, postulated the transduction of a pulsed magnetic field (PMF) signal across the cell membrane and regarded this structure as the primary site of interaction between the oscillating electrical field and the tissue. He suggested that a large amplification of an initial weak trigger can occur as the result of the binding of hormones, antibodies and neurotransmitters to their specific binding sites on the cell membrane due to the effects of magnetic fields.

Other workers, such as Tsong (1989), Westerhoff et al. (1986) and Astumian et al. (1987) have postulated that proteins can undergo conformational changes due to interaction with an oscillating electrical field. For this to occur with any degree of efficiency, the frequency of the field must match the kinetic characteristics of the reaction and be at an optimum field strength (Tsong, 1989). This reaction can lead to pumping effects, with substances being actively transported across the cell membrane, leading to subsequent adenosine triphosphate (ATP) synthesis. Though none of these researchers have specifically examined the effects of pulsed shortwave diathermy, it may be that it also acts upon cells in one or more of these ways.

Mechanical energy may also effect changes in cell membrane behaviour and is thought by some to occur as a result of the use of therapeutic levels of ultrasound. Hill and ter Haar (1989) state that acoustic cavitation results in sound energy being converted into other forms of energy, including shear energy. The sound energy induces the oscillation of minute bubbles within the tissues which in turn induce microstreaming of liquids both around the bubbles themselves and around the cell walls (further details are provided in Chapter 15). Some writers, such as Repacholi (1970) and Repacholi et al. (1971), suggest that microstreaming may alter membrane permeability and secondary messenger activity and be responsible for changes in the surface charge of cells, resulting in the transduction of signals. This view has been reinforced by both Dyson (1985) and Young (1988), who have suggested that microstreaming (at therapeutic doses) may influence cell function by reversibly affecting the integrity of the cell membrane and modifying the local environment through mechanisms such as altered cell metabolite gradients.

Finally, writers such as Smith (1991a, b) have suggested that low-level laser radiation of certain types may initiate reactions at the cell membrane level, possibly through photophysical effects on Ca^{2+} channels.

Intracellular Membranes

Intracellular membranes surround the internal organelles of the cell and exhibit similar electrical characteristics to cell membranes. One of their functions is to exercise control over the movement of substances into and out of these structures (Frohlich, 1988; Alberts et al., 1994) and thereby control the behaviour and actions of the organelles and ultimately of the entire cell. Similar effects to those induced at the cell surface may occur across these membranes, resulting in changes in activity of the organelles.

Microtubules

Microtubules are elongated cylinders made of protein and which are present within cells. Electrically, they consist of dimers, which are charged dipole units — their internal ends are negatively charged relative to the periphery. This arrangement results in the cell having similar electrical properties to electrets, which are insulators carrying a permanent charge analogous to permanent magnets. These properties include the ability to exhibit piezoelectric and electropiezo effects and, in addition, such dipole units rotate under the influence of oscillating fields. However, they do not respond equally to all frequencies of energy, but instead have preferred resonant frequencies which are governed by their moment of rotation (Frohlich, 1988).

Such dipole units may respond to the alternating magnetic and electrical fields produced by shortwave diathermy equipment. In general, it seems likely that such motion will give rise to *microthermal* changes, and Muller (1983) has suggested that an oscillation in temperature might allow a biological system to absorb free energy. Westerhoff *et al.* (1986) note that an electrical field is a 'thermodynamic quantity' and suggest that it may be the oscillation in this parameter which results in changes in the cyclical enzymatic activity of cells.

Mitochondria

It has been suggested that mitochondria may be stimulated directly by the application of electrophysical energy, and a number of researchers have suggested that laser radiation of certain wavelengths may initiate changes at this site in the cell. Karu (1988) has postulated the following sequence of events: certain wavelengths of radiation, when absorbed by components of the respiratory chain within the mitochondria, cause a brief activation of that chain; oxidation of the NAD pool occurs, leading to changes in the redox status of the mitochondria and cytoplasm; these changes lead to altered membrane permeability, and consequently to changes in the transport of ions across the cell wall. For example, changes in the Na^+:H^+ ratio across the membrane occurs, and there are subsequent increases in Na^+K^+–ATPase activity. The Ca^{2+} flux is consequently altered, resulting in modulation of DNA and RNA synthesis and consequent changes in cell growth and proliferation. Smith (1991a, b) has suggested that other wavelengths, not absorbed by mitochondrial cytochromes, may be absorbed by components of the cell membrane, producing direct changes in calcium flux at this site.

Ions

Ions are electrically charged particles that are present in both intracellular and extracellular fluids. Being electrically charged, they respond to oscillating electrical fields and ionic vibration is likely to occur (Frohlich, 1988). Such movement again may lead to changes in ionic distribution within the cells, affecting the cells' activity.

Nucleus

The interaction of electromagnetic fields with the nucleus of the cell has been reviewed by Nicolini (1985) and Frohlich (1988), who note that relatively little is known about these effects. Hisenkamp (1978) and Takahashi *et al.* (1986) are amongst those who believe that direct effects on the nucleus may occur, and they have suggested that pulsed magnetic fields may influence DNA synthesis and transcription. Adey (1988), however, postulates that any changes that have been noted are more likely to be the result of the presence of secondary messengers such as cyclic adenosine monophosphate (cAMP) and Ca^{2+} ions, which may exert such an influence at the membrane level.

Chromophores

Chromophores are molecules that absorb specific wavelengths of electromagnetic radiation. They include melanin, nucleic acids, and proteins, and are therefore distributed widely in the tissues and cells of the body. Ultraviolet radiation, visible light, and infra-red radiation may be absorbed by these structures.

When energy is absorbed by chromophores, an atom of the molecule affected becomes temporarily excited, resulting in the movement of an electron to a higher energy level. It subsequently degrades, releasing energy which may be passed on to other molecules, be used to effect a variety of biochemical changes or to degrade into heat.

Cells

If free to move and subjected to ultrasonically induced standing waves, entire cells can be transported in a predominantly nonthermal fashion to pressure nodes spaced at half-wavelength intervals. Although this is generally a reversible phenomenon, it can be irreversibly damaging in certain circumstances and should therefore be avoided (see Chapter 15).

The Effect of Dosage Parameters

Though it has been suggested that many forms of energy (including electrical, mechanical and chemical) may initiate changes in cell behaviour, it is becoming increasingly clear that the dosage parameters of the energy imparted to the cell are likely to affect the end result. For example, Frohlich (1988) has suggested that ion oscillation and dipole rotation is dependent upon the frequency and amplitude of the electrical field in question. In addition, enzyme activity depends on the availability of specific charge sites on membrane surfaces which, Frohlich (1988) suggests, may be unlocked by the application of electrical signals of an 'appropriate type'. Tsong (1989) states that 'in principle, each class of protein is adapted to respond to an oscillating force field (electrical, sonic or chemical potential) of a defined frequency and strength'. Smith (1991a, b) has suggested that laser radiations of different wavelengths may affect different structures; he postulates that radiation at 633 nm may initiate activity at the mitochondrial level, as suggested by Karu (1987), whereas at 904 nm it may initiate reactions at the cell membrane level, possibly through photophysical effects on Ca^{2+} channels. In addi-

tion, it is known that ultraviolet irradiation of certain frequencies is more likely to produce erythematous changes ('sunburn') and carcinogenic changes than others.

Currently, there is little published information about the precise dosage parameters of many of these agents which are most likely to achieve therapeutic effects in clinical practice. Though there is some evidence that low intensities are adequate to stimulate cell activity *in vitro*, more work is needed to establish the most effective wave bands and pulsing frequencies and to confirm this in clinical environments. It should, however, be appreciated that many therapeutic forms of energy act as stimuli at the cellular level, whether *in vitro* or *in vivo*. The cells transduce these stimuli and amplify them, so the energetic output of the cells far exceeds the energetic input, an extremely efficient mode of activity which would not occur should the changes be of a purely thermal nature.

Conclusion

This overview has highlighted the many theories which are currently being explored with respect to the ways in which the electrotherapy agents used by physiotherapists may effect therapeutically significant change in cell behaviour. As this discussion has shown, it is possible that a number of similarities exist between the mechanisms whereby physiological changes are induced by the use of agents such as low-level ultrasound, pulsed nonthermal levels of shortwave diathermy and laser radiation. However, concrete evidence of both the mechanisms of interaction and physiological effects which occur in living, injured tissue is limited, a fact which should be borne in mind as the various agents are studied and used in clinical practice.

Later chapters in this book will examine in further detail the effects and efficacy of a number of agents used by physiotherapists at nonthermal intensities to treat soft tissue lesions and reduce pain.

References

Adey, WR (1988) Physiological signalling across cell membranes and co-operative influences of extremely low frequency electromagnetic fields, in Frohlich, H (1988) (ed) *Biological coherence and response to external stimuli*. Springer-Verlag, Heidlberg.

Alberts, B, Bray, D, Lewis, J, Raff, M, Roberts, K, Watson, JD (1994) *Molecular biology of the cell*, 2nd edition. Garland Publishing Inc., New York.

Astumian, RD, Chock, PB, Tsong, TY, Westerhoff, HV (1987) Can free energy be transduced from electrical noise? *Proceedings of the National Academy of Science, USA* **84**: 434–438.

Barker, AT (1993) Electricity magnetism and the body. *IEE Science, Education and Technology Division* December, 249–256

Barker, AT, Freestone, IL (1985) Medical applications of electric and magnetic fields. *IEE Electronics and Power* October, 757–760.

Dyson, M (1985) Therapeutic applications of ultrasound, in Nyborg, WL and Ziskin, MC (eds) *Biological Effects of Ultrasound (Clinics in Diagnostic Ultrasound)*. Churchill Livingstone, New York.

Frizzell, LA, Dunn, F (1990) Biophysics of ultrasound, in Lehmann, JF (ed) *Therapeutic Heat and Cold*, 4th ed. Williams and Wilkins. Baltimore, London.

Frohlich, H (1988) *Biological Coherence and Response to External Stimuli*. Springer-Verlag, Heidlberg.

Hill, CR and ter Haar, G (1989) Ultrasound in, Suess MJ, Benwell-Morison, DA (Eds) *Nonionizing Radiation Protection*.

Hiskenkamp, M, Chiabrera, A, Pilla, AA, Bassett, CAL (1978) Cell behaviour and DNA modification in pulsing electromagnetic fields. *Acta Orthopaedica Belgica* **44**: 636–650.

Karu, TI (1987) Photobiological fundamentals of low power laser therapy. *IEEE Quantum Electronics* **23**: 1703–1717.

Karu, TI (1988) Molecular mechanism of the therapeutic effects of low intensity laser radiation. *Lasers in Life Science* **2**: 53–74.

Muller, AWJ (1983) Thermoelectric energy conversion could be an energy source of living organisms. *Physics Letters A* **96**: 319–321.

Nicolini, C (1985) Cell nucleus and EM fields, in Chiabrera, A, Nicolini, C, Schwan, HP (eds) *Interactions between Electromagnetic Fields and Cells*. Plenum Press, London.

Repacholi, MH (1970) Electrophoretic mobility of tumour cells exposed to ultrasound and ionising radiation. *Nature* **227**: 166–167.

Repacholi, MH, Woodcock, JP, Newman, DL and Taylor, KJW (1971) Interaction of low intensity ultrasound and ionising radiation with the tumour cell surface. *Phys Medical Biology* **16**: 221–227.

Smith, KC (1991) The photobiological basis of the therapeutic use of radiation from lasers, in Ohshiro T and Calderhead RG (eds) *Progress in Light Therapy*. John Wiley and Son, Chichister.

Smith, KC (1991b) The photobiological basis of low level laser radiation therapy. *Laser Therapy* **3**: 19–24.

Takahashi, K, Kaneko, I, Date, M, Fukada, E (1986) Effects of pulsing electromagnetic fields on DNA synthesis in mammalian cells in culture. *Experientia* **42**: 185–186.

Tsong, TY (1989) Deciphering the language of cells. *TIBS* **14**: 89–92.

Westerhoff, HV, Tsong, TY, Chock, PB, Chen, Yi-der, Astumian, RD (1986) How enzymes can capture and transmit free energy from an oscillating electrical field. *Proceedings of the National Academy of Science, USA* **83**: 4734–4738.

Young, SR (1988) *The effect of therapeutic ultrasound on the biological mechanisms involved in dermal repair*. PhD Thesis, London University.

8

Stimulative Effects

OONA SCOTT

Basis for the Therapeutic Use of Electrical Stimulation

The excitability of nerve and muscle tissue provides the basis for the therapeutic application of electrical stimulation which has been used throughout the 20th century. Early studies used interrupted galvanic currents to produce contraction in denervated muscles. More recently, electrical stimulation has been used to supplement exercise programmes and, in the past 10 years, the ability of skeletal muscle to alter both its functional and contractile properties in response to long-term or chronic, low-frequency stimulation has been investigated in clinical practice.

To achieve an electrically elicited contraction, two electrodes are placed on the muscle: one electrode (the cathode has proved to be the more comfortable) is placed over the motor point of the muscle (see Chapter 4) and the other (the anode) is placed elsewhere on the body, generally more distally on the muscle belly. The motor point of a muscle is the point on the skin where maximum muscle contraction can be achieved. It is often associated with the point at which the nerve supplying the muscle enters the muscle belly. Frequently located at the junction of the proximal third with the distal two thirds of the muscle belly, it is the position where it is possible to influence the greatest number of motor nerve fibres. If the peripheral nervous system is intact, stimulation is achieved by the intramuscular branches of the nerve supplying that muscle. If not, then direct stimulation can be applied to the muscle, though there are doubts about the efficacy of this procedure in human subjects.

Differences Between Electrical Stimulation and Exercise

In electrical stimulation, activity is restricted to the stimulated muscle and the muscle is less influenced by the other changes that can occur in the body during exercise. Superimposed electrical stimulation bypasses the normal neuronal control mechanisms. Provided that stimuli (pulses) are of sufficient intensity and of long-enough duration to depolarize the nerve membrane, action potentials are generated in the motor nerves and muscle contraction occurs. There is now overwhelming evidence that an important factor in determining a skeletal muscle's properties is the amount of neuronal or impulse activity relative to the activity that is usual for the muscle. Electrical stimulation manipulates the output activity pattern to the motoneurone by adding to its inherent activity whereas, with exercise, the relative activity of each motor unit remains unaltered with respect to the rest of the units due to a relatively rigid pattern of recruitment.

During voluntary exercise, individual motor units are activated in a graded and hierarchical manner (see *Recruitment of Motor Units in Voluntary Contractions* in Chapter 4). Training at high forces i.e. with loads greater than 60–70% of maximum strength, repeated as few as 10 times per day, where each contraction is held for 2–5 s, recruits both high- and low-threshold units, and increases maximum voluntary strength by about 0.5–1% per day. Increases in strength have also been recorded in lower intensity training regimes of about 30% of maximum strength where each contraction is held for longer, say 60 s. This may be because the higher threshold units can be recruited as the lower threshold units fatigue (for review see Edström and Grimby, 1986; Jones *et al.*, 1989; and Lieber 1986).

It has been claimed that, prior to training, muscle cannot be maximally activated by voluntary activity and that large, fast motor units are only recruited at the higher forces. It is possible that some of these fast units are never recruited in the untrained state and there is evidence to show that in trained muscle there is an increased synchronization (see Komi, 1986). In the first 6–8 weeks before changes in muscle size become apparent, activation and therefore strength increases as a result of establishing the correct motor patterns of control of the muscles and of increased neural drive; so far there has been no evidence of fibre type changes after voluntary strength training regimes. If training is continued beyond about 12 weeks, a steady and slow increase occurs in both size and strength of the exercised muscles (for review, see Jones *et al.*, 1989).

Because most training studies have, on the whole, been of short duration (less than 5 weeks) and have been confined to a period when neural adaptations are thought to underlie the increases in strength, it continues to be unclear whether the gains in strength with short-term electromyostimulation are superior to voluntary training.

The order of motor unit activation by electrical stimulation depends on at least three factors:

1 The diameter of the motor axon;
2 The distance between the axon and the active electrode;
3 The effect of input from cutaneous afferents

that have been activated by the artificial stimulus.

Electrical stimulation may facilitate recruitment of the large fast units.

The recruitment order of the motor units is thought to be reversed in electrical stimulation from the natural sequence (Trimble and Enoka, 1991; see section *Recruitment of Motor Units in Voluntary Contractions* in Chapter 4). Because of their large diameter axons and low activation threshold, the larger motor units are recruited first. These fast-contracting, high-tension generating, easily fatiguable motor units are often found in the superficial layers of a muscle and closer to the stimulating electrodes. The stimulation will also be conducted antidromically, that is, going towards the spinal cord, along the motor nerve and by the afferent sensory nerves. This too has been shown to cause a reversal of the order of motor unit recruitment (see Chapter 4) (Garnet *et al.*, 1978).

Low-Frequency Electrical Stimulation

As already stated low frequency electrical stimulation in human studies where the impulses are no greater than 1 000 Hz and usually lower than 100 Hz has traditionally been used to facilitate or to mimic voluntary contractions of skeletal muscle and as a supplement to normal training procedures. Hardly surprisingly, the concentration in animal studies has been on the effect of long-term, low-frequency electrical stimulation where there is no need for active cooperation. More surprising has been the paucity of studies that evaluate any physiological changes which may occur, or that identifing and monitoring aspects of motor performance, such as skill and the

restoration of functional performance in response to electrical stimulation.

Short-Term Electrical Stimulation

This form of electrical stimulation is sometimes known as electromyostimulation or faradic-type stimulation and its rationale is based on the assumption that the output of the motor system is insufficient and needs to be supplemented by artificial means. This seems reasonable, particularly where the function of the nervous system may have been compromised by a traumatic event or some disease process.

Clinically, electrical stimulation is used for strengthening in cases involving immobilization or contraindication to dynamic exercise (e.g. anterior cruciate ligament repairs and reconstructions). In the early stages of rehabilitation after injury or surgery, there can be diminished voluntary control and an inability to exert muscular force. In athletic and sports training regimes, electrical stimulation may be used as an adjunct to voluntary exercise, especially at the end of a session when the motivation to continue exercising may begin to decline.

It is often stated that it is difficult to evaluate the relative effectiveness of the various protocols that have been used because sufficient details are not provided of the parameters that have been used. Most, although not all, studies have shown that it is possible to induce strength gains in both healthy and weakened skeletal muscles with short-term, low-frequency electrical stimulation. The general conclusion to emerge is that strength gains are similar to, but not greater than, those which can be achieved with normal voluntary training.

Gains in strength have been attained with a variety of stimulus parameters ranging from low frequency (25–200 Hz) to trains of high-frequency sinusoidal pulses that are modulated at low frequencies. Enoka (1988), reviewing the training effects underlying neuromuscular stimulation, suggested that an optimum protocol used interferential stimulation (see section on *Interferential therapy* in Chapter 19). The disadvantage of this form of regime is that it requires sophisticated equipment; the advantage of low-frequency stimulation is that it is usually self-applied using a battery driven stimulator. Selkowitz (1989) identified two major categories of electrical stimulation: low-frequency, endurance training programmes, and strength training using interferential stimulation. He suggested that low-frequency, muscle endurance regimes have relatively short intervals between contractions, with contraction durations approximately equal to the rests (usually 4–15 seconds on and off) and last for a total of 6–15 minutes for each treatment session.

Long-Term (Chronic) Electrical Stimulation of Skeletal Muscle

Investigations on animals and recent studies in human muscle have confirmed that it is possible to modify the properties of mammalian skeletal muscle by long-term electrical stimulation. Skeletal muscle has a remarkable ability to change its properties in response to demand, so much so that it is now recognized that every structural characteristic of a muscle can change given the appropriate stimulus. This model has provided the means for researchers to correlate functional changes with changes at the molecular level and has enabled investigations to be undertaken which explore the extent of muscle plasticity. Observation of the time course of changes has led to study of gene expression of different functional elements in muscle fibres (see review, Pette and Vrbová, 1992).

Variation in the parameters used in animal studies, inherent differences between species, and the varying condition of animals prior to stimulation have made it difficult to compare results from different studies. None the less, their findings are largely complementary and an overall pattern of transformation has been established.

A number of reviews have summarized the major effects of long-term, low-frequency electrical stimulation in animal and human muscles (Salmons and Henriksson, 1981; Lieber, 1986; Enoka, 1988; Pette and Vrbová, 1992) and the ability to change the properties of skeletal muscles by chronic, low-frequency stimulation is now well-established in both animal and human muscles.

Although we know that the neuronal control and patterns of activation are different for each activity and for each muscle, and even for the constituent motor units, we do not know yet how best to exploit this ability to change muscle properties. Reversal of the induced changes upon discontinuing the stimulation appears to have different time courses for different properties but, in general terms, the time course of reversal is comparable to that of transformation.

CHANGES IN CONTRACTILE PROPERTIES

The first effect noted in response to chronic, low-frequency stimulation in both rabbit and cat fast-contracting muscles was an increase in both contraction and relaxation times of the stimulated muscles when compared to those of the control muscles (Vrbová, 1966; Salmons and Vrbová, 1969; Pette et al., 1973). There was also an alteration in the twitch-to-tetanic force ratio, in that the twitch tension was very similar to that of the control muscle but the maximal tetanic tension was considerably reduced. The slowing effect became apparent after 9–12 days of stimulation. Similar changes within 3 weeks of superimposed stimulation have been reported in chronically stimulated tibialis anterior, adductor pollicis human adult muscles (Scott *et al.*, 1985; Rutherford *et al.*, 1988) and now more recently in quadriceps femoris (Cramp *et al.*, 1994).

A consistent finding in both animal and human studies in response to long-term stimulation has been an increased resistance to fatigue. This had been described in a large number of animal studies and it was first demonstrated in adult human muscle in a study of the tibialis anterior muscle by Scott *et al.* (1985), then in adductor pollicis by Rutherford *et al.* (1988), and latterly in quadriceps femoris muscle by Cramp *et al.* (1994).

Metabolic Changes In animal muscles, the increased resistance to fatigue has been associated with increases in aerobic–oxidative capacity with a marked decrease in glycolytic enzyme activities. Transformation of fast-twitch muscle fibres into slow ones (see section *Classification – Matching Motoneurones to the Muscle Fibres* in Chapter 4) by chronic stimulation at 10 Hz is well documented, with changes of contractile characteristics, shifts of metabolic enzyme patterns, Ca^{2+} uptake by the sacroplasmic reticulum, and eventual changes in myosin heavy and light chains. These changes of metabolic, histochemical and structural properties have been extensively reviewed (Pette, 1980; Salmons and Henrikson, 1984; Vrbová and Pette, 1984; Enoka, 1988; Pette and Vrbová, 1992) and are shown schematically in Figure 8.1.

Circulatory Changes The earliest changes recorded can be identified as changes in the sacroplasmic reticulum, an increase in blood supply followed by an increase in capillary density surrounding the stimulated muscle fibres (Cotter *et al.*, 1973), and a decrease in muscle fibre diameter. It was found (Hudlická *et al.*, 1977) that, after 4 days, the stimulated muscles fatigued less than the control muscles, suggesting

that the increased capillary density provided a more homogeneous distribution of blood and better diffusion of oxygen. It was suggested that this might be because a greater number of muscle fibres would have access to oxygen which would facilitate rephosphorylation of ATP and creatine phosphate (see section *The Sliding Filament Hypothesis* in Chapter 4).

Structural Changes Heilmann and Pette (1979) investigating the effect of continuous 10 Hz stimulation on rabbit fast-twitch muscles found that one of the earliest changes was a reduction in both the initial and total Ca^{2+} uptake, accompanied by a change in the polypeptide patterns of the sacroplasmic reticulum. Stimulation-induced changes in the muscle fibres include a more homogeneous population of fibres with a smaller cross-sectional area, but no loss of muscle fibres.

Myofibrillar ATPase histochemistry has shown a stimulation-induced increase in the number of Type I muscle fibres in many species, and detailed analysis on chronically stimulated extensor digitorum longus and tibialis anterior in the rabbit muscles have shown an overall transition of fast-muscle type to slow, including changes in the myosin molecule.

Particular attention has been paid to changes in the myofibrillar protein myosin, and to the regulatory proteins tropomyosin and troponin, which are associated with actin. Changes in the myosin molecule were first observed after 2–4 weeks, but the complete fast-to-slow transition of the myosin light chains appears to take several months (for further details see Pette and Vrbová, 1992).

Different Patterns of Stimulation Much less research has been carried out into transformation of slow muscle to fast (apart from early work on the soleus muscle – Vrbová, 1963), but in recent years more work has been done on the

Figure 8.1   Schematic representation of effects of chronic low-frequency stimulation on fast muscle fibres.

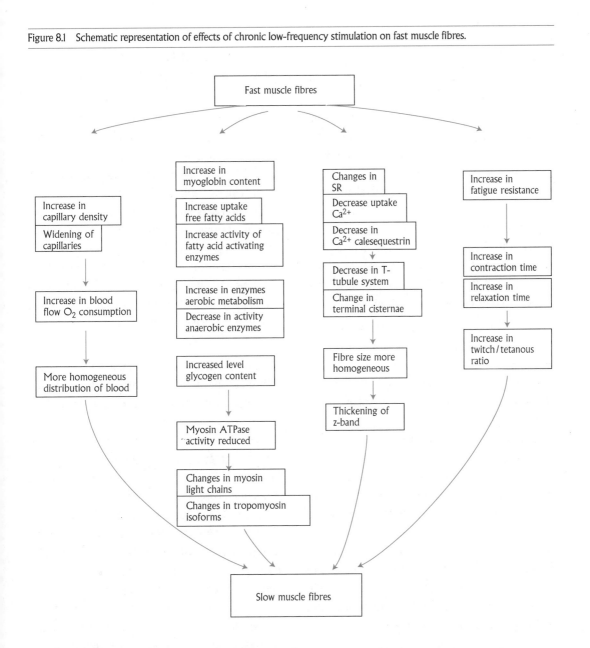

effect of different patterns of stimulation in human muscle.

Throughout many of the studies, investigators have been concerned to consider the effect of external factors on the changes that have been observed in response to stimulation. Such external factors may be of importance when consider-ing the possible effect of long-term stimulation in human muscles. In animal studies, it is usual for the muscle to be stimulated using implanted electrodes and for the entire muscle to be stimu-lated. In human studies, because muscles are often stimulated using surface electrodes (rather than through implants), it is important to be aware of the percentage of the muscle that is being stimulated.

The position and loading of the muscle during stimulation has already been observed to be likely to affect the changes that occur (Williams and Goldspink, 1984). Recent studies on muscle protein metabolism by Williams and Goldspink (1986 and 1988) show the importance of stretch on muscle proteins. Cotter and Phillips (1986) showed that the transition from fast to slow muscle was accelerated in rabbit tibialis anterior muscle with immobilization in the neutral position; Williams et al. (1986) found greater increases in Type I and Type IIa fibres when a muscle was immobilized in a stretched position.

In 1985, Scott and her colleagues investigated the effect on contractile properties of stimulating the intramuscular branches of the lateral popliteal nerve at 10 Hz for an hour, three times a day for six weeks. Using an asymmetrical biphasic waveform of sufficient intensity to give a visible contraction of the tibialis anterior accompanied by movement of the foot, they monitored the effect of chronic low frequency showing that it was possible to change the contractile characteristics of this muscle in human subjects. As in animal studies, long-term, low-frequency stimulation induced a significant increase in resistance to fatigue in the stimulated muscles when compared to the unstimulated controls, suggesting a change in properties of the Type II, fast-contracting, easily fatiguable, glycolytic fibres.

Comparing the effect of long-term, low-frequency stimulation with a non-uniform pattern of stimulation incorporating a range of low through to high frequencies (5–40 Hz) Rutherford and her co-workers (1986) showed similar changes in the fatigue characteristics in response to both patterns of stimulation, but those subjects who stimulated their muscles with a low-frequency pattern lost muscle strength, whereas those subjects who had stimulated their muscles using a mixed pattern of stimulation became stronger.

Since then, investigators have examined both maximum voluntary strength and changes in contractile characteristics of various groups of normal subjects, ranging from the very young to fit, active, elderly subjects. Comparative studies have been undertaken to monitor these changes in patient groups with multiple sclerosis, spinal cord lesions and children with neuromuscular diseases (Lenman et al., 1989; Scott et al., 1990). Changes in the contractile properties often accompany loss of muscle strength, and these changes may well be associated with alterations in neuronal activity.

In some studies, attempts were made to simulate motoneurone discharge patterns on the basis that the natural pattern of discharge of a single, slow motor unit is not a uniform one. Farraher and her associates (1987) described this form of stimulation as 'eutrophic stimulation', identifying a 'neurotrophic effect' of the simulated pattern, and reporting considerable clinical merit for patients suffering from intractable Bell's palsy. Kidd and Oldham in 1988, and then Oldham and Stanley in 1989, gave accounts of the benefits of using eutrophic stimulation on the small muscles of the hand in patients with rheumatoid arthritis and reported significant improvement in functional ability and voluntary fatigue in the hand muscles of these patients. Their pattern of stimulation was derived from a fatigued motor unit from the first dorsal interosseus in a normal hand.

There is still uncertainty concerning optimum patterns of stimulation. The effect of different patterns of stimulation may, of course, be a key factor, but there are additional considerations of patient compliance and acceptability that need to be considered (Baker, 1987). Studies in animals have highlighted the need to consider the effect of loading and normal use of the muscle during periods of stimulation, and another focus of attention has been the possible damaging effect of high frequencies of stimulation on young developing muscles (for further information see Ciba Foundation symposium, 1988).

FUNCTIONAL ELECTRICAL STIMULATION (FES)

Functional electrical stimulation is the electrical stimulation of muscle deprived of normal control to produce a functionally useful contraction (see Singer, 1987). The first portable stimulator was developed in 1960 by Wladimir Liberson to provide a foot assist in hemiplegic patients. It was triggered with a foot switch in the shoe of the affected leg.

FES serves to provoke contraction of a paralysed muscle and to affects the sensory pathways contributing to the normalization of basic reflex motor activities. It has been used primarily in the rehabilitation of:

1 Hemiplegics;
2 Paraplegics and quadriplegics;
3 Children with cerebral palsy,
4 Other patients suffering from impairment or disease of the central nervous system (multiple sclerosis, head injuries etc.) (Vodovnik, 1981).

Patient Tolerance

Comparative comfort is a key issue and tends to limit the widespread application of electrical stimulation (Baker, 1988; Delitto *et al.*, 1992). Surface stimulation activates the sensory receptors on the surface of the skin (see section *Sensory-moto-neurone Activation* in Chapter 4). The resulting discomfort and pain can often limit the effectiveness of the applied stimulation. Subjects adapt to this sensory experience relatively quickly, developing an increased tolerance to all types of stimulation over a number of sessions. The sensation of stimulated muscle contraction can be disconcerting and subjects often comment that a relatively low percentage of their maximum voluntary contraction (MVC) feels like a very strong contraction.

Stimulus waveform and pulse duration play a major role in subject comfort. It is often stated that the level of pain and unpleasant sensation are minimized by the use of short pulse widths (50 µs is often chosen) and high frequencies (40–50 Hz or higher). There is a need for continual reassessment of the therapeutic level of contraction for each muscle that is stimulated to ensure that optimum effects are being obtained.

Monitoring and Measurement

Singer and his colleagues (1987) recommended minimum requirements when reporting muscle strength testing, the stimulus parameters and the design of training programmes. These criteria are as relevant to the clinician recording details of patient progress and requiring a sound basis for therapeutic evaluation as they are for the researchers in their investigative studies. Their objective was to provide a guide toward more appropriate protocols for further research and clinical practice.

References

Baker, L, Bowman, BR, McNeal, DR (1988) Effects of waveform on comfort during neuromuscular electrical simulation. *Clinical Orthopaedics and Related Research* 233: 75-85.

Bélanger, AY (1991) Neuromuscular electrostimulation in physiotherapy: A critical appraisal of controversial issues. *Physiotherapy Theory and Practice* 7: 83-89.+

Ciba Foundation (1988) *Plasticity of the Nervous system*. Wiley & Sons.

Cotter, M, Hudlická, O, Vrbová, G (1973) Growth of capillaries during long-term activity in skeletal muscle. *Bibl Anat* 11: 395-398.

Cotter, M, Hudlická, O (1977) Effects of chronic stimulation on muscles in ageing rats. *Journal of Physiology (Lond)* 266: 102P–103P

Cotter, M, Phillips, P (1986) Rapid fast to slow fiber transformation in response to chronic stimulation of immobilized muscles of the rabbit. *Experimental Neurology* 93: 53–545

Cramp, MC, Manuel, JA, Scott, OM (1995) Effects of different patterns of long-term electrical stimulation on human quadriceps femos muscle. *Journal of Physiology (Lond)* 483: 82P

Davis, HL (1983) Is electrostimulation beneficial to denervated muscles? A review of results from basic research. *Physiotherapy Canada* 35(6): 306–312.

Delitto, A, Strube, MJ, Shulman, AD, Minor, SD (1992) A study of discomfort with electrical stimulation. *Physical Therapy* 72: 410–424.

Edstrom, L, Grimby, L (1986) Effect of exercise on the motor unit. *Muscle and Nerve* 9: 104–126

Enoka, RM (1988) Muscle strength and its development: New perspectives. *Sports Medicine* 6: 146–168.

Farraher, D, Kidd, GL, Tallis, RC (1987) Eutrophic electrical stimulation for Bell's palsy. *Clinical Rehabilitation* 1: 265–271.

Garnett, RAF, O'Donnovan, MJ, Stephens, JA, Taylor, A (1978) Motor unit organisation of human medial gastrochemius. *Journal of Physiology (Lond)* 287, 33-43.

Heilmann, C, Pette, D (1979) Molecular transformations in sacroplasmic reticulum of fast twitch muscle by electro-stimulation. *European Journal of Biochemistry* 93: 437–446.

Hudlická, O, Brown, M, Cotter, M, Smith, M, Vrbová, G (1977) The effect of long-term stimulation on fast muscles on their blood flow, metabolism and ability to withstand fatigue. *Pflugers Arch* 369: 141–149.

Jones, DA, Rutherford, OM, Parker, DF (1989) Physiological changes in skeletal muscle as a result of strength training. *Quarterly Journal of Experimental Physiology* 74: 233–256.

Kidd, GL, Oldham, JA (1988) Eutrophic electrotherapy and atrophied muscle: a pilot clinical study. *Clinical Rehabilitation* 2: 219–230.

Heilmann, C, Pette, D (1979) Molecular transformations in sacroplasmic reticulum of fast-twitch muscle by electro-stimulation. *European Journal of Biochemistry* 93: 437–446.

Lai, HS, De Domenico, G, Strauss, GR (1988) The effect of different electro-motor stimulation training intensities on strength improvement. *Australian Journal of Physiotherapy* 34(3): 151–164.

Lenman, AJR, Tulley, FM, Vrbová, G (1989) Muscle fatigue in some neurological disorders. *Muscle and Nerve* 12: 938–942.

Lieber, RL (1986) Skeletal muscle adatability III: Muscle properties following chronic electrical stimulation. *Developmental Medicine and Child Neurology* 28: 662–670.

Nix, WA, Vrbová, G (1985) *Electrical stimulation and neuromuscular disorders*. Springer-Verlag.

Oldham, JA, Stanley, JK (1989) Rehabilitation of atrophied muscle in the rheumatoid arthritic hand: a comparison of two methods of electrical stimulation. *Journal of Hand Surgery (British Volume)* 14B: 294–297.

Pette, D, Smith, ME, Staudte, HW, Vrbová, G (1973) Effects of long-term electrical stimulation on some contractile and metabolic characteristics of fast rabbit muscles. *Pflugers Arch*, 338, 257–272.

Pette, D, Vrbová, G (1992) Adaptation of mammalian skeletal muscle fibres to chronic electrical stimulation. *Rev Physiol Biochem* 120: 116–202

Rutherford, OM, Jones, DA (1988) Contractile properties and fatiguability of the human adductor muscle and first dorsal interosseus: a comparison of the effects of two chronic stimulation patterns. *Journal of Neurological Science* 85: 319–331.

Salmons, S, Vrbová, V (1969) The influence of activity on some contractile characteristics of mammalian fast and slow muscles. *Journal of Physiology* 201: 535–549

Salmons, S, Henriksson, J (1981) The adaptive response of of skeletal muscle to increased use. *Muscle and Nerve* 4: 94–105.

Scott, OM, Vrbová, G, Hyde, SA, Dubowitz, D (1985) Effects of chronic, low-frequency electrical stimulation on normal tibialis anterior muscle. *Journal of Neurology Neurosurgery and Psychiatry* 48: 774–81.

Scott, OM, Hyde, SA, Vrbová, G, Dubowitz, V (1990) Therapeutic possibilities of chronic low frequency electrical stimulation in children with Duchenne muscular dystrophy. *Journal of Neurological Sciences* 95: 171–182.

Selkowitz, DM (1989) High frequency electrical stimulation in muscle strengthening: A review and discussion. *American Journal of Sports Medicine* 17(1): 103–111.

Singer, B (1987) Functional electrical stimulation of the extremities in the neurological patient: A review. *Australian Journal of Physiotherapy* 33(1): 33–42.

Snyder-Mackler, L, Delitto, A, Stralka, SW, Bailey, SL (1994) Use of electrical stimulation to enhance recovery of quadriceps femoris muscle force production in patients following anterior cruciate ligament reconstruction. *Physical Therapy* 74(10): 901–907.

St Pierre, D, Gardiner, PF (1987) The effect of immobilisation and exercise on muscle function: a review. *Physiotherapy Canada* 39(1): 24–36.

Trimble, MH, Enoka, RM (1991) Mechanisms underlying the training effects associated with neuromuscular electrical stimulation. *Physical Therapy* 71(4): 273–282.

Vodovnik, L (1971) Functional electrical stimulation of extremities, in *Advances in Electronics and Electron Physics*, Academic Press

Vrbová, G (1963) The effect of motoneurone activity on the speed of contraction of striated muscle. *Journal of Physiology (Lond)* 169: 513–526.

Vrbová, G (1966) Factors determining the speed of contraction of striated muscle. *Journal of Physiology (Lond)* 185: 17P–18P.

Williams, PE, Goldspink, G (1984) Connective tissue changes in immobilized muscle. *Journal of Anatomy* 138(2): 343–350

Williams, PE, Catanese, T, Lucky, EG, Goldspink, G (1988) The importance of stretch and contractile activity in the prevention of connective tissue accumulation in muscle. *Journal of Anatomy* 158: 109–114

Williams, PE, Goldspink, G (1986) Effects of stretch combined with electrical stimulation on the type of sarcomeres produced at the ends of muscle fibres. *Experimental Neurology* 93: 500–509

Wong, RA (1986) High voltage versus low voltage electrical stimulation: Force of induced muscle contraction and perceived discomfort in healthy subjects. *Physical Therapy* 66(8): 1209–1214.

C

Conductive Agents

9

Heat and Cold: Conduction Methods

LORNA JOHNSON AND SHEILA KITCHEN

Introduction
•
Heat: Contact Techniques
•
Cold: Contact Techniques (Cryotherapy)

Introduction

Both heat and cold can be effective forms of treatment for a number of conditions and problems, such as musculoskeletal lesions, pain and spasticity. Chapter 6 has described in some detail the nature of the physical and physiological changes which can arise in the human body due to thermal variation. This chapter will expand on some of these areas as consideration is given to the use of therapeutic agents which effect temperature changes through direct physical contact with tissue, predominantly the superficial tissues. Forms of heating that produce thermal changes at a deeper level will be addressed in Chapter 6.

Heat and Cold?

Many, though not all, of the clinical benefits produced by both heat and cold in treatment are similar. Selection is therefore based on a number of factors which may, on occasion, be empirical, but are nevertheless of importance.

- *Stage of inflammation* – generally, cold is preferable during the acute stage of inflammation to relieve pain and possibly reduce swelling. Heat, in contrast, can exacerbate the early inflammatory process. However, it should be remembered that cold can retard the basic healing process.
- *Collagen extensibility* – this is more likely to be

affected by a rise in temperature; stiffness of collagen is increased by cold.

- *Spasm* – both heat and cold can decrease the muscle spasm associated with musculoskeletal injuries and nerve root irritation. Similarly, both will reduce spasticity due to upper motoneurone dysfunction, though heat will do so only for a short period of time; cold is more effective under these circumstances as return to normal temperatures takes longer.
- *Muscle contraction* – moderate cooling to approximately 27°C leads to an increase in the ability of a muscle to sustain a contraction. However, there appears to be a slight increase in the strength of contraction with a rise in temperature.
- *Area to be treated* – in some subjects the application of cold to the hands and feet leads to considerable discomfort and may therefore be an indication for heat therapy.
- *Ease of use* – this can be especially important when considering home therapy administered by the patient.
- *Patient preference* – some subjects find cold intolerable and the use of heat to relieve both pain and muscle spasm may be more acceptable and lead to greater compliance with treatment.

Wet or Dry?

A second important factor to be considered when selecting contact treatment is that of choosing between wet and dry contact techniques. Little is known about the relative efficacy of one or other; however, Abramson (1967) has suggested that dry heat can elevate surface temperature to a slightly greater degree, whilst wet heat can lead to rises in temperature at slightly deeper levels.

Contact Techniques

Contact methods of heating and cooling require, by definition, physical contact between the therapeutic agent and the tissues. Changes in temperature are the result of heat transfer through conduction.

Heat: Contact Techniques

The physiological and therapeutic effects of local heating depend to some extent on whether the method of applying the treatment results in superficial or deep temperature changes. When superficial contact heat is applied, the surface tissue temperature change will depend on:

- The intensity of the heat (measured in watts/cm^2);
- The length of exposure to the heat (measured in minutes);
- The thermal medium for surface heat; this is a product of the thermal conductivity, density and specific heat characteristics of the tissue (Hendler *et al.*, 1958).

In order to achieve therapeutic levels of heating, the temperature attained in the tissues should be between 40 and 45°C (Lehman and de Lateur, 1990). Burning is likely to occur above this level, and below 40°C the effects of heating are considered too mild to be of therapeutic use.

Maximal elevation of the temperature of the skin and very superficial tissue will occur within 6–8 minutes. The underlying muscle will respond to a lesser extent and more slowly, and, at tolerable temperatures, muscle temperature can be expected to be raised by about 1°C at a depth of 3 cm. Another factor that must be considered is the presence of subcutaneous fat which influences the level of heating to deeper tissues by acting as insulation. Conversely, areas such as the hands and feet have little fat and even superficial heat will reach deeper structures. Where a greater depth of penetration is required, deep-heat modalities should be considered.

PHYSIOLOGICAL EFFECTS

The therapeutic effects of locally applied heat include pain relief, muscle relaxation, promotion of blood flow, facilitation of tissue healing and a reduction in joint stiffness. The underlying physiological responses of the body to an elevation in temperature have already been discussed in Chapter 6. These will be discussed here only in relation to an examination of the clinical uses and efficacy of superficial heating.

Pain Relief The application of local heat to alleviate pain is a well-accepted therapeutic technique. It is perhaps surprising that the underlying physiology is poorly understood and that supporting research evidence is scant. There is strong empirical evidence that painful muscle spasm is ameliorated by heat and this may be explained by a reduction in muscle spindle excitability due to reduced γ-efferent activity which occurs with heating (Lehmann and de Lateur, 1990). The application of local heat has been shown to increase the pain threshold in several studies (Lehman *et al.*, 1958; Benson and Copp, 1974). In the latter study, which examined the application of shortwave diathermy in normal subjects, heating was compared to cold. Although there was an increase in the pain threshold following both treatments, cold was more effective. Alterations in nerve conduction velocity (Currier *et al.*, 1982) and changes in the muscle spindle firing rate are also possible mechanisms for the analgesic effects of heat.

In addition, heat is a form of home treatment used and valued by many subjects; Barbour *et al.* (1986) reported that people suffering pain due to a variety of cancers viewed heat as an effective method of pain relief.

Muscle Relaxation Muscle relaxation and pain relief are closely interrelated, and the possible mechanisms responsible for improvement in muscle spasm associated with lower motoneurone activity have been discussed above. Spasticity associated with upper motoneurone lesions can be reduced by heating, but these effects are only short-term and, therefore, the use of cold may be a more effective method of treatment in this instance; this is discussed further later in the chapter.

Muscle Strength and Endurance Both muscle strength and endurance may be affected by an increase in temperature. Following immersion of the lower limbs in a water bath at 44°C for 45 minutes, Edwards *et al.* (1970) demonstrated a reduction in the ability of subjects to sustain an isometric contraction. Similarly, an immediate reduction in the strength of the quadriceps muscle following the application of heat through the use of short-wave diathermy has also been demonstrated (Chastain, 1978). In this study, a temperature of 42.4°C at a depth of 3.22 cm was reported. However, Chastain (1978) also noted that over the ensuing two hours muscle strength increased and remained above pretreatment levels. These finding are important in clinical practice, and should be considered both when making objective measurements of muscle strength in order to evaluate treatment efficacy and when implementing exercise programmes.

Increase in Blood Flow The mechanisms underlying the increase in blood flow associated with heating have been discussed in some detail in Chapter 6. It is unlikely that skeletal blood flow will be influenced by superficial heating methods, but the presence of chemical mediators such as bradykinin and histamine which are associated with heating may affect capillary and post-capillary venule permeability. This, together with the increase in capillary hydrostatic pressure, may result in oedema. It is for this reason that the application of local heat in the early stages of trauma should be avoided (Feibel and Fast, 1976). This view is further supported by experimental evidence derived from animal models; acute and chronic inflammatory conditions were created in the paws of rats. It was found that the application of heat depressed the chronic inflammatory response but aggravated acute inflammation (Schmidt et al., 1979). Similarly, clinical research has demonstrated an increase in oedema together with a prolonged healing time in acute injuries treated with heat (Wallace et al., 1979).

Tissue Healing There are positive affects of the increase in the chemical reaction rates which occur with heating. There is an increase in oxygen uptake associated with a muscle temperature of about 38.6°C (Abramson et al., 1958). The right-sided shift of the oxygen dissociation curve that occurs with an increase in temperature means that oxygen is more readily available for tissue repair. Haemoglobin releases twice as much oxygen at 41°C than at 36°C, and this also occurs twice as quickly (Barcroft and King, 1909). The increase in blood flow means that there are likely to be a greater number of white cells and more nutrients available for the healing process.

There is conflicting evidence arising from animal studies regarding the efficacy of heating in the management of haematomas. Fenn (1969) showed a greater resolution of artificially induced haematomas in rabbit ears accompanying the application of shortwave diathermy compared to a control

group. In contrast, Lehmann et al. (1983) investigated the clearance of radioactively labelled red cells which had been injected into the gluteal muscle of pigs, and found no difference in clearance rates between the control group and those treated with microwave diathermy.

Extensibility of Collagen A number of researchers suggested that an increase in temperature alters the behaviour of collagen when under stress and, therefore, is of value prior to the application of passive or active stretch designed to mobilize scars or lengthen contractures. Most have examined the behaviour of animal collagen tissue under passive stretch and have used a variety of heating methods, including hot-water baths.

Gersten (1955) showed an increase in the extensibility of frog Achilles' tendon following heating with ultrasound, whilst Lehmann et al. (1970) heated rat-tail tendon to a temperature of 41–45°C, using a hot-water bath. At these temperatures the viscous properties of tendon were evident, leading to a reduction in tensile strength. The stress–strain relationship was altered and residual elongation occurred following the application of a designated force at temperatures of 45°C. No such effects occurred at normal body temperatures. Similarly, Warren et al. (1971, 1976), using rat-tail collagen heated in a water bath, demonstrated that tissue rupture occurred at similar levels of stress in collagen heated to 45°C and in material tested at normal body temperatures; at 39°C, however, rupture occurred at loads of 30–50% of normal. This temperature relates to the transition phase of collagen.

Such studies provide useful information about the behaviour of collagen under stress at different temperatures, but it is important to remember that caution must be used when attempting to extrapolate from the experimental to clinical environments. The passive stretch applied by a physiotherapist on tissue is probably in the region of about one third of the force used *in vitro* to produce deformation. Similarly, stresses applied during active exercise vary widely, but are also unlikely to reach experimental levels. In addition, the role of played by reflexes, especially when pain is present, and the behaviour of muscle under stretch must also be taken into account. Thus, clinical results may not mimic experimental data.

METHODS OF APPLICATION

Surface heat may be applied to the tissues in a number of ways, and through the use of a variety of media. Whereas all methods perform the same basic function of raising superficial tissue temperatures, some may be more suitable in given situations due to the nature of the material used (e.g. wet or dry heat) and the practicalities of application.

Wax This method of heat treatment is normally restricted to the extremities for practical reasons. Paraffin wax is melted to allow the subject to dip the part in the liquid. Such wax has a melting point of approximately 54°C, a temperature which is too high for therapeutic purposes; however, the addition of a mineral oil such as liquid paraffin reduces the melting point and facilitates the development of a bath at a temperature of between 42°C and 50°C. The temperature of the molten wax is maintained by the use of a thermostatically controlled bath.

These temperatures are slightly higher than would be tolerated if the part was placed in hot water. This is because the specific heat of paraffin wax is less than that of water (2.72 kJ/kg/°C for wax and 4.2 kJ/kg/°C for water). Wax therefore releases

less energy than water when cooling. In addition, Griffin and Karselis (1988) have suggested that the first layer of wax to form on the part acts as an insulator to the hotter surrounding wax. Selkins and Emery (1982) suggest that the amount of heat imparted to the tissue due the solidification of the wax — the latent heat of fusion — is small. At the same time, heat loss is prevented due to the insulating nature of the material. The net result is a well-insulated, low-temperature method of heating tissue.

Slightly higher temperatures may be used for the upper extremities (generally the hand) and lower temperatures for the lower extremities (the feet) and newly healed tissue such as that after burns (Burns and Conin, 1987; Head and Helms, 1977).

Prior to the application of wax, the part to be treated is inspected for any contraindications (see the following section), and washed. In the *dip and wrap method* (Figure 9.1) of application, the part is immersed in the warm wax. It is then withdrawn

Figure 9.1 Wax applied to hand and wrist using dip and wrap method.

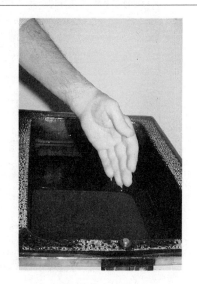

and the wax allowed to set. The procedure is repeated, normally six to twelve times, to develop a wax glove. The whole is then wrapped in plastic or waxed paper and an insulating layer of material such as a towel. The application is retained for up to 20 minutes.

Alternatively, the part may be retained in the bath following the development of the wax glove, in a

Figure 9.2 (a) Shows hydrocollator moist steam packs with terry towelling covers (b). (Photography courtesy of Chatanooga Group Ltd., Bicester.)

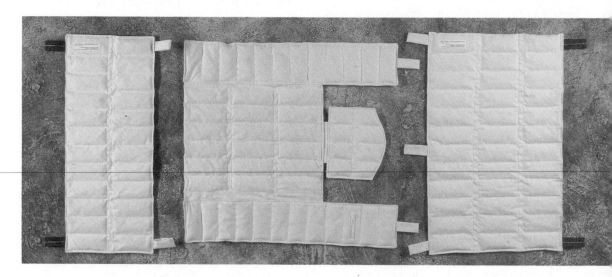

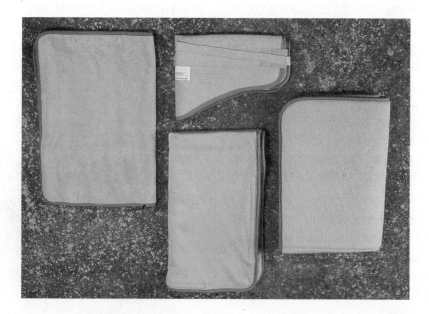

method sometimes referred to as the *dip and reimmerse method*. This technique results in a greater increase in temperature (Abramson *et al.*, 1964; Abramson *et al.*, 1965). However, the part must be dependent during such a treatment, a situation which may lead to the exacerbation or development of oedema.

Heated pads and packs A variety of heated pads may be used to provide heat to small areas. Hydrocollated pads, pads which have been immersed in hot water, and electrically heated pads may all be used. The first comes in a variety of sizes and consists of a hydrophillic silicate gel within a cotton wrapping (Figure 9.2a and b). The gel absorbs water, which, when warm, may be used to impart thermal energy to the tissues. The temperature of the pack is raised to approximately 75°C in a hot bath, wrapped in a material such as towelling, and then applied to the part. Again, the pack should generally remain *in situ* for about 20 minutes, during which time gradual cooling will occur. Lehmann *et al.* (1966) reported that such packs might be replaced during treatment and noted that this resulted in prolonged heating but that no significant differences in subcutaneous temperatures.

Pads immersed in hot water perform a similar function but tend to cool more quickly as it is not practical to provide an insulation layer. Such pads need to be replaced after approximately 5 minutes. Electrically heated pads vary in size from small pads to blankets. Electrical resistance wire lies within the structure and the design allows the temperature to be controlled thermostatically.

Hydrotherapy The use of hot water to heat the body has a long history and is still an effective way of increasing body temperature. Whilst hydrotherapy can include exercising and moving the whole body in water, this text addresses the use of water to heat small parts only. Whirlpools and still water baths are most commonly used.

Whirlpool baths involve both water movement and temperature increases. Temperatures are usually between 36 and 41°C (lower than wax temperature for the reasons discussed above). Borell *et al.* (1980) confirmed that, again, treatment at these temperatures results in an increase in subcutaneous temperature. In addition, it is possible that the motion of the water can stimulate receptors in the skin surface, giving rise to stimuli which act through the pain gate mechanism.

However, care should be taken in the use of whirlpool treatment in some cases as it has been shown that it can result in an increase in oedema, possibly due to a limb being in a dependent position whilst immersed (Magness *et al.*, 1970).

Heated air Hot air, both dry and moist, can be used to warm the tissues. Though whole-body cabinets may be found, it is more usual for smaller designs to be used. The air is circulated within the cabinet and maintained at a temperature of around 70°C. Due to the low conductivity of air, the tissue temperature remains lower than this. The two primary advantages of the method lie in the possibility of moving the part during treatment and the lack of body contact with wet materials such as water or wax.

Fluidotherapy This form of treatment involves placing the part in a cabinet which contains a suspension of cellulose particles which are kept in motion by air movement. It is a form of dry heating but makes use of convection forces to transfer energy (see Chapter 6). Temperatures are generally maintained at between 38 and

45°C. It has been suggested that the low viscosity of such an arrangement may facilitate exercise (Borell, 1977).

HAZARDS

There are few hazards with the use of surface heating methods *provided* care is taken to ensure that the temperatures used are not greater than those recommended. Temperatures should therefore always be checked.

Burns Burns are the main hazard associated with contact heating methods. However, they will only arise if there is inadequate testing of materials and equipment, the patient has severely impaired circulation, or the tissue is devitalized for some reason.

Foreign material Contact methods carry with them the possibility of foreign material being introduced into open wounds. Particles of wax may remain in lesions, and water and wet materials may carry infection if not carefully controlled. In addition, the materials used in fluidotherapy may adhere to tissue.

CONTRAINDICATIONS TO SURFACE HEATING

The following may either fully contraindicate treatment or may indicate that extra care is needed in its application:

- Lack of local thermal sensitivity on the part of the patient;
- Impaired circulation;
- Areas of recent bleeding or haemorrhaging;
- Devitalized skin, e.g. after deep x-ray treatment;
- Open wounds;
- Certain skin conditions, e.g. skin carcinomas;
- Subject with cardiovascular impairment may be inappropriate for immersion in warm liquids if a large part is the to be treated;
- Moisture may encourage damaged or infected tissues to break down.

Cold: Contact Techniques (Cryotherapy)

Contact techniques may also be used to cool tissue with a view to producing physiological changes which bring about therapeutic benefits. The changes in temperature that are achieved with cooling have been reported in many studies and vary enormously. This variation can be attributed to:

- The different methods of application;
- The length of time over which cooling has been applied;
- The initial temperature of the technique used, e.g. water temperature.

Studies have shown that the drop in *skin temperatures* can vary enormously. Greatest changes in temperature reported in a variety of studies for the different methods of application are shown below.

- Immersion in water: a drop of 29.5°C at a water temperature of 4°C after 193 minutes;
- Ice massage: a drop of 26.6°C at ice temperature of 2°C after 10 minutes application;
- Evaporation sprays: a drop of 2°C with spraying over 15–30 seconds;
- Ice packs: a drop of 20.3°C at a contact temperature of 0–3°C after 10 minutes;
- Ice towels: a drop of 13°C after a 7-minute period.

The associated drop in *intramuscular temperature* depends on the duration of the treatment, the depth of the muscle from the surface and the initial temperature of the treatment agent. Intramuscular temperatures have been evaluated in both animal and human subjects, and it has been shown that they may be as low as 2°C. Intramuscular temperatures continue to decline after the removal of the agent, and cooling persists for several hours (Meussen and Lievens, 1986). *Joint temperature* appears to remain low after the application of cold, although some investigators have reported an initial brief rise in temperature (Kern *et al.*, 1984).

PHYSIOLOGICAL EFFECTS

The physiological effects of cooling have been outlined in Chapter 6 and these will now be discussed in the light of the therapeutic effects. The generally accepted effects which are thought to be of benefit in clinical practice are: a reduction in bleeding and/or swelling at the site of acute trauma; pain relief; a reduction in muscle spasm and a reduction in spasticity which may occur in upper motoneurone lesions. Additional effects, such as the effects on muscle strength, joint stiffness and safety must also be considered. Evidence to support the use of cold therapy in these situations is often empirical but, where possible, relevant clinical research findings will be discussed.

Reduction in Swelling and Bleeding The reduction in swelling that accompanies the application of cold therapy following acute injury can be attributed to the immediate vasoconstriction of the arterioles and venules which reduces the circulation to the area and therefore reduces the extravasation of fluid into the interstitum. This effect is enhanced by the reduction in both cell metabolism and vasoactive substances, such as histamine, which are also associated with cooling. It is important to note that the period of vasoconstriction lasts between 10 and 15 minutes and is then followed by the cycle of cold-induced vasodilation (CIVD) followed

by vasoconstriction known as the 'hunting reaction'. This means that the beneficial aspects of vasoconstriction may be utilized only for a limited period of time.

It is of interest that experimentally induced swelling in animals has shown a variable response to the application of cooling, although the techniques used to produce cooling are not necessarily representative of current practice. Several of these studies have demonstrated an increase in swelling following ice therapy (e.g. Farry and Prentice, 1980) and it may be that this is due to the effects cold-induced vasodilation or possibly due to thermal injury of the lymphatic system (Meeusen and Lievens, 1986). In contrast, a number of clinical studies support the empirical evidence for the use of ice to reduce swelling (e.g. Basur *et al.*, 1976). It is, however, important to note that cooling in clinical practice is often accompanied by compression which means that it is difficult to ascribe the benefits to cooling alone.

In addition, it is possible that cooling may lead to a reduction in bleeding; again this may be due to a reduction in blood flow and is most likely to occur during the early phase of treatment.

Reduction in Pain The reduction in pain that accompanies cooling can be due to either direct or indirect factors such as a reduction in swelling and a reduction in muscle spasm as discussed earlier in this chapter. The elevation of the pain threshold in normal subjects (Benson and Copp, 1974) and in patients with rheumatoid arthritis (Curkovic *et al.*, 1993) occurs immediately following treatment but declines within 30 minutes; it may be due to a direct effect on the sensory nerve endings and to changes in the action of pain receptors and fibres (see Chapter 5 for further details of pain). It has been demonstrated that peripheral nerve conduction is slowed by cold (Lee *et al.,* 1978) and that fibres vary in their sensitivity according to their diameter and whether they are myelinated. Animal studies have demonstrated that the small diameter myelinated fibres, i.e. Aδ fibres, which conduct pain, are most responsive to cold, and it is possible that this is a mechanism for the analgesic effects of cooling, although it would be unwise to extrapolate these findings directly to humans. Finally, cold may be also be used as a counter-irritant, acting through the pain gate mechanism.

Pain may sometimes be due to particular tissue irritants. For example, a number of studies have suggested that patients with arthritis may experience pain relief due to the adverse effects of cooling on the activity of destructive enzymes within the joints (Pegg *et al.,* 1969; Harris and McCroskery, 1974).

Reduction in Muscle Spasm/spasticity In an acute injury a reduction in muscle spasm may be attributed partly to the reduction of pain which has been described above and may also be due to a reduction in the sensitivity of the muscle spindle afferents.

It has been demonstrated both in experimental studies and in clinical practice (Figure 9.3) that cooling a muscle reduces spasticity, and this has proved a useful therapeutic tool in the rehabilitation of patients with upper motoneurone lesions (Miglietta *et al.,* 1973; Price *et al.,* 1993). In the latter study, there was a statistically significant reduction in spasticity at the ankle (secondary to head injury) following the application of liquid ice in a bag to the gastrocnemius muscle for 20 minutes. However, it should be noted that two of the patients exhibited an aggravated response which was attributed to the effects of tactile stimulation.

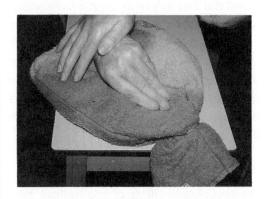

Figure 9.3 Appplication of ice to reduce spasticity.

As has already been stated in Chapter 6, the underlying physiology is not totally understood. It may be due to a slowing of conduction in both the muscle and motor nerves, a reduction in the sensitivity of the muscle spindle, or impaired conduction in the γ efferents which are more susceptible to cooling than the α efferents. The response is rapid, occurring in a matter of seconds, and it is clinically important that the muscle is cooled thoroughly and for at least 30 minutes in order to achieve a longer-lasting effect.

Muscle Strength The effect of temperature on muscle strength is a complex issue involving the effects of cold on the contractile process and the effects of temperature on neuromuscular transmission and circulatory oxygen. Some muscle properties have a large thermal dependence while others are barely influenced by temperature (Bennett, 1985). An additional point to consider is the actual temperature achieved in the muscle, as this will vary enormously.

A number of experimental studies have been conducted to examine these effects. For example, Davies and Young (1983) examined the effects of cooling the triceps surae muscle by immersion at 0°C for 30 minutes which resulted in a deep muscle temperature drop of 8.4°C. They reported a reduction in maximal voluntary contraction and peak power output, components of muscle performance which are thought to be most temperature sensitive. Clinical studies support these findings (e.g. Oliver *et al.*, 1979) but there is evidence that muscle performance improves above pretreatment levels over the hours following cooling.

The ability to sustain a maximal muscle contraction is also temperature dependent and is optimum at 27°C. Above 27°C the increase in muscle metabolism leads to a build up in metabolites which produces an early onset of fatigue. Below this temperature, the mechanisms described above come into play and the muscle may be further impaired by an increase in viscosity which hampers repetitive exercise (Clarke *et al.*, 1958). Short-term increases in strength have been reported following brief application of ice, but the mechanism for this remains unclear.

DETRIMENTAL EFFECTS OF COOLING

When considering the beneficial effects of cooling it is important that other, less therapeutically useful effects are not underestimated. The immediate increase in peripheral vascular resistance associated with vasoconstriction that occurs with cooling causes an increase in blood pressure. This may preclude the safe use of this modality in patients who have a history of hypertension. Ice should not be applied to areas affected by peripheral vascular disease as vasoconstriction will only impair the blood supply to an area which is already compromised. The later vasodilation, which occurs as part of the 'hunting reaction', is also of limited value as the left-sided shift of the O_2-dissociation curve which also occurs with cooling means that O_2 is not readily available to the tissues.

As mentioned in Chapter 6, some of the circula-

tory responses are mediated by the sympathetic nervous system, so the associated therapeutic effects will not occur in patients who have sympathetic dysfunction.

The effects on muscle strength discussed above should be considered when making objective measures of muscle strength, as such measures may be unreliable if made after cooling.

The effects of temperature on collagen have been discussed in the section on collagen heating. It is important to note, however, that a reduction in temperature is likely to increase the mechanical stiffness of collagenous tissue and therefore increase joint stiffness (Hunter *et al.*, 1952).

METHODS OF APPLICATION

Cold may be applied in a number of ways, including wet and dry packs and the use of evaporating sprays. During the application of cold therapy, the subject will experience a number of sensations; these may include:

- Intense cold;
- Burning;
- Aching;
- Analgesia.

Cold packs Cold packs (Figure 9.4) may either be either 'home-made' by the clinician or

Figure 9.4 Application of a 'home-made' ice pack to the elbow in the treatment of tennis elbow.

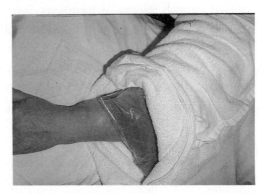

purchased. Satisfactory packs may be made by wrapping flaked ice in damp terry towels. These can be applied to the part to be treated for anything up to 20 minutes. Initial cooling is rapid but slows down as a film of water forms between the pack and the skin; this means that the temperature of the skin is usually above that of melting ice and is generally in the region of 5–10°C.

Ice packs produced commercially are of two types. First, bags which contain a mixture of water and an antifreeze substance are available. These may be cooled in a freezer and then moulded to the part. Care should be taken on initial application as the temperature of the pack can be below 0°C and can therefore lead to very rapid, surface tissue cooling. Placing a damp towel between the skin and the pack can ensure that the contact temperature remains about 0°C. Second, packs are available that rely on a chemical reaction for their cooling properties. Such packs may be used only once. Though both types of pack are effective in reducing tissue temperatures, McMaster et al. (1978) demonstrated that chemical packs are more effective in lowering subcutaneous temperatures. However, as suggested earlier in this section, the final temperature developed depends on a variety of factors.

Ice towels Very superficial cooling may be achieved through the use of ice towels. Terry towelling is placed in a mush of flaked ice and water, wrung out, and applied to the part. Large areas may be covered but the towel will need to be replaced frequently as it warms up rapidly. Treatment may be given for up to twenty minutes.

Cold baths One of the simplest methods of cooling tissue is to place the part in cold water or a mixture of ice and water. The temperature can be controlled by varying the ratio of ice to water. Lee et al. (1978) suggest that a temperature of 16–18°C may be tolerated for 15–20 minutes. Lower temperatures may be used, but will require intermittent immersion of the part.

Vaporizing sprays Chapter 6 discusses the role of evaporation in producing cooling of the skin. Techniques which use this method of reducing skin temperature result in effective but short-lived tissue cooling. A volatile liquid is sprayed directly onto the area to be treated. It is important that the spray should be both non-flammable and non-toxic for safety reasons. It should be applied over the area in a number of short bursts (approximately 5 s each). Generally, three to five bursts are adequate.

Ice massage Ice 'lollipops' or blocks may be used for this technique. First, ice massage may be used to produce analgesia. It is normally performed over a small area such as a muscle belly or trigger point and may be used prior to other techniques such as deep massage. Waylonis (1967) discusses the physiological effects of ice massage and suggests that an area of 10 × 15 cm should be treated for up to 10 minutes or until analgesia occurs. A slow circular motion over a small area is used. Temperatures do not drop to levels below 15°C with this method. Second, ice massage may be used to facilitate muscle activity. In this case, ice is applied briskly and briefly over the skin dermatome of the same nerve root as the muscle in question.

HAZARDS

Damage due to the therapeutic use of cold therapy is rare. However, *ice burns* can arise if the use of cold is excessive or the pathology of the patient is such as to predispose to damage at temperature which are normally acceptable. Damage appears, a few hours after the application of cold, in the form of erythema and tenderness. More severe damage can lead to fatty necrosis and the appearance of bruising, and ultimately, severe cooling can lead to frost bite; these last two are very unlikely using the methods described above.

CONTRAINDICATIONS

The following conditions contraindicate the use of cryotherapy:

- Arteriosclerosis;
- Peripheral vascular disease – cold will compromise the already inadequate blood supply in the area;
- Vasospasm – conditions such as Raynaud's disease which are associated with excessive vasospasm;
- Cryoglobinaemia – abnormal blood proteins can precipitate at low temperatures. This can lead to vessel blockage. The condition may be associated with rheumatoid arthritis and system lupus erythematosus;
- Cold urticaria – histamine, released by mast cells, leads to local weal formation, itching and the development of an erythema; changes in blood pressure (lowered) and pulse rate (raised) occur occasionally.

Caution should be exercised when treating patients with the following problems:

- Cardiac disease and altered arterial blood pressure – this may be important factors if a large area of tissue is to be cooled.
- Defective skin sensation – whilst most ice therapy leads to analgesia and it is therefore unnecessary for patient to be sensorily aware during treatment, loss of sensory awareness may indicate other neuromuscular and auto-

nomic problems which may preclude the use of cold therapy;

- Skin hypersensitivity;
- Psychological factors – some subjects have a strong dislike of cold and it should therefore not be used in these cases.

In addition, care should be taken when applying cooling agents to areas in which nervous tissue is very superficial. A number of authors have reported neural damage, including confirmed axonotmesis, following cooling of the peroneal nerve, the lateral cutaneous femoral nerve and the cutaneous femoral nerve (Parker et al., 1983; Green et al., 1989; Covington and Bassett, 1993).

References

Abramson, DI, Kahn, A, Tuck, S et al. (1958) Relationship between a range of tissue temperature and local oxygen uptake in the human forearm. I. Changes observed under resting conditions. Journal of Clinical Investigation 37: 1031–1038.

Abramson, DI, Tuck, S, Chu, L et al. (1964) Effect of paraffin bath and hot fomentations on local tissue temperature. Archives of Physical Medicine in Rehabilitation 45: 87–94.

Abramson, I et al. (1965) Indirect vasodilation in thermotherapy. Archives of Physical Medicine in Rehabilitation 46: 412.

Abramson, DI (1967) Comparison of wet and dry heat in raising temperature of tissue. Archives of Physical Medicine in Rehabilitation 48: 654.

Barbour, LA, McGuire, DB, Kirchhoff, KT (1986) Nonanalgesic methods of pain control used by cancer patients. Oncology Nursing Forum 13(6): 56–60.

Barcroft, J, King, W (1909) The effect of temperature on the dissociation curve of blood. Journal of Physiology 39: 374–384.

Basur, R, Shephard, E, Mouzos, G (1976) A cooling method in the treatment of ankle sprains. Practitioner 216: 708.

Bennett, AF (1985) Temperature and muscle. Journal of Experimental Biology 115: 333–344.

Benson, TB, Copp, EP (1974) The effects of therapeutic forms of heat and ice on the pain threshold of the normal shoulder. Rheumatology and Rehabilitation 13: 101–104.

Borell, RM et al. (1977) Fluidotherapy: evaluation of a new heat modality. Archives of Physical Medicine in Rehabilitation 58: 69.

Borell, PM, Parker, R, Henley, EJ et al. (1980) Comparison of in vivo temperatures produced by hydrotherapy, paraffin wax treatment and fluidotherapy. Physical Therapy 60: 1273–1276.

Burns, SP, Conin, TA (1987) The use of paraffin wax in the treatment of burns. Physiotherapy Canada 39: 258.

Chastain, PB (1978) The effect of deep heat on isometric strength. *Physical Therapy* 58: 543.

Clarke, RSJ, Hellon, RF, Lind, AR (1958) The duration of sustained contractions of the human forearm at different temperatures. *Journal of Physiology* 143: 454–473.

Covington, DB, Bassett, FH (1993) When cryotherapy injures. *The Physician and Sports Medicine* 21(3): 78–93.

Curkovic, B, Vitulic, V, Babic-Naglic, D, Durrigl, T (1993) The influence of heat and cold on the pain threshold in rheumatoid arthritis. *Zeitschrift fur Rheumatologie* 52: 289–91.

Currier, DP, Kramer, JF (1982) Sensory nerve conduction: heating effects of ultrasound and infrared. *Physiotherapy Canada* 34: 241.

Davies, CTM, Young, K (1983) Effect of temperature on the contractile properties and muscle power of triceps surae in humans. *Journal of Applied Physiology* 55: 191–195.

Edwards, R, Harris, R, Hultman, E *et al.* (1970) Energy metabolism during isometric exercise at different temperatures of m. quadriceps femoris in man. *Acta Physiologica Scandinavica* 80: 17–18.

Farry, PJ, Prentice, NG (1980) Ice treatment of injured ligaments: an experimental model. *New Zealand Medical Journal* 9: 12.

Fenn, JE (1969) Effect of pulsed electromagnetic energy (Diapulse) on experimental haematomas. *Canadian Medical Association Journal* 100: 251.

Feibel, A, Fast, A (1976) Deep heating of joints: a reconsideration. *Archives of Physical Medicine in Rehabilitation* 57: 513.

Gersten, JW (1955) Effect of ultrasound on tendon extensibility. *American Journal of Physical Medicine* 34: 362–369.

Green, GA, Zachazewski, JE, Jordan, SE (1989) Peroneal nerve palsy induced by cryotherapy. *The Physician and Sports Medicine* 17(9): 63–70.

Griffin, JE, Karselis, TC (1988) *Physical Agents for Physical Therapists*, 3rd edition. Charles C Thomas, Springfield, Illinois.

Harris, ED, McCroskery, PA (1974) The influence of temperature and fibril stability on degradation of cartilage collagen by rheumatoid synovial collegenase. *New England Journal of Medicine* 290: 1–6.

Head, MD, Helms, PS (1977) Paraffin and sustained stretching in the treatment of burns contracture. *Burns* 4: 136.

Hendler, E, Crosby, R, Hardy, JD (1958) Measurement of heating of the skin during exposure to infrared radiation. *Journal of Applied Physiology* 12: 177.

Hunter, J, Kerr, EH, Whillans, MG (1952) The relation between joint stiffness upon exposure to cold and the characteristics of synovial fluid. *Canadian Journal of Medical Science* 30: 367–377.

Kern, H, Fessl, L, Trnavsky, G, Hertz, H (1984) Das Verhalten der Gelenkstemperatur unter Eisapplikation – Grundlage fur die praktische Anwendung. *Weiner Klinische Wochenschrift* 96: 832–837.

Lee, JM, Warren, MP, Mason, SM (1978) Effects of ice on nerve conduction velocity. *Physiotherapy* 64: 2–6.

Lehmann, JF, Brunner, GD, Stow, RW (1958) Pain threshold measurements after therapeutic application of ultrasound, microwaves and infrared. *Archives of Physical Medicine in Rehabilitation,* 39: 560–565.

Lehmann, JF, Silvermann, DR, Baum, B *et al.* (1966) Temperature distribution in the human thigh produced by infrared, hot pack and microwave applications. *Archives of Physical Medicine in Rehabilitation* 47: 291–299.

Lehmann, JF, Masock, AJ, Warren, CG, Koblanski, JN (1970) Effects of therapeutic temperatures on tendon extensibility. *Archives of Physical Medicine in Rehabilitation* 51: 481–487.

Lehmann, JF, Dundore, DR, Esselmann, PC (1983) Microwave diathermy: effects on experimental haematoma resolution. *Archives of Physical Medicine in Rehabilitation* 64: 127–129.

Lehmann, JF, de Lateur, JB (1990) Therapeutic heat, in Lehman JF (ed): *Therapeutic Heat and Cold*, 4th edition. Williams and Wilkins, Baltimore.

Magness, J, Garret, T, Erickson, D (1970) Swelling of the upper extremity during whirlpool baths. *Archives of Physical Medicine in Rehabilitation* 51: 297.

McMaster, WC, Liddle, S, Waugh, TR (1978) Laboratory evaluation of various cold therapy modalities. *The American Journal of Sports Medicine* 6: 5, 291–294.

Meussen, R, Lievens, P (1986) The use of cryotherapy in sports injuries. *Sports Medicine* 3: 398–414.

Miglietta, O (1973) Action of cold on spasticity. *American Journal of Physical Medicine* 52: 198–205.

Oliver, RA, Johnson, DJ, Wheelhouse, WW, *et al.* (1979) Isometric muscle contraction response during recovery from reduced intramuscular temperature. *Archives of Physical Medicine in Rehabilitation* 60: 126.

Parker, JT, Small, NC, Davis, DG (1983) Cold induced nerve palsy. *Athletic Training* 18: 76.

Pegg, SMH, Littler, TR, Littler, EN (1969) A trial of ice therapy and exercise in chronic arthritis. *Physiotherapy* 55: 51–56.

Price, R, Lehmann, JF, Boswell-Bessette, S, Burleigh, S, de Lateur, B (1993) Influence of cryotherapy on spasticity at the human ankle. *Archives of Physical Medicine in Rehabilitation* 74: 300–304.

Schmidt, KL *et al.* (1979) Heat, cold and inflammation. *Rheumatology* 38: 391.

Selkins, KM, Emery, AF (1982) Thermal science for physical medicine, in Lehmann, JF (ed) *Therapeutic Heat and Cold*, 4th edition. Williams and Wilkins, Baltimore.

Wallace, L *et al.* (1979) Immediate care of ankle injuries. *Journal of Orthopaedic and Sports Physical Therapy* 1: 46.

Warren, CG, Lehmann, JF, Koblanski, JN (1971) Elongation of rat tail tendon: effect of load and temperature. *Archives of Physical Medicine in Rehabilitation* 52: 465–475.

Warren, CG, Lehmann, JF and Koblanski, JN (1976) Heat and stretch procedures: an evaluation using rat tail tendon. *Archives of Physical Medicine in Rehabilitation* 57: 122–126.

Waylonis GW (1967) The physiological effect of ice massage. *Archives of Physical Medicine in Rehabilitation* 48, 37–41.

D

Electromagnetic Agents

10

Infrared Irradiation

SHEILA KITCHEN

Introduction
•
Physical Characteristics
•
Dosage
•
Biological Effects
•
Clinical Efficacy
•
Clinical Application

Introduction

The use of infrared irradiation in the treatment of a variety of medical conditions has a long history. As a modern therapeutic agent it has a history that reaches back to the beginning of the century. A report presented by Fleck (1952) suggested that infrared irradiation was then being used in the management of a wide variety of conditions such as tuberculosis, elephantiasis and a range of soft tissue lesions. Infrared (IR) has continued to be used in clinical practice for the relief of pain and stiffness, to increase joint motion and to enhance the healing of soft tissue lesions and skin conditions (Michlovitz, 1986; Kitchen and Partridge, 1991). Its popularity in clinical practice in Britain appears at present, however, to be on the wane, along with other thermal agents such as continuous shortwave diathermy and microwave diathermy.

Physical Characteristics

Infrared (IR) radiations lie within that part of the electromagnetic spectrum which gives rise to heating when absorbed by matter (see page 19). The radiations are characterized by wavelengths of 0.78–1000 µm and lie between microwaves and visible light on the spectrum. It is important to note that many sources which emit visible light or ultraviolet radiation also emit IR.

The International Commission on Illumination (CIE) describes infrared irradiation in terms of three biologically significant bands which differ in the degree to which they are absorbed by tissues and therefore their effect upon tissues:

- IR-A: spectral values of 0.78–1.4 μm;
- IR-B: spectral values of 1.4–3.0 μm;
- IR-C: spectral values of 3.0–1.0 mm.

The wavelengths mainly used in clinical practice are between 0.7 μm and 1.5 μm, and are therefore concentrated in the IR-A band.

Production of Heat

Infrared irradiation is produced as a result of molecular motion within heated materials. An increase in temperature above absolute zero results in the vibration or rotation of molecules within matter, which leads to the emission of infrared irradiation. All hot bodies and materials therefore emit IR, albeit to differing degrees. The temperature of the body affects the wavelength of the radiation emitted, with the mean frequency of emitted radiation rising with an increase in temperature. Thus, the higher the temperature of the body the higher the mean frequency output and, consequently, the shorter the wavelength. Most bodies do not, however, emit IR of a single wave band. A number of different wavelengths may be emitted due to interplay between the emission and absorption of radiations affecting the behaviour of molecules.

Sources of Infrared Irradiation

Infrared sources can be either natural or artificial. By far the most significant natural source is the sun, which emits vast quantities of radiant energy. However, this source is both unreliable in Britain and not easily controlled, with the result that artificial sources are used predominantly in both the home and medical practice. Such sources include domestic space heaters, hair dryers, industrial furnaces and ovens.

Artificial sources are used by physiotherapists in clinical practice and may be divided into luminous or nonluminous generators. The most usual method of producing IR is passing an electrical current through a coiled resistance wire (Figure 10.1). Luminous generators (which may also be called radiant heaters) consist of a tungsten filament within a glass bulb which contains an inert gas at low pressure (Figure 10.2). They emit both infrared and visible radiations with a peak wavelength of 1 μm. Filters may be used to limit the output to particular wave bands, such as when a

Figure 10.1 Shows a nonluminous infrared unit. (Photograph courtesy of Chatanooga Group Ltd, Bicester.)

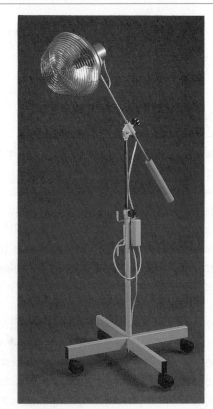

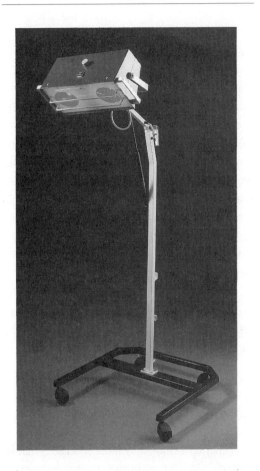

Figure 10.2   Shows a luminous infrared unit. (Photograph courtesy of Electro-Medical Supplies (Greenham) Ltd, Wantage.)

red filter is used to filter out blue and green light waves.

Nonluminous generators normally consist of a coiled resistance wire which may be wound around or embedded within a ceramic insulating material; less frequently, the heated wiring may be placed behind or within a metal shield or tube. Infrared irradiation will therefore be emitted by both the wire and the heated materials surrounding it, resulting in the emission of radiations of a number of different frequencies. Nonluminous generators, however, produce radiations which peak at a wavelength of 4 µm.

Both luminous and nonluminous lamps are available with different power ratings. Luminous lamps are generally available with power levels of between 250 and 1500 W, and nonluminous lamps normally range between 250 and 1000 W. Both experience and research have shown that a period of time should be allowed for the lamp to heat up prior to treatment, as the energy emitted by the source increases over a period of time (Orenberg et al., 1986; Ward, 1986); the time required will vary according to the type of lamp. Nonluminous lamps will take longer than luminous lamps to reach a stable, peak level of heat emission as the molecular oscillation causing heating spreads through the body of the heater.

Physical Behaviour of Infrared Radiations

Infrared radiations can be reflected, absorbed, transmitted, refracted and diffracted by matter. All of these parameters are of importance when measuring IR radiations, but reflection and absorption are of most biological and clinical significance when considering the effects of IR on tissues of a patient. These effects will moderate the penetration of energy into the tissues and thus affect the biological changes which may take place in the tissues.

REFLECTION

Jacques et al. (1955) examined the reflection characteristics of the human skin and noted that maximum reflectivity occurs at IR wavelengths of between 0.7 and 1.2 µm, the range of many therapeutic lamps. Maximum penetration occurs with wavelengths of 1.2 µm, whilst the skin is virtually opaque to wavelengths of 2 µm and more (Moss et al., 1989). Hardy (1956) showed that at least 50% of radiations of 1.2 µm penetrated to a depth of 0.8 mm, allowing interaction with capillaries and nerve endings. As the energy penetration decreases exponentially with depth, most heating due to IR will occur superficially. Selkins and Emery (1982) demonstrated that almost all energy was absorbed at a depth of 2.5 mm and Harlen (1980) noted penetration depths of 0.1 mm for long IR wavelengths and up to 3 mm for the shorter wavelengths.

ABSORPTION

Radiation must be absorbed in order to facilitate changes within the body tissues and, therefore, the greater the level of penetration the more extensive these effects are likely to be.

Penetration of energy into a medium is dependent upon the intensity of the source of infrared, the wavelength (and consequent frequency of the radiation), the angle at which the radiation hits the surface, and the coefficient of absorption of the material. Skin is a complex material and consequently its reflective and absorptive characteristics are not uniform; they depend primarily on the blood supply to the area and skin pigmentation (Moss et al., 1989). Hardy (1956) points out that short wavelengths are scattered more than long and that the differences are minimized as the thickness of the skin increases. Penetration therefore depends both on the absorptive properties of the constituents of the skin and on the degree of scattering brought about by the skin microstructure.

HEATING DUE TO CONDUCTION

Some further heating may occur at a greater depth due to the conduction of heat from the superficial tissue due to both direct conduction and the increased local circulation. Infrared should, however, be regarded as a surface heating modality. Further information about the transfer of heat by conduction is to be found in Chapter 6.

Dosage

The degree of heating produced in the tissues of a patient as a result of the application of IR may be calculated mathematically (Selkins and Emery, 1982; Orenberg et al., 1986) or may be recorded in the tissues by the use of heat sensors of varying types (Westerhof et al., 1987; Kramer, 1984; Moss et al., 1989). Whilst both practices may be suitable in research situations, it is normal clinical practice to gauge the level of heating developed in the surface tissues by the sensory report of the patient. The amount of energy received by the patient will be governed by the intensity of the output of the lamp (usually measured in watts), the distance of the lamp from the patient and the duration of the treatment.

Biological Effects

It is generally assumed by most specialists that IR photons do not give rise to photochemical effects. The main physiological effects claimed for infrared are, therefore, the result of local tissue heating, which has been discussed in detail in Chapters 6 and 9. These effects include alterations in metabolic and circulatory behaviour, in neural function and in cellular activity.

Metabolic Changes

An increase in temperature will result in an increase in the metabolic activities in the superficial tissues due to the direct effect of heat on chemical processes.

Circulatory Changes

Infrared radiation has been shown to cause an increase in blood flow in the cutaneous circulation (Crockford and Hellon, 1959; Millard, 1961; Wyper and McNiven, 1976). This increase is due to vasodilation of the blood vessels of the skin, and the effect may be mediated through the direct effect of heat on the vessels themselves or via their vasomotor nerve supply. Increased levels of certain metabolites in the blood — the result of increased metabolic activity arising from the increased temperatures — also have a direct effect on vessel walls, stimulating vasodilation.

These changes are not reflected in the deeper tissues of the body such as the underlying muscle tissue and no significant changes are seen in body core temperature and blood pressure, even when the whole of one aspect of the body is exposed to a source of infrared.

Neurological Effects

Melzack and Wall (1982) state that 'despite widespread use of heat to relieve pain, we do not know why it works'. They suggest two possible mechanisms of pain relief. First, vasodilation must bring cells and chemicals to the area to assist healing and remove the breakdown products of injury. Second, the pain gate control theory might indicate that the transmission of thermal sensations may take precedence over nociceptive impulses (see Chapter 5 for further details).

Lehmann et al. reported work in 1958 which demonstrated that when IR was applied to the ulna nerve region at the elbow, an analgesic effect was noted distal to the point of application. Kramer (1984) utilized infrared as a control when evaluating the heating effect of ultrasound in nerve conduction tests on normal subjects. Both infrared and ultrasound were applied separately to the distal humeral segment of the ulna nerve in dosages that generated a rise in tissue temperature of 0.8°C. An increase in the post-treatment ulna nerve conduction velocity was found in both cases. The workers attributed this velocity change directly to the increases in temperature.

The studies of Halle et al. (1981) and Currier and Kramer (1982), again on human subjects, supported this work. Though infrared irradiation was again used as a control for work on ultrasound, evidence suggests that IR can cause an increase in the conduction velocity of normal nerves in man. This could have implications both in terms of motor and sensory conduction; an increase in motor conduction can result in an increase in speed of a reflex response and possibly the speed of muscle contraction. Current theories suggest that an increase in sensory conduction may influence sensory responses via an increase in endorphins which could affect the pain gate mechanism, though there is no firm evidence for this view at present.

Barbour et al. (1986) conducted a subjective evaluation of methods of pain relief used by patients suffering from cancer. He found that 68% used heat in some form to help control pain. Despite difficulties in establishing mechanisms it is interesting to note that patients regard heating as an effective method of pain relief.

Clinical observation suggests that heat may relieve muscle spasm, but there is currently little experimental evidence to substantiate or explain this phenomenon. Lehmann and de Lateur (1990) describe work which demonstrated that heating tissue to therapeutic temperatures of between 40°C and 45°C results in a reduction of spasm and that stimulation of skin in the neck region could result in increased muscle relaxation. Little is known about the mechanisms which may initiate such changes, though the reduction of pain has been suggested as one possible mechanism which may lead to the relief of pain (for further discussion see Chapter 5).

Cellular Effects

Kligman (1982) showed that prolonged exposure (15 minutes, three times a week over 45 weeks) of guinea pigs to infrared at an intensity of 12.45 J/cm^2 (giving rise to a skin temperature of about 40°C) can result in an increase in elastic fibres in the upper dermis and a large increase in ground substance. This effect is particularly noticeable when the infrared is combined with ultraviolet light.

Infrared radiation may cause an alteration in the amino acid composition of proteins which then appear to become more resistant to heat. This means that thermal tolerance develops and results in a reduction in the physiological effects of subsequent doses (Westerhof et al., 1987). This effect can be overcome by allowing a period of between 36 and 72 hours to elapse between treatments.

Whilst normal cells are unaffected, the effects of mild hyperthermia (41–45°C) on cancer cells can include the inhibition of the synthesis of RNA, DNA and proteins (Westerhof et al., 1987). This can cause irreversible structural damage to cell membranes and the disruption of organelles.

Clinical Efficacy

A number of authors have suggested that infrared radiation can be effective in a variety of clinical settings. It has been suggested that IR may be used for the following purposes:

- The reduction of pain;
- The reduction of muscle spasm;
- The reduction of joint stiffness;
- The acceleration of healing;
- The improvement of the circulation;
- The reduction of oedema;
- The treatment of certain skin conditions.

In order for these therapeutic effects to occur it has been suggested that there is a need for a temperature of between 40 and 45°C which should be maintained for at least five minutes (Lehmann and de Lateur, 1990). Crockford and Hellon (1959) demonstrated a gradual rise in temperature which occurred during the first ten minutes of irradiation, with the return to normal taking an average of 35 minutes.

Pain

Infrared may be used in the clinical situation for the relief of both chronic and acute pain; relief of chronic pain, such as that arising from joint disease, is likely to be only temporary. The mechanisms whereby this is thought to occur have been discussed in Chapter 9 and highlighted in the previous section of this chapter.

Muscle Spasm

Muscle spasm arising from pain and stress may be treated using infrared irradiations; that arising due to neurological dysfunction is, however, unlikely to respond. Again, possible mechanisms whereby these effects may occur have been discussed previously.

Joint Stiffness

Joint stiffness encompasses a number of parameters such as the behaviour of ligaments (which tend to degenerate with immobilization), joint capsule and periarticular structures (which tend to stiffen with immobilization), and alterations in fluid pressure. Wright and Johns (1961) applied IR to a normal hand joint *in vivo*, producing a surface temperature of 45°C. They measured a 20% drop in joint stiffness at 45°C when compared to stiffness at a temperature of 33°C. This work was performed with two subjects only and has not been replicated. They also demonstrated that people suffering from rheumatoid arthritis and chronic tophaceous gout exhibited increased stiffness, and suggest that the work on the effects of heat on stiffness in the normal subjects would apply to those with pathological stiffening.

Chapter 9 discusses the known effects of heat on collagen tissue and provides limited evidence of changes in pliability of the tissue following heating. Such limited evidence does not provide a sound basis for the advocacy of the general use of IR to reduce joint stiffness.

Tissue Healing

Infrared irradiation has been used to promote tissue healing by a number of workers (Stillwell, 1971; Hyland and Kirkland, 1980). The latter applied infrared radiation to ulcers with the objective of improving healing by dehydration, increasing the circulation and the metabolic rate, and retarding bacterial growth. Infrared therapy was most successful in ulcers of 5 mm or less in depth. However, this trial was poorly controlled and offers little evidence of the efficacy of this method.

Cummings (1990) suggests that infrared irradiation should no longer be considered an appropriate treatment for open wounds as its tendency to dehydrate the tissue may in fact cause further damage to the lesion and inhibit healing. Closed lesions are unlikely to be greatly affected by heating with IR due to the superficial nature of the agent.

Circulation

Infrared irradiation may be used to increase the local, superficial circulation of an area. IR has been used in clinical practice to increase the blood flow to areas of skin which have been subject to pressure or friction and are vulnerable to breakdown and the development of pressure sores. Such treatment should be repeated at regular intervals in conjunction with steps to reduce or remove the causes of the pressure or friction.

Oedema

Wadsworth and Chanmugan (1980) advocate the use of infrared irradiation in the management of oedema of the extremities; such treatment can only be seen as an adjunct to other procedures such as elevation and exercise of the part. It is claimed that the use of IR will cause vasodilation of the vessels and encourage increased rates of tissue fluid exchange. No studies have been found to substantiate these claims or to indicate that the addition of IR to other treatments actually facilitates the reduction of oedema.

Skin Lesions

A number of skin lesions may benefit from the application of a drying heat. Fungal infections, such as paronychia, may be managed through the regular use of infrared treatment. Psoriatic lesions may also respond to the use of IR. These, though of uncertain origin, may result from the activity of either epidermal keratinocytes or dermal fibroblasts, or both. Both Westerhof *et al.* (1987) and Orenberg *et al.* (1986) examined the use of heat to manage the condition. The former exposed patients with psoriasis to IR for 1 month.

A skin temperature of 42°C was achieved and the resulting vasomotor erythema persisted for half an hour. Eighty per cent of these patients experienced remission, 30% experiencing a dramatic improvement. Care should, however, be taken with such treatment as drying of tissue may be detrimental to the patient.

Orenberg et al. (1986) compared heat delivery systems for the hyperthermic treatment of psoriasis, using ultrasound, hot water and infrared. They concluded that infrared systems provide adequate heating for the treatment of the condition.

Infrared Radiation and Ultraviolet Irradiation

In the past, some therapists have held the belief that the application of IR radiation prior to UVR could increase the absorption of the latter and that the effects of UVR are diminished by the application of infrared following the UVR treatment. There is some evidence to support these beliefs. Work by Kligman (1982) on guinea pigs suggests that the two together may modify cellular activity and both Bain et al. (1943) and Freeman and Knox (1964) report that heat increases the incidence and development of UVR-induced tumours in mice. Montgomery (1973) reported that the application of infrared radiation both before and after UVR treatment could enhance the erythema. When applied before the UVR treatment an increase in erythema always resulted; when given after the UVR it enhanced as often as diminished the erythema.

In contrast, Kaidbey et al. (1982) evaluated the effect of applying infrared to the skin before, during, and after the use of UVR, and reported that infrared irradiation neither enhanced the UVR erythema when given prior to, or reduced it when given after, ultraviolet radiation. These workers draw attention to the large number of variables involved in such trials and point out that these results may not hold if the variables are altered.

Thus, results are mixed and suggest that further work is needed in order to substantiate any claims made for the use of infrared radiation in association with ultraviolet radiation.

Hazards

Infrared irradiation may cause damage to a number of tissues in the body if used at excessive levels over long periods of time or if used at very high intensities. Those tissues most likely to be damaged are the skin or the eyes, with most studies examining the effects of high doses of infrared irradiation on the tissues of the eye.

The effects of both prolonged and excessive exposure to infrared irradiation on the skin have been described by Hyland and Kirkland (1980) and Moss et al. (1989) as increased vasodilation of the arteriolar system leading to:

- An 'erythematous'-type appearance;
- Permanent pigmentation;
- Wheal formation;
- Blistering;
- Oedema;
- Burns.

Kligman (1982) examined the damage caused by prolonged exposure of the skin to infrared of a tolerable temperature and found that epidermal hyperplasia and a large increase in ground substance occurred in guinea pigs. Space heaters such as electric fires, infrared reflector lamps in beauty salons and sunbathing can all have these effects, as can infrared lamps used by subjects for self treatment.

Acute burns following a single exposure to infrared irradiation are possible, but are rare if the sensitivity of the skin to temperature is normal. Skin damage normally occurs at temperatures of 46–47°C and above; pain, however, is usually elicited at a temperature of 44.5 ± 1.3°C and should, therefore, provide protection from acute burns by evoking a withdrawal response (Hardy, 1951; Stevens, 1983).

Others consider *optical damage* to be the most likely hazard to arise from excessive exposure to infrared irradiation, with corneal burns resulting from far-IR and retinal and lenticular injury from near-IR (Moss *et al.* 1989). These latter injuries are normally associated with long-term irradiation at high temperatures such as those found in industrial environments and are unlikely to occur during normal therapeutic use of the agent.

Other tissues and structures that may be damaged through excessive exposure to infrared irradiation are the testicles, the respiratory system and exposed subdermal tissues: heating can result in a temporary lowering of the sperm count in those exposed; infants exposed to radiant warmers may be subject to periods of apnoea; and subdermal tissues exposed to overhead infrared heating lamps during surgical procedures have shown an increased tenancy to develop adhesions. The use of infrared irradiation to treat open wounds may have similar effects, though there is currently no data to confirm this.

Additional hazards include the possibility of dehydration following prolonged treatment to large areas of the body and temporary lowering of the blood pressure. Both of these are rare in clinical practice but should be guarded against in susceptible subjects, such as the elderly. Such people may experience dizziness and headaches following treatment, especially when it is directed at large areas such as the back, neck and shoulders.

Safety Precautions and Contraindications

A number of precautions should be considered when using infrared irradiation to treat patients, and both the equipment to be used, the procedure and the subject should be checked.

The electrical safety of the equipment should be checked regularly by appropriately qualified staff and should meet the standards laid down in BS5274: part 1, *General Requirements for the Safety of Medical Electrical Equipment.* The output of the lamp should be checked, and the mechanical stability, alignment and security of all parts of the lamp should be examined (with particular attention being directed at the security of the heating elements and the effectiveness of the positional locking devices).

The procedure used in the administration of IR treatments should be followed strictly in order to avoid injury to the subject; this procedure is described in the following section.

The patient must also be examined for any characteristics which may contraindicate the use of IR therapy, should be made fully aware of the nature of the treatment, the possible hazards associated with it, and be aware of the need to immediately report any inappropriate heating.

The following is a commonly agreed list of contraindications to the use of infrared irradiation by physiotherapist in clinical practice; whilst not all factors have been substantiated fully through research, such a list has resulted in minimal damage to patients in clinical practice:

- Areas with poor or deficient cutaneous thermal sensitivity;
- Subjects with advanced cardiovascular disease;
- Local areas of impaired peripheral circulation;
- Scar tissue or tissue devitalized by deep x-ray

treatment or other ionizing radiations (which may be more subject to burning);

- Malignant tissue of the skin (though such tissue may occasionally be treated through the use of infrared irradiation);
- Subjects with a reduced level of consciousness or understanding of the dangers of treatment;
- Subjects with acute febrile illness;
- Some acute skin diseases such as dermatitis or eczema;
- The testes.

Clinical Application

The following procedure should be used when giving infrared therapy to a patient.

- *Select equipment*: either a luminous (radiant) or nonluminous lamp may be used. The energy from a luminous lamp will tend to penetrate slightly further into the tissues than that of a nonluminous generator due to the frequency of the peak emissions and may therefore be preferable when maximum penetration of energy is required. Some sources suggest that a nonluminous generator provides greater sensory stimulation to the skin and may therefore be selected for this purpose.
- *Warm-up*: allow an adequate 'warm-up' period for each piece of equipment prior to use. This provides time for the output of the machine to reach its maximum before usage. A nonluminous lamp will require approximately 15 minutes to stabilize, whereas a luminous lamp requires a few minutes only.
- *The Subject*: the patient should be positioned in a comfortable, supported position which will allow them to remain still for the duration of the treatment. The part should be uncovered and the skin examined for lesions of all types.

The skin should be clean and dry, all liniments and creams being removed.

- *Safety Precautions*: the nature, effects and possible dangers of the treatment should be explained to the patient fully. The patient should be examined for any contraindications to the treatment and the thermal sensitivity of the skin should be examined. The eyes should be shielded if they are likely to be irradiated in order to prevent drying of the surface. The patient should also be warned of the dangers inherent in touching the lamp during treatment.
- *Lamp positioning*: the lamp is positioned in such as way as to allow the radiations to strike the skin at a right angle; this facilitates maximum absorption of energy by the skin. The distance of the lamp from the part will vary according to the output of the lamp, but is usually between 50 and 75 cm.
- *Dosage*: The intensity of the dosage is determined by the response of the subject to the perceived thermal stimulus. It is therefore important that the subject is advised of the appropriate level of heating to be felt and should understand the importance of reporting any changes to the perceived temperature both when the equipment is initially set up and during the course of the treatment. The intensity is altered by either changing the distance of the lamp from the part or by altering a resistance which controls the current passing to the element in a luminous generator. By the end of a treatment, a mild dose should generate skin temperatures in the region of between 36–38°C, and a moderate dose should produce temperatures of between 38–40°C. Infrared treatment is normally continued for a period of between 10 and 20 minutes, depending on the size and vascularity of the part, the chronicity of the lesion and the nature of the lesion.

Small avascular parts, acute conditions, and skin lesions tend to be treated for shorter periods of time.

- *Follow up*: Following the cessation of treatment, the temperature of the skin should feel mildly or moderately warm to touch. The degree of erythema induced should be noted and any unexpected changes evaluated. Records should be kept of each treatment, and the changes induced by the radiation.

References

Bain, J, Rusch, H, Kline, B (1943) The effect of temperature on ultraviolet carcinogenesis with wavelengths 2800–3400 Å. *Cancer* 3: 610–612.

Barbour, LA, McGuire, DB, Kirchhoff, KT (1986) Nonanalgesic methods of pain control used by cancer patients. *Oncology Nursing Forum* 13(6): 56–60.

Crockford, GW, Hellon, RF (1959) Vascular responses of human skin to infra-red radiation. *Journal of Physiology* 149: 424–432.

Cummings, J (1990) Role of light in wound healing, in Kloth, L, McCullock, JM, Feedar, JA (eds) *Wound healing: alternatives in management*. F A Davies Company, Philadelphia.

Currier, DP, Kramer, JF (1982) Sensory nerve conduction: heating effects of ultrasound and infrared. *Physiotherapy Canada* 34: 241–246.

Fleck, U (1952) *Infrared in relation to skin and underlying tissue: A bibliography*. Technical Information Division, Library of Congress, Washington DC.

Freeman, R, Knox, J (1964) Influence of temperature on ultraviolet injury. *Archives of Dermatology* 89: 858–864.

Forster, A, Palastanga, N (1985) *Clayton's Electrotherapy: Theory and Practice*. Bailliere Tindall, London.

Halle, JS, Scoville, CR, Greathouse, DG (1981) Ultrasound's Effect on the Conduction Latency of the Superficial Radial Nerve in Man. *Physical Therapy* 61: 345–350

Hardy, JD (1951) Influence of skin temperature upon pain threshold as evoked by thermal irradiation. *Science* 114: 149–150.

Hardy, JD (1956) Spectral transmittance and reflectance of excised human skin. *Journal of Applied Physiology* 9: 257–264.

Harlen, F (1980) in Docker, MF (ed) *Physics in Physiotherapy, Conference Report Series – 35*, The Hospital Physicists Association.

Hyland, DB, Kirkland, VJ (1980) Infra Red Therapy for skin ulcers. *American Journal of Nursing* October, 1800–1801.

Jacques, JA, Kuppenheim, HF (1955) Spectral reflectance of human skin in the region of 0.7–2.6 µm. *Journal of Applied Physiology* 8: 297–299.

Kahn, J (1987) *Principles and Practice of Electrotherapy*. Churchill Livingstone, London.

Kaidbey, K, Witkowski, T, Kligman, A (1982) The influence of infrared irradiation on short term ultraviolet irradiation induced injuries. *Archives of Dermatology* 118: 315–318.

Kitchen, SS, Partridge, CJ (1991) Infrared therapy. *Physiotherapy* 77: 4, 249–254.

Kligman, LH (1982) Intensification of ultraviolet-induced dermal damage by infrared radiation. *Archives of Dermatological Research* 272: 229–238.

Kramer, JF (1984) Ultrasound: evaluation of its mechanical and thermal effects. *Archives of Physical Medicine and Rehabilitation* 65: 223–227.

Lehmann, JF, de Lateur, BJ (1990) in Lehmann, JF (ed) *Therapeutic Heat and Cold*, 4th edition. Williams and Wilkins, Baltimore, London.

Low, J, Reed, A (1990) *Electrotherapy Explained: Principles and Practice*. Butterworth Heinemann, London

Melzack, R, Wall, PD (1982) *The Challenge of Pain*. Penguin Books, London.

Michlovitz, SL (1986) *Thermal Agents in Rehabilitation, Contemporary Perspectives in Rehabilitation*, Volume 1. F A Davies Company, Philadelphia.

Millard, JB (1961) Effects of high frequency currents and infrared rays on the circulation of the lower limb in man. *Annals of Physical Medicine* 6(2): 45–65.

Montgomery, PC (1973) The compounding effects of infrared and ultraviolet irradiation upon normal human skin. *Physical Therapy* 53(5): 489–495.

Moss, C, Ellis, R, Murray, W and Parr, W (1989) *Infrared Radiation, Nonionising Radiation Protection*, 2nd edn, WHO Regional Publications, European Series, No 25.

Orenberg, EK, Noodleman, FR, Koperski, JA, Pounds, D, Farber, EM (1986) Comparison of heat delivery systems for hyperthermia treatment of psoriasis. *International Journal Hyperthermia* 2(3): 231–241.

Selkins, KM, Emery, AF (1982) in Lehmann, JF (ed) *Therapeutic Heat and Cold* 3rd edn. Williams and Wilkins, Baltimore, London.

Stevens, J (1983) Thermal sensation: infrared and microwaves, in Adair E (ed) *Microwaves and Thermal Regulation*. Academic Press, London.

Stillwell, GK (1971) Therapeutic heat and cold, in Krusen, FH (ed) *Handbook of Physical Medicine and Rehabilitation*, 2nd edition. W B Saunders, Philadelphia.

Wadsworth, H, Chanmugan, APP (1980) *Electrophysical Agents in Physiotherapy: Therapeutic and Diagnostic Use*. Science Press, Mackerville, NSW, Australia.

Ward, AR (1986) *Electricity Fields and Waves in Therapy*. Science Press, Mackerville, NSW, Australia.

Westerhof, W, Siddiqui, AH, Cormane, RH and Scholten, A (1987) Infrared hyperthermia and Psoriasis. *Archives of Dermatological Research* 279: 209–210.

Wright, V, Johns, RJ (1961) Quantitative and Qualitative analysis of Joint Stiffness in normal Subjects and in Patients with Connective Tissue Disease. *Annals of Rheumatological Disease* 20: 26–36.

Wyper, DJ, McNiven, DR (1976) Effects of some physiotherapeutic agents on skeletal muscle blood flow. *Physiotherapy* 62(3): 83–85.

11

Shortwave Diathermy

SHONA SCOTT

Brief History

Reference to the medical use of high frequency electrical currents can be traced as far back as the 1890s. In Paris, d'Arsonval passed a 1 AMP current at high frequency through himself and an assistant. While similar amounts of electricity at low frequencies were known to be potentially fatal, he reported feeling only a sensation of warmth (Guy, 1984). Subsequent work led to the development of inductive and capacitive methods of applying high frequency currents to the body to produce what was claimed to be non-superficial heating (Guy, 1984). These methods became known as 'diathermy' from the Greek meaning 'through heating'.

To prevent interference with high frequencies used in communications, international convention has allocated three high frequency bands for medical uses. By far the most widespread use is made of the frequency band at 27.12 MHz ± 160 kHz, with a corresponding wavelength of around 11.062 m. Application of this type of electromagnetic energy for therapeutic purposes is referred to as shortwave diathermy (PSWD).

PSWD is a widely used clinical modality. Figure 11.1 shows a modern shortwave diathermy machine. However, the understanding of the mechanisms leading to the clinical effects are still poorly understood for whether or not suggestion can account for the clinically reported response to treatment 157is still a matter for debate.

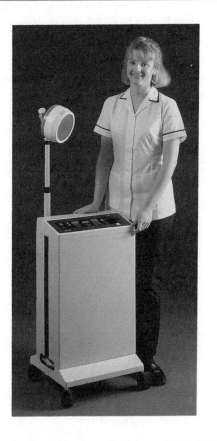

Figure II.I   A pulsed shortwave diathermy machine. (Photograph courtesy of Central Medical Equipment Ltd, Nottingham.)

Physical Characteristics

Shortwave electromagnetic radiations range in frequency from 10–100 MHz; known as radio-frequency waves, the shortest wave band is used in therapeutic diathermy. Short wavelength radio waves lie between microwaves and medium wavelength radio waves on the electromagnetic spectrum, as shown in Figure 1.20 in Chapter 1). Shortwave energy can be delivered in either a continuous or pulsed mode. Whilst continuous shortwave diathermy may be confined to a frequency of 27.12 MHz, pulsing results in the development of side bands which can mean that the energy used ranges in frequency from 26.95–27.28 MHz, with little, if any, of the energy being in the parent band.

Radio waves have the longest wavelength of any region of the electromagnetic spectrum and therefore the lowest frequency; they thus also have the lowest energy per quantum. They are produced as the result of electrical oscillations and both electric and magnetic fields may be set up as a result of their action.

An electric field (E) is set up as the result of the presence of electrical charges; this field is characterized by both direction and magnitude. An electrical charge, such as an electron or proton, placed within this field will experience a force (F). E and F are related as follows:

$$F = qE,$$

where q is the strength of the charge placed in the field.

In electrically conductive materials, such as living tissues, the forces will result in the production of electrical currents.

A magnetic field is produced by a moving electrical charge and, since magnetic fields exert forces on other charges in motion, an alternating electrical current (i.e. a moving charge) will initiate the production of a magnetic field which in turn may initiate the production of an *induced* current. Magnetic fields are specified by two quantities: the magnetic flux density (B) and magnetic field strength (H), having units of tesla (T) and amperes per meter (amp / m) respectively.

Both electric and magnetic fields can be set up in human tissues subjected to shortwave diathermy (Delpizzo and Joiner, 1987; Guy, 1990). In the application of this agent, the patient is made part of the electrical circuit by the use of an inductive coil or capacitive type electrodes; this is shown in Figure 11.2. The resonator (or patient circuit) and generator circuit are tuned by use of a variable capacitor in order to match the parameters of each circuit and thus generate maximum power transfer.

The interaction of the field with the tissues is affected by the macroscopic property of the tissue called the 'complex permittivity'; this represents the dielectric constant and the loss factor of the tissue (Delpizzo and Joiner, 1987). The dielectric constant is a factor representing the depolarization characteristics of a tissue, and is primarily dependent upon water content. Complex permittivity is a function of frequency and, therefore, the propagation and attenuation of the electromagnetic waves are dependent upon frequency (Johnson and Guy, 1972).

The use of a *capacitive circuit* to treat a tissue requires that it lies within an oscillating electrical field; this causes vibration of tissue molecules and thus heating of tissues. The tissue acts as a dialectric and the level of heating is thus partially dependent on the dielectric constant of that structure (Guy, 1990). Such a high-frequency alternating voltage applied to tissues gives rise to two types of current.

Conduction Current (I_R)

Heat develops in relation to the following equation:

$$Q = I^2\, R\, t,$$

where Q = heat in joules, I_R = the amplitude of the current in amperes, R = ohmic resistance, and t = time.

Figure 11.2 Block diagram to show shortwave diathermy generation. (Modified from Low & Reed: Electrotherapy Explained. Second edition. Butterworth Heinemann. Reproduced with permission.)

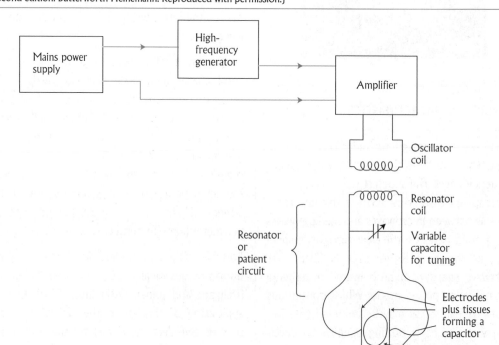

Displacement Current (I$_C$)

A displacement of electrical energy occurs as the result of polarization of the tissue, and its magnitude depends upon the capacitance of the tissue and the frequency of the alternating current.

The use of an *inductive applicator* relies on the tissue being placed within a rapidly alternating magnetic field which is generated by passing the high-frequency current through a coil; this results in the creation of eddy currents within the tissue, induced by the oscillating electromagnetic field.

The level of heat generated depends on the conductivity of the tissues, with those rich in water and ions being heated most readily.

Shortwave diathermy can be delivered in either in a continuous mode or by a pulsed mode. Whereas the continuous mode almost always results in the production of clinically perceptible thermal changes in the tissue, this may not be so when the beam is pulsed. High pulse rates and intensities can lead to thermal change whereas low pulse frequencies and intensities do not.

Absorption of Radiofrequency Energy

Shortwave Diathermy: Thermal Application

The traditional reason for applying high frequency currents to living tissues is to cause heating. The rise in tissue temperature during the application of SWD depends on a factor known as the specific absorption rate (SAR). The SAR is defined as the rate at which energy is absorbed by a unit tissue mass, and is calculated in units of watts per kilogram (W/kg). SAR is a function of tissue conductivity and the electrical field magnitude in tissue. *Tissue conductivity* is a measure of the ease with which an electric field can be set up in tissue. The SAR and, therefore, the heating produced by SWD is dependent upon the electrical properties of tissue within the electromagnetic field (Kloth and Ziskin, 1990). The concentration of the electric field will be highest in the tissues with the greatest conductivity. Living tissues can be considered to consist of three molecular types: charged molecules, dipolar molecules and non-polar molecules (Ward, 1980). Different tissues contain varying proportions of these molecules, influencing the conductivity and hence the SAR and heating pattern when irradiated by SWD.

Heat Production in Tissue

CHARGED MOLECULES

Within living tissue there is an abundance of charged molecules — mainly ions and certain proteins. In response to the forces of repulsion and attraction that occur between charged molecules, exposure to an SWD field causes the charged molecules to be accelerated along lines of electric force. The high-frequency field induces the charged molecules to oscillate about a mean position (Figure 11.3), and kinetic energy is converted into heat (Ward, 1980). Oscillation of charged molecules is an efficient means of heat production (Ward, 1980; Low and Reed, 1990). Tissue containing high proportions of charged molecules will in theory be heated most during SWD treatment.

Figure 11.3   Charged ions move to and fro in response to an oscillating electric field.

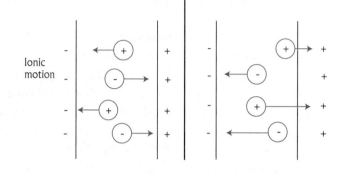

Ionic motion

DIPOLAR MOLECULES

The dipolar molecules found in living tissues consist principally of water and some proteins. They are also affected by electric fields. The positive pole of the molecule aligns itself towards the negative pole of the electric field, and so the alternating SWD field causes rotation of these molecules as the charge of the plates alters rapidly (Figure 11.4). Heating results from the frictional drag between adjacent molecules. Ward (1980) describes this process as a moderately efficient means of heating.

NON-POLAR MOLECULES

Fat cells are an example of non-polar molecules. Although non-polar molecules do not have free ions or charged poles, they still respond to the influence of the SWD field. During exposure to SWD the electron cloud becomes distorted, but negligible heat is produced.

Tissues that have a high ionic content in solution or a large number of free ions (an example of which is blood) are the best conductors; any highly vascular tissue, therefore, is a good conductor. Similarly, both metal and sweat are good

Figure 11.4   Dipolar molecules rotate as the electric field oscillates.

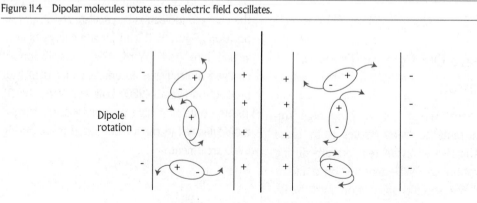

Dipole rotation

conductors. This is important because if a metal implant or drop of sweat are within the electric field they will create an area of high field density and adjacent tissues may be exposed to a large thermal load which may be sufficient to cause a burn. Adipose tissue, on the other hand, is a poor conductor and, therefore, the magnitude of current set up in fat will be minimal.

Heating Patterns Produced with Different Application Techniques

At present there is some debate as to which tissues are heated most during SWD treatments. Tissues which have a high dielectric content and good conductivity tend to absorb more energy from the SWD field. Muscle tissue and blood contain a high proportion of ions compared to adipose tissue. Thus, Kloth and Ziskin (1990) conclude that 'clinically, diathermy can be used to increase the temperature of skeletal muscle'. However, both Goats (1989b) and Ward (1980) do not concur with this view. Both have suggested that SWD may cause excessive heating of superficial adipose tissue. Although adipose tissue contains few ions for the efficient conversion of Electromagnetic Radiation energy into heat energy, they point out that living adipose tissue is permeated with many small blood vessels. These blood vessels provide appropriate conditions for the absorption of EM radiation, and the adipose tissue surrounding the blood vessels insulates and prevents the dissipation of heat produced and, thus, areas of intense heat production within adipose tissue have been suggested.

A similar controversy exists as to where the different techniques of applying SWD cause most heating. A selective heating based on the technique of application has been proposed. For example, Guy (1990) states that inductive shortwave diathermy applications elevate the temperatures of deeper tissues selectively, with relatively smaller effects in surface tissues. van der Esch and Hoogland (1991) consider the effect of the capacitive technique to occur mainly in superficial tissue.

Some figures are available that estimate the ratio of superficial to deep heating for capacitive and inductive methods (Table 11.1). They suggest that the inductive method is more likely to produce an effect in deep tissue. Also, any deep effects with the capacitive method will be associated with extremely large effects in superficial tissue.

This information is important because, as Guy (1990) has stated, 'the most desirable heating or absorption patterns for therapeutic purposes correspond to the minimum relative heating in fat with maximum relative heating and depth of penetration into muscle'. Thus, the physiotherapist needs to be able to apply SWD or PSWD in a

Table 11.1

Figures estimating the ratio of superficial to deep heating for the capacitive and inductive methods

Application Method	Superficial:Deep	Reference
Capacitive	13:1	van der Esch and Hoogland, 1990
	10:1	van der Esch and Hoogland, 1990
	12-18:1	Hand et al., 1990
Inductive	1:1	van der Esch and Hoogland, 1990
	1:4	Hand et al., 1990

manner that will allow the treatment to be specific to the damaged tissues.

Several studies have investigated the heating produced by SWD. In summary, there is conclusive evidence that SWD can cause both deep and superficial tissue heating. Depending on the dosage, it may be possible to raise superficial temperature by as much as 6°C. However, there is still considerable debate as to the pattern of heating produced with different application techniques. For example Abramson *et al.* (1960) failed to demonstrate selective heating of either fat or muscle when SWD was applied with a longitudinal capacitive technique. However, the results need to be interpreted with caution as the SWD was interrupted every 3–4 minutes for readings to be taken because the SWD interfered with the instrumentation that was used for recording temperature. This interruption to the treatment may have allowed an unequal dissipation of heat from the tissues and may not reflect the true heating pattern seen during continuous treatment.

Fortunately, the work of Verrier *et al.* (1977) provides some evidence to substantiate this work. Under carefully controlled conditions, SWD was applied for 20 minutes at the maximum tolerable dose. The capacitive (longitudinal

contraplanar technique — see later) and inductothermy applications were studied. Both applications led to a significant increase in cutaneous and intramuscular (IM) temperature. In addition, a minimal dose of SWD was also studied and inductothermy application was found to produce significantly more heating than the capacitive technique.

Finally, SWD has been shown to raise the temperature of deep tissues, whereas a superficial heating technique that relies on the conduction of heat to deeper tissues is unable to raise the deep tissues by a similar amount (Verrier *et al.*, 1978).

In conclusion, SWD is able to heat deeper tissues than conductive heating agents. However, there is still some controversy as to whether fat or muscle is heated more during the treatment and also whether the application technique alters the heating pattern.

Pulsing Shortwave Diathermy (PSWD)

Pulsed SWD is the application of a series of short bursts (pulses) of SWD. This means that there are

Figure 11.5 The paths of orbiting electrons are distorted in alternate directions as the electric field oscillates. (Modified from Low & Reed: Electrotherapy Explained. Second edition. Butterworth Heinemann. Reproduced with permission.)

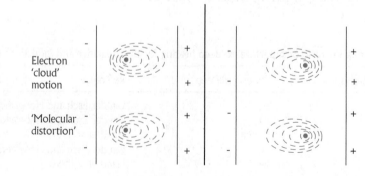

Table 11.2
Summary of the studies that have reported the heating effect that can be produced by SWD.

	Method	Skin	Subcutaneous	IM	Intraartic
Hollander and Hovarth (1950), n=5 Dose: just perceptible	I	7.4F	7.02F	–	–
Abramson (1960), n=14 Dose: comfortably warm	C	1.3	1.5	1.9	–
Verrier et al. (1977), n=20	I	5.05	–	4.40	–
Dose Maximum tolerable dose	C	2.24	–	3.28	–
Verrier et al. (1978) Dose: comfortable	I	6.60	–	6.36	–
Oosterveld et al. (1992) Dose: just perceptible warmth	C	2.4	–	–	1.4

– indicate variables are not reported in paper

Figure 11.6 Diagramatic illustration of the differences between continuous shortwave diathermy (SWD) (a) and pulsed shortwave diathermy (PSWD) (b).

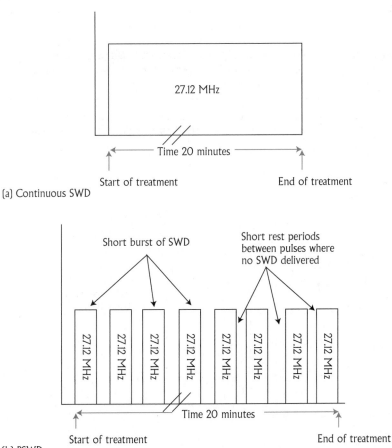

short periods of SWD interspersed with gaps where there is no SWD (Figure 11.6). During the 'on' pulses of SWD the frequency of the electromagnetic radiation is still approximately 27.12 MHz. Pulsing the delivery of SWD means that the patient will receive a lower dose of SWD energy if the treatment is applied for the same length of time as a continuous treatment. The tissues will receive a lower thermal load.

There are three principal variables that are under the control of the therapist:

- Pulse repetition rate;
- Pulse duration;
- Peak pulse power.

Depending on the machine, it may be possible to modify one or more of the variables. Table 11.3 gives a brief explanation of each variable; a knowledge of a number of these parameters provides information about the energy delivered. The mean power can be calculated as in the example below (Figure 11.7):

Table 11.3
Pulse SWD parameters.

Parameters	Explanation	Range
Pulse repetition rate (PRR)	The number of pulses delivered in 1 Second	15–800 Hz
Pulse duration (PD)	The length of each pulse or 'on' period	25–400 μs
Peak pulse power (PPP)	The amplitude of the pulse (often referred to as intensity)	100–1000w
Mean power (MP)	Gives a measure of the dose of PSWD that a patient receives, as illustrated in Figure 7	

Figure 11.7   Illustration of the parameters required for calculating the mean power of PSWD treatments.

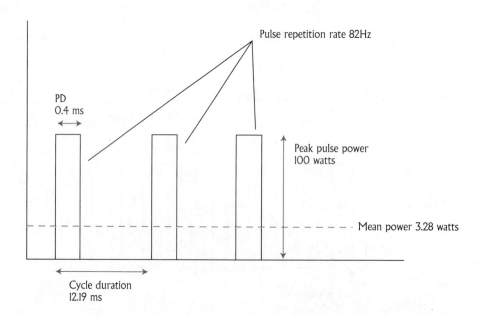

Pulse repetition rate 82Hz

PD
0.4 ms

Peak pulse power
100 watts

Mean power 3.28 watts

Cycle duration
12.19 ms

Pulse repetition rate $= 82\ Hz$

Pulse duration $= 0.4\ ms$

Peak pulse power $= 100\ W$

Cycle duration $= \dfrac{1000}{PRR}$

$= \dfrac{1000}{82}$

$= 12.19\ ms$

% cycle SWD delivered $= \dfrac{PD}{Cycle\ duration}$

$= \dfrac{0.40 \times 100}{12.19}$

$= 3.28\%$

Mean power delivered $= PPP \times \%\ cycle\ SWD$

$= 100 \times 3.28$

$= 3.28\ W$

Therapeutic Effects of SWD and PSWD

The main effect of SWD application is heating of the tissues. The response to tissue heating is similar no matter the modality used to produce the heating, and the only difference with SWD and conductive heating agents is the depth at which the thermal effect occurs. The decision to use SWD is appropriate if the desired treatment outcome is to produce heating within deep tissues. SWD has been reported to:

- Increase blood flow;
- Assist in the resolution of inflammation;
- Increase the extensibility of deep collagen tissue;
- Decrease joint stiffness;
- Relieve deep muscle pain and spasm (Kloth and Ziskin, 1990).

Further details of the effects of heating are to be found in Chapters 6, 9 and 10.

Some authors suggest that the clinical results produced with PSWD can also be attributed to a mild rise in tissue temperature (O'Dowd et al., 1989; Lehman, 1990). The only difference between SWD and PSWD is that PSWD tends to deliver a lower mean power to the patient and therefore causing less heating occurs.

However, a different effect has also been proposed – the athermal effect (Hayne, 1984). What is meant by the athermal effect is that there is a physiological response to PSWD irradiation that is not due to the thermal effect. However, several comprehensive reviews of the PSWD literature have concluded that there is currently little evidence to support the athermal theory (Ward, 1986; Kloth and Ziskin, 1990; Lehman, 1990). PSWD has been shown to cause orientation of fat and red blood cells at right angles to the lines of force of the field (known as the pearl formation of particles). However, it is worth noting that the pearl-chain formation of particles can be produced by either PSWD or SWD if the same average power is used (Lehman, 1990). The clinical implications, if any, of this phenomenom have not yet been proven (Kloth and Ziskin, 1990; Lehman, 1990).

Increased Blood Flow and Metabolism

Blood flow increases in response to heating to help dissipate the local heating effect and prevent tissue damage. Changes in blood flow, in response to SWD treatment, are proportional to the average power delivered to the patient's tissues (Silverman and Pendleton, 1968). During PSWD treatment, friction, displacement and collisions of small particles within the tissues are likely to occur as the short bursts of PSWD are absorbed by the exposed tissues, but the long rest period before the next pulse, in theory, allows the dissipation of any heat (Bouwhuijsen, 1985).

However, Table 11.4 summarizes three studies that have all shown that PSWD is able to produce small increases in tissue temperature, particularly if a high mean power is used. Clinically, a high mean power will be achieved if a long pulse duration, high pulse repetition rate and peak pulse power are used.

Clinical Effects of SWD and PSWD

Although there is still considerable debate as to the mode of action of SWD and PSWD, these modalities are still used extensively in the clinical setting to treat a wide variety of conditions and pathologies. Similarly, there are many opinions on the pathologies that will benefit from SWD and PSWD. Hayne (1984) suggested that PSWD may be useful for recent injuries, post-operative and severely traumatised hands, recent burns, plastic surgery, Bell's palsy, post-laminectomy pain, sinusitis, chronic arthritis and degenerative complaints. PSWD was felt to be beneficial to over 80% of conditions treated. Wright (1973) describes the benefit of PSWD in conjunction with other physiotherapy treatments in the management of soft tissue football injuries. Ginsberg (1961) describes SWD as a beneficial treatment for subdeltoid bursitis associated with calcification. SWD has been recommended as part of a treatment regime for patients suffering from temporomandibular joint disorders (Selsby, 1985). Comorosan et al. (1991) suggest PSWD for the treatment of post-traumatic algoneurodystrophy. The positive outcome of SWD for a patient suffering from pelvic inflammatory disease was described by Balogun and Okonofua (1988). Allbery et al. (1974) suggested that SWD could be used to reduce the pain associated with herpes zoster infection. There are many more similar accounts, but there is insufficient scientific evidence to support such claims. In the absence of adequate clinical measurement no conclusions can be built on these observations. Thus, the following section provides a review of the scientific articles and attempts to summarize the current status of the evidence to support the use of SWD and PSWD in the clinical setting.

Soft Tissue Healing

Several trials, using animals as subjects, have investigated the possible effect of SWD and PSWD on

Table 11.4
Summary of the changes in tissue temperature that have been recorded during PWSD treatments.

	PRR (Hz)	PD (μs)	PPP (W)	MP (W)	Temperature increase (°C)
Erdman, 1960	400	65	–	16	0.5 (below treatment head) 2.0 (dorsum of foot)
Morrisey, 1966	600	50	–	40	2.2 (below treatment head)
	–	50	–	80	10.6 (below treatment head)
Silverman and Pendelton (1968)	–	–	–	15	3.1 (below treatment head) (no change on foot)
	–	–	–	65	5.3 (below treatment head) 1.9 (on foot)
				placebo	NS change

– indicates variables are not reported in paper.

the rate of healing; there is conflicting evidence. In a study of 20 dogs, Bansal *et al.* (1990) concluded that SWD stimulated earlier maturation of the collagen fibres and more rapid regeneration of damaged muscle fibres. Also, in a similar study, Cameron (1961) credited PSWD with causing more rapid activity in collagen formation, white blood cell infiltration, phagocytosis, histocyte activity, fat activity and haematoma canalization in the rate of healing an incision in the thigh of twenty dogs. In contrast to these findings, Constable *et al.* (1971) conducted a series of three experiments to establish whether or not PSWD accelerated experimental wound healing in rabbits and guinea pigs; no benefit was reported. Finally, similar results were reported from a study using a well-controlled double-blind experimental design (Krag *et al.*, 1979). PSWD had no effect on the survival of experimental skin flaps in rats.

The different findings reported in these studies may be attributed to poor methodologies or to differences in the doses used (none of the trials described the dose of SWD used in sufficient detail to allow the trial to be repeated).

On the other hand, trials that have used humans as subjects tend to suggest that PSWD enhances the rate of skin healing. Cameron (1964) studied the effect of PSWD on the rate of healing of surgical wounds. A double-blind protocol was used and one group received PSWD; however, little detail of the treatment parameters are provided. The other group received sham PSWD. Twenty two of the sham-treated and 32 of the PSWD-treated group were rated by their surgeon as being better. Regrettably, no statistical analysis of the results was undertaken. However, supporting this trend, PSWD has been reported to have increased the rate of healing of the donor site wound following medium-thickness skin grafts (Goldin *et al.*, 1981). Again, a randomized dou-

ble-blind procedure was used. The stage of healing was assessed on the seventh day and it was found that 59% of the active group compared with 29% of the sham group were more than 90% healed ($p < 0.05$). Similarly, Itoh *et al.* (1991) produced evidence to suggest that PSWD enhanced the rate of resolution of chronic pressure ulcers. In addition to the normal management, the ulcers were treated with PSWD. Unfortunately, the PSWD details were not described fully and this last result must be interpreted with caution as there were neither control or placebo groups.

Resolution of Haematomas

Two studies, reporting conflicting results, evaluated the effect of PSWD on the resolution of haematomas. A study by Fenn (1969) produced experimental haematomas by injecting a known volume of autogenous blood into the ears of 60 rabbits. The treatment group received twice-daily PSWD. By the sixth day of the experiment the treated haematomas were significantly smaller and exhibited more advanced colour changes than the sham treated haematomas. Thus, a clear effect on the resolution of a haematoma was demonstrated. It should be noted that the clinical implications of this study are limited because the method used to produce haematomas did not involve any trauma or tissue damage.

However, the carefully designed study by Brown and Baker (1987) produced experimental haematomas by injecting a myotoxic drug into the lateral head of gastrocnemeus of 32 rabbits. Pulsed SWD was given to half of the animals with the rest acting as controls. Unfortunately, only a few details of the PSWD dose are provided, and one machine was used to treat two animals simultaneously. No differences in the rate of healing between the treated and control animals were found. However, the clinical relevance of this study must be questioned as treating two animals with one machine must have distorted the PSWD field shape, and thus the distribution of imparted energy.

The rate of healing, pain and swelling following oral surgery procedures were found to respond favourably to PSWD treatment (Aronofsky, 1971). Assessment of recovery was based on clinical judgement and indicated considerably earlier recovery in the 60 treated patients over the control patients. Furthermore, the group of patients who received preoperative PSWD showed even better recovery than the group who received only postoperative treatment.

The effect of PSWD on swelling, disability and pain from recent hand injuries was studied, and PSWD was found to be a beneficial treatment (Barclay et al., 1983). However, in similarity to the previous study, a subjective assessment scale was used and the assessors were not blind to the treatment group. No conclusions can therefore be drawn from these two results.

In contrast, a well-controlled double-blind study by Grant et al. (1989) compared the effect of PSWD, ultrasound, placebo PSWD and placebo ultrasound on the recovery from perineal trauma in a trial of 414 postpartum women. Only a few details of the PSWD treatment parameters are given, but the treatment was applied for 10 minutes between 12 and 36 hours post delivery. The mothers and the midwives did not know the treatment groups and made assessments of the extent of bruising, oedema, use of analgesics and pain (on a VAS). Analysis revealed that for all the parameters assessed there were no differences between the groups either immediately after the treatment, 10 days post partum or 3 months

follow-up. If a control group had been used the extent of the placebo effect associated with these treatments could have been assessed.

A study by Livesly et al. (1992), evaluated the effectiveness of PSWD in 48 patients with minimally displaced fractured neck of humerus. The trial was double-blind and the patients were assigned randomly to either sham or active PSWD (0.4 ms, 35 Hz, 300 W, mean power = 4.2 W, 30 minutes daily for 10 consecutive working days). The results showed no significant difference between the pain levels at one, two and six months. However, it should be noted that 4.2 W is a low mean power.

A clinical trial by Gray et al. (1994) compared four different physiotherapy treatment modalities on the symptoms of temporomandibular joint disorders. This was a double-blind trial and 176 patients were allocated randomly to five groups: SWD, mild thermal setting for 10 minutes; PSWD for 20 minutes; US; laser; and placebo. Treatment was given three times a week for four weeks. The measured outcomes were: range of movement, palpation of joints and muscles, and presence of joint sounds. No difference between the groups was found immediately after the treatments had finished, but at the three month post treatment review the actively treated patients were significantly more improved than the placebo group.

In conclusion, there is only limited experimental evidence to make judgements on the anecdotal claims that SWD or PSWD has a positive effect on the rate of healing after soft tissue trauma. The studies based on poorer experimental design did tend to suggest a positive effect of SWD, which highlights the problems that may be encountered if suggestion and observer bias are not eliminated. The results of the well-controlled studies (Grant et al., 1989; Livesly et al., 1992) indicate that SWD had little beneficial effect on the resolution of soft tissue damage. However, each study used only one of the many possible treatment doses. It is quite possible that damaged cells or different tissues respond to a particular frequency or peak power (Kitchen and Partridge, 1992). It may be that too high a dose will cause a worsening of a condition or that too low a dose will have no effect. There is an urgent need for well-designed trials, so that the effects of different treatment parameters can be investigated. The work that has been done to date does point the way for future work in this area.

The effect of PSWD and SWD on the resolution of several clinical conditions have been studied.

Recent Ankle Injuries

Recent ankle injuries are a condition that have received some attention from SWD and PSWD investigators. Five studies appear to have been undertaken, all using a fairly homogeneous group of patients.

A clinical trial by Wilson (1972), found that active PSWD produced a significantly greater improvement in pain, swelling and disability than placebo treatment of recent ankle injuries. A second study, of a similar group of subjects, compared SWD treatment with PSWD (Wilson, 1974). PSWD was found to be a more effective treatment than SWD.

The effectiveness of two different SWD machines were compared by Pasila et al. (1976). This was a large study of 321 patients with recent ankle injuries. No difference in strength, weight bearing, range of movement, and volumetric measurements were found. However, post treatment, the ankle circumference of those treated with Curapulse was significantly less than the placebo group, and the Diapulse group showed a significant improvement in gait compared to the placebo group.

In another study, Barker et al. (1985) investigated the effect of PSWD on the resolution of 73 recent ankle injuries which were uncomplicated by bone injury. Patients received 45 minutes treatment on three consecutive days. A double-blind protocol was used, and patients were allocated randomly to active or dummy treatment. Assessments were made of range of movement, gait, swelling and pain relief. No significant difference between the groups was identified post treatment.

Finally, McGill (1988) found no difference in the pain, swelling, or time to weight bearing in 31 patients receiving PSWD or placebo treatment; a double-blind protocol was used.

Of the five trials discussed, only three reported using a double-blind protocol (Wilson, 1972; Barker et al., 1985; McGill, 1988). However, the results of these three are inconclusive and even contradictory. An explanation for this may lie in the doses used. In Wilson's 1972 study, a mean power of 40 watts was used and the treatment lasted for an hour. McGill (1988) on the other hand used a mean power of 19.6 watts for 15 minutes. Finally, the Barker (1985) trial was certainly flawed as it describes the peak pulse power only as 'high'. Thus, it could be that the far higher dose used by Wilson (1974) may have been sufficient to produce an effect compared to the lower dose used by McGill.

Pain

In the clinical environment, SWD and PSWD may be used to relieve the pain associated with various conditions. In a review of physiotherapy modalities used in pain control, Chapman (1991) summarizes that PSWD produces a significant relief of pain associated with acute injuries, but its value in the treatment of more chronic conditions remains to be proven. The mechanisms through which SWD and PSWD may alleviate pain are described in Wells, Frampton and Bowsher (1988).

Abramson et al. (1966) reported that SWD treatment, at a maximal tolerated dose, caused an increase in the conduction velocity of median and ulnar motor nerves. Without further work the implications of this observation remain unclear.

A more clinically relevant study was undertaken by Talaat et al. (1986). Patients with myofacial pain dysfunction syndrome were studied and SWD was found to reduce the patients' pain and tenderness compared to a group of patients who received drugs aimed at producing muscle relaxation and analgesia. An obvious problem with the study design is that the group of patients treated with drugs will not have received the same amount of attention as the patients receiving the SWD.

Reed et al. (1987) studied 43 patients who underwent elective repair of reducible inguinal hernia. They wished to evaluate the effect of PSWD on postoperative wound pain. Patients were allocated randomly to either treatment or sham-treatment groups. The PSWD treatment consisted of 15 minutes of treatment twice daily (60 μs, 320 Hz, 1 W, mean power = 0.019 W). The PSWD was reported as having no beneficial effect. However, it must be noted that an extremely low power (0.019 W) of PSWD was used. Finally, SWD was reported to ease the sensitivity of trigger points more so than hot packs (McCray and Patton, 1984). However, this trial did not use a double-blind protocol.

Back Pain

Back pain is a common problem and leads to considerable clinical intervention. Waggstaff et al. (1986) used standardized inclusion criteria to obtain a fairly homogeneous group of patients.

Patients were allocated randomly to SWD or PSWD (82 Hz, 700 W, mean power = 23.2 W) or a second PSWD group (200 Hz, 300 W, mean power = 23.4 W). Treatment was applied for 15 minutes twice a week for three weeks. An independent assessor was used to assess pain before and after each treatment using a 15 cm VAS. The results indicate that all three groups showed a significant decrease in pain by the end of the trial. The PSWD groups showed a significantly greater reduction in pain than the SWD group. There was no difference in the improvement between the PSWD groups. However, limited interpretations can be made from these results because the study did not contain a placebo group; the placebo effect of SWD on back pain has been demonstrated by Gibson et al., (1985) and Koes et al. (1992). They conclude that their studies demonstrate the placebo response which can be induced by health-care professionals showing renewed interest in the patients' condition or the benefits of a technical piece of equipment that is applied with conviction.

A similar problem is evident in the study by Santiesteban and Grant (1985) which found that patients undergoing elective foot surgery who received PSWD required significantly less analgesic medication and were also discharged from hospital an average of eight hours earlier than a control group. However, there was no sham group so the suggestion effect of the PSWD group can not be eliminated.

Very low dose PSWD (60 μs, 450 Hz, mean power = 1.5 mW/cm^2) that was applied for eight hours a day, for 6 weeks, improved the symptoms of patients with persistent neck pain significantly (Foley-Nolan, 1990). The placebo group did not demonstrate the same improvement. The PSWD was delivered from small portable units which were placed inside surgical collars. This was a well-designed trial and this type of unit may warrant further investigation.

In conclusion, the results of the clinical trials that have investigated the effect of PSWD on pain, when taken together, provide some support for the idea that PSWD may induce pain relief for various musculoskeletal pain conditions. However, they also highlight the flaws in the research and further clinical trails are warranted.

Nerve Regeneration

Wilson and Jagadeesh (1976) reported regeneration of axons in the spinal cord of cats treated with PSWD. They also found that PSWD accelerated recovery of nerve conduction in rats. However, no statistical or histological analysis was undertaken in either study. Raji and Bowden (1983) demonstrated a significant acceleration in the recovery of injured peripheral nerves of rats. These studies provide interesting data. However, more work needs to be undertaken before the clinical importance of these findings can be established.

Osteoarthritis

SWD and PSWD often form part of the physiotherapeutic management of patients with osteoarthritis (OA). However, the value of SWD and PSWD for alleviating the symptoms of OA has not yet been established. Vanharanta (1982) found that there was no difference in the radiographic changes between SWD-treated and control rabbits who had OA produced experimentally in their knees. Furthermore, the mobility of the SWD treated animals was poorer than the control animals. The author concluded that more work is required to determine the reason for this apparent negative effect of SWD.

There are also several studies of patients with OA.

Regrettably, there are many methodological problems which may explain the contradictory results.

In a study by Quirk et al. (1985), SWD in combination with exercise was found to significantly decrease the pain and disability experienced by patients with OA. Unfortunately, no details are given of how the SWD was applied. Similarly, patients suffering from OA of the hips and knees were studied by Svarcova et al. (1988). After 10 treatments of low-dose PSWD, the pain experienced by the patients had decreased significantly. A slightly different study by Jan and Lai (1991) involved treating patients with OA, with either SWD or US. Patients were allocated randomly to receive the treatments either with or without exercise. The functional ability of the patients who performed exercises improved significantly more than the patients who had SWD or US in isolation. No further analysis was undertaken.

Finally, a randomized control trial studied the effect of different dosages of PSWD on the symptoms of OA of the hips (Klabber Moffat, 1991). Pain, functional ability and range of movement were monitored over a 3-week treatment period with a 3-month follow-up. No significant difference was found between the three groups at any time, but these results are not supported by any substantial data.

Obviously, there is a need for further trials before the value of PSWD and SWD for alleviating the symptoms of OA is known.

Postoperative

A randomized double-blind trial by Barker et al. (1984) was used to determine if SWD could reduce postoperative illeus after abdominal surgery. Fifty patients were assigned randomly to either active (0.1 ms, 500 Hz, 250 W, mean power = 12 W) or to sham treatment. Treatment was given for one hour every twelve hours postoperatively. The treatment group had a significantly shorter time for the return of bowel sounds, but there was no significant difference in time to tolerate fluids or pass flatus. The benefit of PSWD for this group of patients was felt to be of little clinical importance. This study used a low mean power and it is possible that a higher dose may have produced a more definite effect, but further work would be required before this suggestion could be substantiated.

Conclusion

At the present time, the literature on SWD and PSWD is not sufficiently well-developed to allow unequivocal conclusions to be drawn. The methodologies reported do not allow the exclusion of several variables as possible explanations of the results presented. Many trials even fail to describe the application parameters in sufficient detail to enable comparison between trials or repetition. However, all need not be viewed with a totally negative eye as the literature to date does point the way for future studies.

Application of SWD

During the application of SWD the patient is connected to the electrical circuit of the high frequency generator by means of a capacitive applicator or an inductive coil.

The Capacitive Technique

There are two different types of electrodes for applying the capacitive method of SWD to the patient:

- Flexible metal plates (malleable electrodes) — flexible electrodes are flat metal sheets that are covered with a thick layer of rubber. They are often placed under or around the body part requiring treatment. A felt-like material is used to ensure that a sufficient spacing occurs between the electrode and the patient (Figure 11.8).
- Rigid metal discs — disc electrodes are flat, round, metal electrodes that are encased with a clear plastic cover (Figure 11.9). They are used far more commonly than the flexible electrodes.

The SWD machine has adjustable arms to position the electrodes close to the body part requiring treatment. The SWD field is generated between the two plates and the configuration of the electrodes influences the distribution of the SWD

Figure 11.8 Flexible electrodes: three different sizes are available. Felt spacers are used to ensure suficient electrode to skin distance.

Figure 11.9 Disc electrodes: three different sizes are available. The electrode to skin distance can be altered by sliding the plate inside the plastic case.

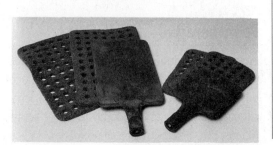

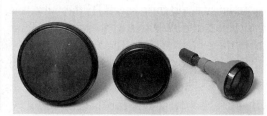

field within the tissues. It is therefore vitally important that the electrodes are positioned appropriately.

GUIDELINES FOR ELECTRODE SELECTION AND PLACEMENT

1 Electrodes should be of equal size. If electrodes of unequal size are used, stronger heating will occur close to the smaller electrode because the field will be concentrated over a small surface area. A very non-uniform electric field may be produced.

2 Electrodes should be slightly larger than the body part because the electric field is less uniform at the edge of the plates. A weak or nonuniform field is not recommended for treatment purposes. Most SWD equipment has a choice of three different sizes of electrode that can be used: small, medium and large.

3 Electrodes should be equidistant and at right angles to the skin surface. When the electrode is close to the skin intense superficial heating may occur. When the electrodes are placed further from the skin the distribution of the field will be more uniform. However, if the distance between the electrode and skin is too great the field strength will be severely reduced. Thus, a balance must be reached to prevent either excessive skin heating or insufficient energy absorption. A skin-to-electrode distance of between 2 and 4 cm is optimum. It is the distance from the metal plate and not the plastic cover that is important. If the electrodes are not parallel to the skin areas of intense heating will occur in the tissues closest to the electrodes and hot spots or burns could result.

Deviation from this ideal electrode configuration can lead to less efficient field distribution or areas of intense heating.

ELECTRODE ARRANGEMENT

There are three principal electrode arrangements used with the capacitive techniques:

1 Contraplanar application (transverse) – an electrode is placed on either side of the limb (Figure 11.10).

2 Coplanar application – both electrodes are placed on the same side of the limb. The field follows the route of least resistance, e.g. through the blood vessels which contain a high proportion of ions. If the electrodes are placed closer together than the distance between the electrodes and the skin, the field will pass directly between the electrodes and no tissue treatment will occur (Figure 11.11 a, b).

3 Longitudinal application – one electrode is placed at each end of the limb. The aim of this electrode placement is to allow the electric field to be oriented in the same direction as the tissues, thus providing good conditions for the current to flow through tissues of low resistance (van den Bouwhuijsen, 1985).

Figure 11.10 Contraplanar application. Note that the electrodes are of equal size, slightly larger than the part to be treated, and equidistant from and parallel to the skin surface.

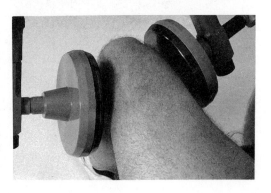

Inductive Application

SWD can also be achieved using the inductive technique. Based on the law of electromagnetic induction, a magnetic field is generated whenever an electric current flows in a material. The lines of force of the magnetic field radiate at right angles to the direction of the current. This process has a converse, termed *magnetic induction*, in that the magnetic field induces secondary currents – eddy currents – in the material. The inductive SWD method uses magnetic induction to produce small eddy currents in the tissues. The eddy currents can result in an increase in tissue temperature.

Inductive SWD can be administered using two different applicators. The most commonly used is an inductive (coil) applicator. Units available commercially include the Circuplode (Figure 11.12) and the Megaplode. The SWD cable is pre-coiled and encased in an insulated drum. The drum is placed close to the part requiring treatment so that the coil is parallel with the skin surface. An electric current is generated inside the machine and passed through the coil. The magnetic field associated with this current is set up at right angles to the direction of current flow, and it is therefore directed into the body part where eddy currents are established.

The second method involves wrapping an insulated cable around the limb to be treated. Again, an electric current is passed through the cable setting up a magnetic field. As before, eddy currents are generated within the tissue. Wooden or plastic clips are used to ensure that sufficient space is maintained between adjacent coils. The correct skin-to-coil distance is achieved by covering the limb with several layers of towelling. If the distance between the coils or the coils and skin is too small then areas of excessive heating may occur.

Conventional wisdom holds that the eddy currents produce the physiological effects. The role of the magnetic field is to act as a carrier medium into the tissues.

Dosage: Thermal Treatments

The parameters used to describe shortwave diathermy should include frequency, power, time of irradiation and method of application

Figure 11.11 Coplanar application (a) correct electrode arrangement, (b) electrodes placed too close together with the result that no tissue treatment will occur.

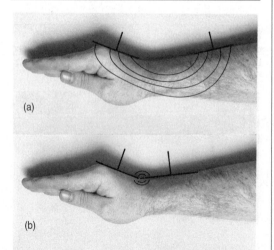

(a)

(b)

Figure 11.12 Circuplode. Inside the drum is a coiled electrode.

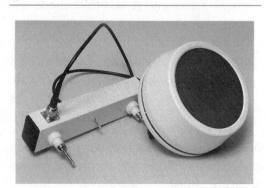

for continuous wave therapy; the type of field used should also be indicated. Peak power, average power, pulse strength, and rest period or number of pulses per second should be added for pulsed therapy.

THE USE OF THERMAL SENSATION FOR ASSESSING SWD DOSE

At present, the therapist or researcher must use their knowledge of the theoretical patterns of heat production and seek information from the patient to determine the qualitative amount of heat that is being produced. This aspect of applying SWD has been described as more of an art than a science (Ward, 1980).

A standard method of determining dose is to ask the patient to report thermal sensation. Low and Reed (1990) suggest five SWD dose levels based on patient perception ranging from an imperceptible heating dose at which the patient reports no sensation of heat, to a maximum tolerable heating dose at which the patient reports the heat to be as much as can be taken. It is, however, practically impossible in the clinical situation to accurately calculate the exact dosimetry of SWD in the different tissues of the body. Monitoring dose by thermal sensation provides an extremely inaccurate measure of dose. The sensitivity to temperature change is vastly superior in the skin when compared to that of deeper tissue. Patient statements of thermal sensation are, therefore, reports of temperature in skin and not deeper tissues. Odia and Aigbogun (1988) have reported that different areas of the body were more sensitive to changes in temperature than others. Subjects were more accurate in reporting increases in temperature of the facial skin than in the skin of the lower limb.

Elder (1989) reports animal work which showed that temperature-induced cell injury occurred at a threshold level (42°C) that was below the threshold of thermally induced pain (45°C). Thus, Delpizzo and Joyner (1987) point out that when the patient is asked to report thermal sensation there is a possibility of high levels of heat and cell damage occurring in areas with low numbers of thermal receptors. As stated above, this can refer to deeper tissue. Elder (ibid) extends this argument to state that cutaneous perception is not reliable in the prevention of potential damage from electromagnetic radiation. This is because electromagnetic radiation can reach tissues deeper than superficial skin structures where most thermal receptors are located.

Such arguments appear to limit the safe dose of SWD to those reported by a patient as *at most* 'a very mild sensation of warmth'. Even then, this dose level may be too high if the thermal sensory discrimination of the patient is less than optimum due to pathology or to anatomical site. This is relevant particularly where the energy absorbed in superficial tissue may be lower than that absorbed in deep tissue. Certainly, the use of doses above this level of 'mild sensation' would appear to have potentially hazardous effects.

Delpizzo and Joyner (1987) divide doses for SWD into three categories — high, medium and low:

- High — clear increase in heat;
- Medium — thermal effects are weak but still apparent;
- Low — thermal effects are not noticeable, although physiological effects have been reported at these doses.

These exposure levels are based on work on recommendations for microwave irradiation, but may also be useful for shortwave frequencies until clearer guidelines are made available.

Thus, at the present time, until more accurate methods of assessing dose are established, the therapist must be aware of the potential risk of causing tissue damage and ensure that the maximum dose that a patient receives causes only a mild sensation of warmth.

PSWD Dose

In theory, it is suggested that acute conditions should be treated with a low dose and more chronic conditions with a high dose (van der Esch and Hoogland, 1990). To give a patient a low dose of PSWD, the pulse repetition rate, the pulse duration and the peak pulse power should all be as low as possible. If the intention is to apply a high dose of PSWD, the above variables should be at their maximum (Table 11.5). However, the same mean power of PSWD can be delivered by using different combinations of the above variables (Table 11.6). Unfortunately, there is little data available to allow the importance of this to be determined. It is therefore essential that when PSWD treatments are recorded, sufficient information is given so that the treatment can be accurately repeated (Table 11.7).

Very few research trials investigating PSWD gave sufficient details of the treatment parameters, and comparing studies is very difficult when such important detail is absent. Also, it is impossible to evaluate if there is a trend where a variable, such as mean power, influences the results.

Table 11.5
Examples of low dose and high dose PSWD

	Low dose	High dose
Pulse repetition rate	26 Hz	200 Hz
Pulse duration	0.065 ms	0.4 ms
Peak pulse power	100 W	1000 W
Mean power	1.7 W	80 W

Table 11.6
An example of how the same mean power (PSWD) can be delivered by using different pulse parameters

	Low dose	High dose
Pulse repetition rate	82 Hz	20 Hz
Pulse duration	0.4 ms	0.4 ms
Peak pulse power	200 W	800 W
Mean power	6.6 W	6.4 W

Table 11.7
Information required when recording PSWD treatments

Pulse repetition rate
Pulse duration
Peak pulse power
Length of treatment
Mode of delivery
Electrode type, spacing and size

Treatment Procedures

The treatment procedure should ensure optimum safety for both patient and operator. The following procedure as outlined by the National Health and Medical Research Council of Australia in 1985 is suggested.

Prepare the patient:

The operator should examine the thermal and pain sensitivity of the patient for signs of impairment;

- The operator should exclude any contraindications;
- The operator should ensure that all metal objects (rings, jewellery, metal spectacles, etc.) are removed from the treatment area;

- Ensure that any hearing aid is removed;
- All bandages and clothing should be removed from the treatment area;
- Ensure that the skin is dry;
- Ask the patient to report immediately any sensation felt during treatment.

Prepare the machine:

- Ensure that cables are connected correctly;
- Ensure that cables or applicators are not rested on metal surfaces;
- Ensure appropriate alignment of the applicator for maximum energy transfer;
- Ensure that the gonads are not subject to irradiation;
- Ensure that the cables are not placed close to the patient's non-targeted tissue;
- Ensure that the patient support (e.g. chair or bed) is not metallic and that all metal objects are kept at least 3 m away from the applicator and cables.

Once the unit has been activated the operator should:

- Remain at least 1 m from the electrodes and 0.5 m from the cables;
- Ensure that the patient maintains the correct position throughout the duration of the treatment;
- Ensure that the patient is not left alone during treatment unless supplied with a reliable cut-off switch;
- Ensure that the patient does not touch the machine;
- Ensure that no other person is in the vicinity of the machine.

Contraindications

The following factors contraindicate the use of SWD:

- Implanted pacemakers (because the electromagnetic field may interfere if there is insufficient screening);
- Metal in the tissues or external fixators (because metal concentrates the magnetic field);
- Impaired thermal sensation (because burns and scalds may occur);
- Uncooperative patients (e.g. uncooperative physically due to movement disorders or uncooperative mentally due to disability or age);
- Pregnancy;
- Haemorrhaging areas (women who are menstruating should be warned that a temporary increase in bleeding may occur if the pelvis is irradiated);
- Ischaemic tissue;
- Malignant tumours (Burr (1974) in Kitchen and Partridge (1992) state that cancer cells proliferate in response to heating and the temperature in tumours tends to rise more than surrounding cells therefore not even a low dose of PSWD should be given);
- Active tuberculosis;
- Recent venous thrombosis;
- Patient pyrexia;
- Areas of skin affected by courses of x-ray.

The following should be treated with caution:

- A study by Doyle and Smart (1963) demonstrated that repeated exposure of the growing epiphysis of the femur of rats to SWD increased the rate of growth compared to the untreated legs. No histological abnormalities were identified.

Safety of Operator

An aspect of SWD which is often overlooked is the safety of the operator. Bearing in mind the presence of the electromagnetic field in the vicinity of the machine, the listed contraindications should apply to the machine operator as well as to the patient. Some studies suggest that this part of SWD should be taken more seriously. Hamburger *et al.* (1983, no.135 in Elder) investigated the association between non-ionizing radiation and heart disease. Using a questionnaire to survey 3004 male physiotherapists they showed a link between heart disease (notably ischaemic heart disease) and high exposure to SWD. This incidence of heart disease was smaller than in the general population compared for sex, age and race. This was supposed due to higher socioeconomic status and proposed better health in the physiotherapist population.

Kallen *et al.* (1983) carried out an epidemiological study of birth outcomes in physiotherapists in Sweden. They reported an above-normal incidence of death or malformations in babies born to those involved in operating SWD machines.

References

Abramson, DI, Bell, Y, Rejal, H *et al.* (1960) Changes in blood flow, oxygen uptake and tissue temperatures produced by therapeutic physical agents. II effect of short-wave diathermy. *American Journal of Physical Medicine* **39**: 87–95.

Abramson, DI, Chu, LSW, Tuck, S (1966) Effect of tissue temperatures and bloodflow on motor nerve conduction velocity. *Journal of the American Medical Association* **198**(10): 1082–1088.

Allberry, J, Manning, FRC, Smith, EE, (1974) Short-wave diathermy for herpes zoster. *Physiotherapy* **60**: 12, 386.

Aronofsky, DH (1971) Reduction of dental postsurgical symptoms using non thermal pulsed high-peak-power electromagnetic energy. *Oral Surgery* **32**(5): 688–696.

Balogun, JA, Okonofau, FE, (1988) Management of chronic pelvic inflammatory disease with shortwave diathermy. *Physical Therapy* **68**(10): 1541–1545.

Bansal, PS, Sobti, VK, Roy, KS (1990) Histomorphochemical effects of shortwave diathermy on healing of experimental muscular injury in dogs. *Indian Journal of Experimental Biology* **28**: 766–770.

Barclay, V, Collier, RJ, Jones, A (1983) Treatment of various hand injuries by pulsed electromagnetic energy (diapulse). *Physiotherapy* **69**(6): 186–188.

Barker, AT, Barlow, PS, Porter, J *et al.* (1985) A double blind clinical trial of low power pulsed shortwave therapy in the treatment of a soft tissue injury. *Physiotherapy* **71**(12): 500–504.

Barker, P, Allcut, D, McCollum, CN (1984) Pulsed electromagnetic

energy fails to prevent postoperative ileus. *Journal of the Royal College of Surgeons of Edinburgh* **29**(3): 147–150.

van den Bouwhuijsen, F, Maassen, V, Meijer, M *et al.* (1985) *Pulsed and Continuous Short-wave Therapy.* Enraf-Nonius, Delft.

Brown, M, Baker, RD (1987) Effect of pulsed short-wave diathermy on skeletal muscle injury in rabbits. *Physical Therapy* **67**(2): 208–214.

Burr, B (1974) Heat as a therapeutic modality against cancer. Report 16 US National Cancer Institute, Bethesda, Maryland.

Cameron, B (1961) Experimental acceleration of wound healing. *American Journal of Othopaedics* **3**: 336–343

Cameron, BM (1964) A three-phase evaluation of pulsed, high frequency, radio short waves (Diapulse) on 646 patients. *American Journal of Orthopaedics* **6**: 72–78.

Chapman, EC (1991) Can the use of physical modalities for pain control be rationalized by the research evidence? *Canadian Journal of Physiology and Pharmacology* **69**: 704–712.

Comorosan, S, Pana, L, Pop, L *et al.* (1991) The influence of pulsed high peek power electromagnetic energy (Diapulse) treatment on posttraumatic algoneurodystrophies. *Rev. Rheum. Physiol* **28**(3-4): 77-81.

Constable, JD, Scapicchio, AP, Opitz, B (1971) Studies of the effects of diapulse treatment on various aspects of wound healing in experimental animals. *Journal of Surgical Research* **11**: 254–257.

Delpizzo, V and Joyner, KH (1987) On the safe use of microwave and shortwave diathermy units. *Australian Journal of Physiotherapy* **33**(3): 152–162.

Doyle, JR, Smart, BW (1963) Stimulation of bone growth by shortwave diathermy. *Journal of Bone and Joint Surgery* **45**(AI): 15–23.

Elder, JA, Czerski, PA, Stuchly, MA *et al.* (1989) Radiofrequency radiation, in Suess, MJ, Benwell-Morison, DA (1989) *Nonionizing radiation protection*, 2nd edition. WHO Regional Publications, European Series, no 25, Ottawa.

Erdman, WJ (1960) Peripheral blood flow measures during application of pulsed high frequency currents. *American Journal of Orthopaedics* **2**: 196–197.

van der Esch, M, Hoogland, R (1990) *Pulsed Shortwave diathermy with the curapuls 419.* Delft Instruments Physical Medicine BV, Delft.

Fenn, JE (1969) Effect of electromagnetic energy (diapulse) on experimental haematomas. *Canadian Medical Association Journal* **100**: 251–253.

Foley-Nolan, D, Barry, C, Coughlan, RJ *et al.* (1990) Pulsed high frequency (27MHz) electromagnetic therapy for persistent neck pain. A double blind, placebo-controlled study of 20 patients. *Orthopedics* **13**(4): 445–451.

Forster, A, Palastanga, N (1985) *Clayton's Electrotherapy.* Bailliere-Tindall, London.

Gibson, T, Harkness, J, Blagrave, P *et al.* (1985) Controlled comparison of short wave diathermy treatment with osteopathic treatment in non-specific low back pain. *The Lancet* June 1, 1258–61.

Ginsberg, AJ (1961) Pulsed short wave in the treatment of bursitis with calsification. *International Record of Medicine* **174**(2): 2936, 71–75.

Goats, CG (1989a) Continuous short-wave (radio frequency) diathermy. *British Jouranl of Sports Medicine* **23**(2): 123–127.

Goats, CG, (1989b) Pulsed electromagnetic (short-wave) energy therapy. *British Journal of Sports Medicine* **23**(4): 213–216.

Goldin, JH, Broadbent, NRG, Nancarrow, JD et al. (1981) The effects of diapulse on the healing of wounds: a double blind randomised control trial in man. Brtitish Journal of Plastic Surgery 34: 267–270.

Grant, A, Sleep, J, McIntosh, et al. (1989) Ultrasound and electro-magnetic energy treatment for the perineal trauma. A randomised placebo control trial. British Journal of Obstetrics and Gynaecology 96: 434–439.

Gray, RJ, Quayle, AA, Hall, CA, Schofield, MA (1994) Physiotherapy in the treatment of temporal mandibular joint disorders: a comparative study of four treatment methods. The British Dental Journal (ASW) April 9, 176 (7: 257–261)

Guy, AW et al. (1984) Average SAR and distribution in man exposed to 450 Mhz radiofrequency radiation. IEEE transactions on microwave theory and techniques. MTT-32: 752–762.

Hamburger, S et al. (1983) Occupational exposure to non-ionising radiation and an association with heart disease. An exploratory study. Journal of Chronic Diseases 36: 791–802.

Hand, JW (1990) Biophysics and technology of electromagnetic hypothermia, in Gautherie, M [ed] (1990) Methods of External Hyperthermic Heating. Springer-Verlag, Berlin.

Hayne, CR (1984) Pulsed High frequency energy — its place in physiotherapy. Physiotherapy 70(12): 459–66.

Hollander, JL, Hovarth, SM (1949) The influence of physical therapy procedures on the intra-articular temperature of normal and arthritic subjects. American Journal of Medical Science 218: 543–548.

Hovind, H, Nielson, SL (1974) The effects of short-wave and microwave on blood flow in subcutaneous and muscle tissue in man. Proceedings of the 7th WCPT Montreal Canada 147–151.

Itoh, M, Montemayor, JS, Matsumoto, E et al. (1991) Accelerated wound healing of pressure ulcers by pulsed high peak power electromagnetic energy (Diapulse). Decubitus 4(1): 24–34.

Jan, MH, Lai, JS (1991) The effect of physiotherapy on osteoarthritic knees of females. Journal of the Formosan Medical Association. 90(10): 1008–1013.

Kallen, B et al. (1982) Delivery outcome among physiotherapists in Sweden: is non-ionising radiation a fetal hazard? Archives of Environmental Health 37: 81–85.

Kitchen, S, Partridge, C (1992) Review of shortwave diathermy. Continuous and pulsed patterns. Physiotherapy 78: 4, 243–252

Klabber Moffett, JA, Frost, H, Richardson, PH (1991) Controlled study to measure the effectiveness of pulsed short wave for pain relief in osteoarthritic hips. Proceedings of the World Confederation for Physiotherapy, 11th International Congress. Book 2: 760–762.

Kloth, LC, Ziskin, MC (1990) Diathermy and Pulsed Electromagnetic Fields, in Michlovitz, SL (1990) Thermal Agents in Rehabilitation, 2nd edition. FA Davis Company, Philadelphia.

Koes, BW, Bouter, LM, van Maneren, H et al. (1992) The effectiveness of manual therapy physiotherapy and treatment by the general practitioner for nonspecific back and neck complaints. Spine 17(1): 28–35.

Koes, BW, Bouter, LM, van Mameren, H et al. (1992) Randomised clinical trial of manipulative therapy and physiotherapy for persistent back and neck complaints: results of one year follow up. British Medical Journal 304: 601–605.

Krag, C, Taudorf, U, Siim, E, Bolund, S (1979) The effect of pulsed electromagnetic energy (Diapulse) on the survival of experimental skin flaps. A study on rats. Scandinavian Journal of Plast Reconstr Surg. 13: 377–380.

Lehmann, JF (1990) Therapeutic Heat and Cold, 4th edition. Williams and Wilkins, Baltimore.

Livesley, PJ, Mugglestone A, Whitton J (1992) Electrotherapy and the management of minimally displaced fracture of the neck of the humerus. Injury 23(5): 323–327.

Low, J, Reed, A (1990) Electrotherapy Explained, Principles and Practice. Butterworth-Heinemann, London.

McGill, SN (1988) The effects of pulsed shortwave therapy on lateral ligament ankle sprains. New Zealand Journal of Physiotherapy December 21–24.

McCray, RE, Patton, NJ (1984) Pain relief at trigger points; a comparison of moist heat and shortwave diathermy. The Journal of Orthopaedic and Sports Physical Therapy 5(4): 175–178.

Michlovitz, SL (1990) Thermal Agents in Rehabilitation, 2nd edition. FA Davis company, Philadelphia.

Morrissey, LJ (1966) Effect of pulsed short-wave diathermy upon volume blood flow through the calf of the leg. Journal of the American Physical Therapy Association 46(9): 946–952.

Odia, GI, Aigogun, OS (1988) Thermal sensation and the skin sensation test: regional differences and their effects on the issue of reliability of temperature ranges. The Australian Journal of Physiotherapy 34(2): 89–93.

O'Dowd, WJ (1989) Pulse mythology. Physiotherapy 75: 3, 97–8.

Oliver, DE (1984) Pulsed electro-magnetic energy - what is it? Physiotherapy 70(12): 458–459.

Oosterveld, FGJ, Rasker, JJ, Jacobs, JWG et al. (1992) The effects of local heat and cold therapy on the inraarticular and skin surface temperature of the knee. Arthritis and Rheumatism. 35(2): 146–151.

Paslia, M, Visuri, T, Sundholm, A (1978) Pulsating shortwave diathermy; Value in treatment of recent ankle and foot sprains. Archives of Physical Medicine and Rehabilitation 59: 383–386.

Quirk, AS, Newman, R, Newman, KJ (1985) An evaluation of interferential therapy, shortwave diathermy and exercise in the treatment of osteoarthritis of the knee. Physiotherapy 71(2): 55–57.

Raji, ARM, Bowden, REM (1983) Effects of high-peak pulsed electromagnetic field on the degeneration and regeneration of the common peroneal nerve in rats. The Journal of Bone and Joint Surgery 65B(4): 478–492.

Raji, AM (1984) An experimental study of the effects of pulsed electromegnetic field (Diapulse) on nerve repair. The Journal of Hand Surgery 9B(2): 105–112.

Reed, MWR, Bickerstaff, DR, Hayne, CR et al. (1987) Pain relief after iginal herniorrhaphy. Ineffectiveness of pulsed electromagentic energy. The British Journal of Clinical Practice 41(6): 782–784.

Santiesteban, AJ, Grant, C (1985) Post-surgical effect of pulsed short-wave therapy. Journal of the American Pediatric Association 75(6): 306–309.

Selsby, A (1985) Physiotherapy in the management of temporomandibular joint disorders. Australian Dental Journal 30(4): 273–80.

Silverman, DR, Pendleton, L (1968) A comparison of the effects of continuous and pulsed shortwave diathermy on circulation. Archives of Physical Medicine Rehabilitation 49: 429–436.

Svarcova, J, Trnavsky, K, Zvarova, J (1988) The influence of ultrasound, galvanic currents and shortwave diathermy on pain intensity in patients with osteoarthritis. *Scandinavian Journal of Rheumatology (suppl.)* **67**: 83–85.

Talaat, AM, El-Dibany, MM, El-Garf, A (1986) Physical therapy in the management of myofacial pain dysfunction syndrome. *Annals of Otology, Rhinology and Laryngology* **95**: 225–228.

Vanheranta, H (1982) Effect of short-wave diathermy on mobility and radiological stage of the knee in the development of experimental osteoarthritis. *American Journal of Physical Medicine* **61**(2): 59–65.

Verrier, M, Ashby, P, Crawford, JS (1978) Effects of thermotherapy on the electrical and mechanical properties of human skeletal muscle. *Physiotherapy Canada* **30**(3): 117–120.

Wagstaff, P, Wagstaff, S, Downey, M (1986) A pilot study to compare the efficacy of continuous and pulsed magnetic energy (shortwave diathermy) on the releif of low back pain. *Physiotherapy* **72**(11): 563–566.

Ward, AR (1980) *Electricity, Fields and Waves in Therapy.* Science Press, Marrickville.

Wells, PE, Frampton, V, Bowsher, D (1988) *Pain Management and Control in Physiotherapy.* Heinman Physiotherapy, London.

Wilson, DH, (1972) Treatment of soft-tissue injuries by pulsed electrical energy. *The British Medical Journal* **2**: 269–270.

Wilson, DH (1974) Comparison of shortwave diathermy and pulsed electromagnetic energy in treatment of soft tissue injuries. *Physiotherapy* **60**(10): 309–310.

Wilson, DH, Jagadessh, P (1976) Experimental regeneration in peripheral nerves and the spinal cord in laboratory animals exposed to a pulsed electromagnetic field. *Paraplegia* **14**: 12–20.

Wright, GG (1973) Treatment of soft tissue and ligamentous injuries in professional footballers. *Physiotherapy* **59**(12): 385–387.

Wyper, DJ, McNiven, DR (1976) Effects of some physiotherapeutic agents on skeletal muscle bloodflow. *Physiotherapy* **62**(3): 83–85.

12

Microwave Diathermy

JOAN McMEEKEN AND BARRY STILLMAN

Introduction

Magnetron valves, the basis for microwave production, were first described in 1921 (Licht, 1982). Later, development of the multicavity magnetron valve accelerated the use of microwave in radar installations during World War II. The potential therapeutic value of microwave was realized with its capacity to increase temperature and induce an increase in blood flow. Today's community is largely aware of microwave use in the preparation of food and in communication systems, but may not be aware of its medical uses. Hyperthermia in management of tumours is the predominant medical use of microwaves outside physiotherapy, whereas the principal physiotherapeutic application, as with all other physiotherapy heating modalities, is to promote soft tissue healing through increased blood flow, to facilitate mobilization and to relieve pain.

In order to address concerns regarding hazardous exposure to electromagnetic radiation, standards of exposure have been developed by international and national authorities, including the Canadian Department of Health and Welfare (1983), Australian National Health and Medical Research Council (1985) (reproduced in Delpizzo and Joiner, 1987), National Radiation Protection Board (1989) and Australian Standards Association (1992). In Australia, these standards 'promote the basis for uniformity in design, safety, performance, purchase and application of equipment in health-care facilities and institutions . . ..' Many of the Standards listed are used in the accreditation scheme operated by the Australian Council of Hospital Accreditation. These standards are embodied in 'Clinical standards for the use of electrophysical agents' (Electromedical Committee of the Australian Physiotherapy Association, 1990) and are encompassed in the remainder of this chapter.

Nature of Microwaves

Microwaves fall within a range of physiotherapeutic heating modalities that are broadly divisible into *surface* or *superficial* heating — where energy is first absorbed at the surface of the body (skin) — and *deep, volume* or *diathermy* heating (Gk. dia = through, therm = heat) where a significant proportion of the energy penetrates the surface before absorption in the deeper tissues. As the title of this chapter suggests, microwaves are a form of diathermy, although not as deep a form of heating as capacitive shortwave or ultrasonic heating. In addition, some nonthermal effects may occur.

From an energetics point of view, microwaves are a form of *electromagnetic radiations* and are therefore part of the electromagnetic spectrum (Table 1.20, Chapter 1). Microwaves are positioned between the radiations generated during short-wave diathermy and the radiations from infrared lamps. The microwave spectrum ranges from 1 m (300 MHz) to 1 mm (300 GHz). The operating specification for apparatus in Australia, the United Kingdom and Europe is 122.5 mm (2450 MHz), whilst in North America physiotherapeutic microwaves at 327 mm (915 MHz) and 690 mm (433.9 MHz) may also be available. Physiotherapeutic microwave devices are relatively expensive compared to simple heating apparatus such as hot packs and infrared lamps, but are a convenient source of volume heating. In contrast to most shortwave applications, the single microwave director and few operating controls provides simplicity of operation.

Microwave Production

The apparatus used to produce microwaves (Figure 12.1) has three main components:

1 A multicavity magnetron valve;
2 A coaxial cable to transmit the high frequency energy to an antenna; and
3 A director for transmitting the energy (through air) to the patient.

Direct current is shunted to the cathode in the magnetron valve, and electrons are released from the cathode towards the multicavity anode block of the magnetron. The electrons oscillate within the cavities at the predetermined frequency, thereby generating the high frequency current which is transmitted along a coaxial cable comprising a copper core surrounded by a braided copper shield. The magnetic fields generated by the currents in the copper core and braid cancel

Figure 12.1 Control panel of microwave (above) and general outline of key microwave components (below).

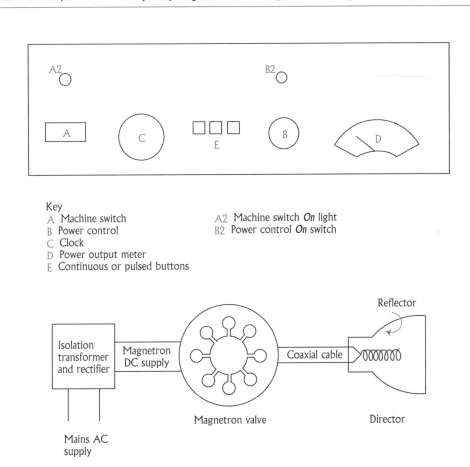

Key
A Machine switch
B Power control
C Clock
D Power output meter
E Continuous or pulsed buttons

A2 Machine switch *On* light
B2 Power control *On* switch

one another so there is no field around a coaxial cable.

The coaxial cable transmits the energy to a director where a radiating system comprising an antenna within a reflector is used to direct the microwaves to the patient. The high frequency alternating current in the antenna produces electromagnetic waves. By placing the antenna within a director with a suitably curved reflecting surface, divergence of the microwave radiations can be controlled in their transmission to the patient.

Different shaped reflectors produce different beam profiles. Several different shapes and sizes of directors are available for use:

1 A circular director with a parabolic reflecting surface reduces the divergence of the microwave beam to 100–200 mm in order to localize energy to the part [Ward, 1986; Delpizzo and Joiner, 1987]. The circular microwave director produces a doughnut-shaped pattern of heat distribution, with minimum heating occurring in the central area. This director is preferred for treating an area with a bony prominence or a superficial joint, because the central part of the director can be positioned over the area requiring less heating;

2 Rectangular directors, which may vary considerably in size, have an oval-shaped heat

distribution with greatest intensity in the centre;

3 Direct-contact applicators with in-built power limitations are also available in some countries. These were designed for the treatment of small areas such as the temporomandibular joint. The safety and effectiveness of such small ceramic contact applicators has been questioned (Scowcroft et al., 1977; Forster and Palastanga, 1985);

4 Air-cooled applicators operating at 915 MHz are used in contact with the skin and are considered to be more efficient at deep tissue heating. This may be at the expense of an enhanced risk of burning as skin temperature receptors are deliberately cooled by the circulating air;

5 Small power-delimited electrodes, usually rectangular-shaped, have been designed for use in treatment of sinusitis, however, as will be elaborated below, use of microwaves in the treatment of sinusitis is strongly condemned.

Radiant energy, including that from microwave apparatus, is characterized by its capacity to travel through a vacuum. In practical terms this means that microwave can be directed at the part to be treated without need for direct contact between the equipment and the subject, thus contributing to the practical simplicity of the apparatus.

Physical Behaviour

On reaching the surface of the body or any other material, radiant energy may be *absorbed* – i.e. the energy is taken up by the material it encounters, *transmitted* – i.e. pass through the material without being absorbed, *refracted* – i.e. altered in its direction of propagation (either leading to scattering or convergence) as it passes through the surface, or *reflected* – i.e. turned back from the surface.

The propagation characteristics of microwaves are first determined by the wavelength and frequency of the energy. Whilst the penetration of microwave energy (that is the proportion of energy transmitted relative to the proportion absorbed) is inversely proportional to microwave wavelength, this is not a simple (linear) relationship (see depth efficiency and Figure 12.3), and a number of other factors also contribute to the final pattern of absorption and effects of the energy. The most important of these is the composition, determining the electrical properties of the tissue to be heated.

Tissue Composition and Microwave Absorption

Heat in solids is produced by the vibrational movement of atoms and molecules about their equilibrium position. Adding energy usually increases motion and the solid becomes hotter. In liquids, atoms and molecules move more quickly, more randomly and over greater distances because of the added energy. The constituent atoms and molecules of gases move more rapidly with added energy. Heat therefore has the capacity to increase volume and pressure, to change the physical state of a substance and to increase its temperature.

Microwave energy has a tendency to penetrate tissues with low electrical conductivity and be absorbed in tissues with high conductivity. In essence, high electrical conductivity equates with high fluid content; typically blood vessels, muscle, moist skin, internal organs and eyes. In such tissues the water molecules are referred to as *dipoles* since each molecule of water has a different electrical charge at each end — positive at one, negative at the other (Figure 12.2). Muscle tissue contains more dipole molecules than does fatty tissue leading to a greater rise in muscle temperature when microwave diathermy is used (McMeeken and Bell, 1990a). When subjected to the microwave energy, the dipoles are caused to rotate, first one way, then the other, in concert

with the frequency of the microwaves. Under the influence of the high frequency oscillating field, charged ions which are also present in these tissues, will move to and fro. The resultant frictional energy is the cause of the heat which is thus generated. Indeed all generation of heat in the tissues, no matter what the source, is ultimately due to frictional release of thermal energy — the greater the movement, the greater the heating. This explains the propensity for microwave to selectively heat moist over dry tissues.

In tissues with low fluid content such as fat, the effect of microwave energy is to distort the electron shells of the molecules into an oval shape with resulting accumulation of negative and positive charge at each end of the molecule (Figure 12.2). This effect, termed *molecular distortion*, leads to some heating in these relatively avascular tissues, but not of the magnitude associated with dipole rotation. Little energy is absorbed in ceramics, plastic and wood which contain nonpolar molecules, and therefore such materials do not become hot in a microwave beam.

Reflection of energy at the junction of tissues with relatively large differences in dielectric properties also influences the distribution of microwave absorption, and hence that of the heating. There are three particular interfaces of this type: skin and air, muscle and overlying fat, and bone and any of the adjacent soft tissues. Each of these surfaces behaves like a mirror, causing a proportion of the microwaves to reflect back into the overlying tissues. The proportion of energy which is reflected is determined by the magnitude of the difference in dielectric properties of the two surfaces, and by the angle of the incident microwave radiations (Figure 12.4).

The skin—air interface is the first and most significant interface limiting the deep heating

Figure 12.2 The effect of the alternating microwave beam on tissue molecules.

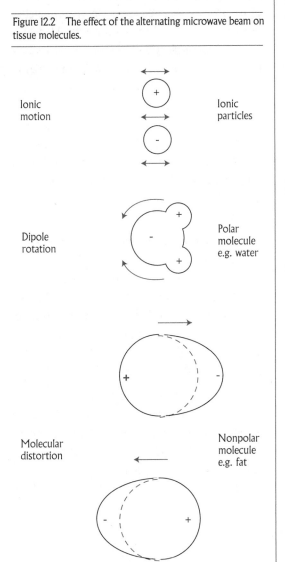

Ionic motion

Ionic particles

Dipole rotation

Polar molecule e.g. water

Molecular distortion

Nonpolar molecule e.g. fat

capacity of microwaves (Schwan and Piersol, 1954, 1955). The 122.5 mm (2450 MHz) microwaves heat the skin at least to the extent of the deeper tissues, thus ensuring patient safety (Low and Reed, 1990). Consequently, some efforts have been made to minimize the reflection-based surface heating by using direct-contact and air-cooled directors. All such methods of minimizing skin heating, whilst facilitating deep heating, at the same time increase the danger of burns. They diminish skin heating and thereby remove or minimize the basis for dosage — the patient's perception of warmth on the skin. Although incongruous, it is the relative inefficiency of heating apparatus, that is the skin heating effects, that constitutes the foremost protection of patients against burns by deep and superficial heating apparatus.

A further consequence of reflection of microwaves at tissue interfaces is that fat immediately overlying muscle may be increased in temperature to a greater extent than would be expected on the basis of fat's primary absorption characteristics. Lehmann et al. (1962) found that a subcutaneous fat layer thicker than 20 mm may be heated even more than muscle.

Significant reflection also occurs in relation to bone. Whilst in theory microwaves are capable of passing through solid bone, in practice the energy is largely prevented from entering bone due to reflection at its surface. Such an effect might prove beneficial when applying microwaves around some joints such as the knee, where reflection of energy into and absorption by the periarticular tissues occurs. By contrast, microwaves delivered over the cheek bone or forehead, ostensibly for the purpose of treating sinusitis, is reflected back from the bone with negligible penetration through to the intraosseous maxillary and frontal sinuses. Leaving aside questions of safety, microwave treatment of sinusitis is at best ineffective.

Relation Between Wavelength and Microwave Absorption

The penetration of microwaves is proportional to the wavelength of the radiations and hence inversely proportional to frequency. As the wavelength of electromagnetic radiation increases, penetration increases and absorption occurs in deeper tissues. Two wavelengths have been made available for physiotherapeutic use, 122.5 mm (2450 MHz) and 327 mm (915 MHz). The former produces more superficial heating because of diminished penetration. It is a paradox that microwave radiation at 690 mm (433.9 MHz), which has the greatest penetration and the least reflection at tissue interfaces (see below) is not available for unrestricted physiotherapeutic use in a number of countries.

The ratio of heat developed in muscle to the total heating of fat and muscle, *penetration depth*, is a convenient means of measuring the capacity of apparatus for deep heating. Perfect deep heating exists when the depth efficiency equals 1.0 (Ward, 1986). Representative examples are shown in Figure 12.3 which also reveals that there is an interactive effect with fat thickness.

The *specific absorption rate* describes the rate of absorption per unit mass of tissues. Its calculation requires the assumption of a number of unmeasurable variables and is not practical for clinical purposes (Delpizzo and Joiner, 1987).

Figure 12.3 The relationship of efficiency of penetration (where maximum = 1) for microwaves at 2450 and 450 MHz at three different thicknesses of superficial fat.

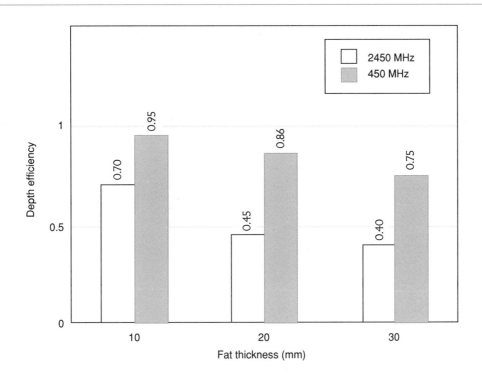

Laws of Microwave Radiations

The optical laws of microwaves have been listed earlier in this chapter. Here it should be stressed that it is only the microwave radiations which are absorbed that can be considered to have any potential for therapeutic effect. Transmitted, refracted and reflected microwaves have no effect other than to change where the energy is eventually absorbed. One important example concerns what are termed *standing waves*. When microwaves are reflected at an interface such as the surface of bone, a proportion of the energy may be reflected back from the surface and coincide, and be superimposed on the incident rays. This will lead to amplification of energy in some areas and reduction in some others.

With a perfect plane reflecting surface and a point source of energy, electromagnetic radiations, including microwaves, obey the cosine law (Figure 12.4):

The intensity of radiation falling on unit surface area of the body is proportional to the cosine of the angle of incidence; i.e. the angle formed between the incident ray and the perpendicular to the surface at the point of incidence. This is expressed by the formula: $I = I_o \cos \varnothing$ where $I =$ intensity, $I_o =$ original intensity and $\varnothing =$ The angle of incidence.

In practice, the director is always placed at a short fixed distance from the part, and hence the tendency to tilt the director is relatively small; none the less care should be taken to position the director so that the energy beam is perpendicular to the surface.

Curved surfaces within the body, notably curved metallic implants (see Hazards of Microwave), may

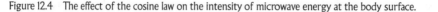

Figure 12.4   The effect of the cosine law on the intensity of microwave energy at the body surface.

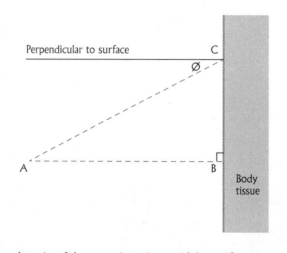

Perpendicular to surface

C

Ø

A   B

Body
tissue

Intensity of the energy is maximum with beam AB
Intensity of beam AC = cos Ø x maximum

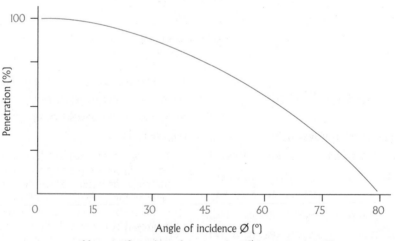

100

Penetration (%)

0   15   30   45   60   75   80

Angle of incidence Ø (°)

Note significant loss of energy when Ø is greater than 15°

serve to converge (concave surfaces) or diverge (convex surfaces) microwave energy in surrounding tissues. In addition to reflection, Ho (1976) has suggested that the curved skin surface may refract the microwave beam to produce convergence leading to increased efficiency for heating deeper tissues including muscle (Figure 12.5).

A further optical law influencing the intensity of microwaves is the inverse square law of distance (Figure 12.6):

The intensity of radiation falling on unit surface area of the body is inversely proportional to the square of the distance of the source of energy from the surface, provided the source of energy is a point source (*Figure 12.6*). This is expressed

Figure 12.5   Refraction of the microwave beam at a curved skin surface producing convergence of the beam.

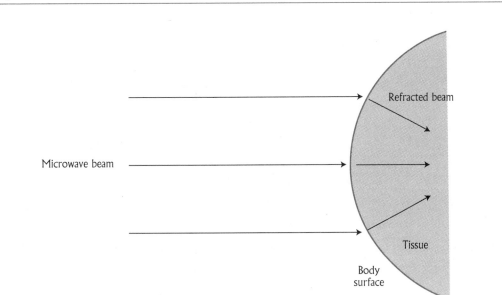

Refracted beam

Microwave beam

Tissue

Body
surface

by the formula: $I = 1/d^2$, where I = intensity and d = distance.

As previously indicated, the microwave director is placed close to the part and the intensity is varied by adjusting the variable power control. Because of the squaring of distance in the formula, small changes in the patient's position with correspondingly small changes in the distance between the director and the part will result in a marked increase or decrease in power; accordingly, appropriate precautions should be taken. Also, when using powerful microwave apparatus where a small advance of the power control leads to a marked change in intensity of heating, there should be no hesitation in applying the inverse square law by increasing the distance between the director and the part, thereby effectively reducing the sensitivity of the power control.

Physiological Influences on the Effects of Microwave

Having outlined a number of the properties of microwave radiations and related issues concerned with the composition of the tissues, it remains to consider the significance of delivering microwaves into living tissue. Chapter 6 and 7 consider the principles both to underlying thermal and non thermal effects of electrophysical agents.

Regardless of the many different types of equipment used to produce a variety of forms of thermogenic energy, once the energy is absorbed it is immaterial as to how the heat was delivered. There are no *different* heats, only different means of generating the same heat. The different effects of heating are the consequence of such factors as:

1 The volume of tissue absorbing the energy;
2 The composition of the absorbing tissue;

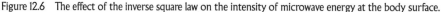

Figure 12.6   The effect of the inverse square law on the intensity of microwave energy at the body surface.

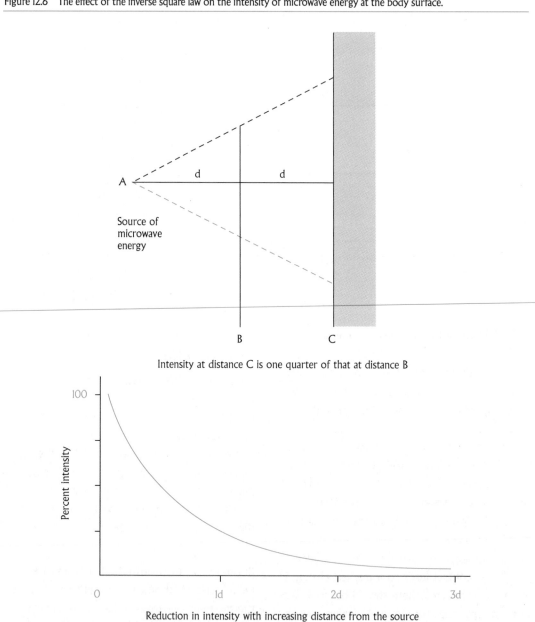

3 The capacity of the tissue to dissipate heat —
   largely a factor of blood supply;

4 The temperature to which the tissue is raised;
   and

5 The rate of rise of temperature.

The first two points have been discussed earlier.

Microwave irradiation has been shown to significantly increase skin and muscle temperature and
blood flow in dogs (Kemp *et al.*, 1948; Siems *et al.*,
1948; Richardson *et al.*, 1950; McMeeken and Bell,

1990a), pigs (Sekins *et al.*, 1980) and man (de Lateur *et al.*, 1970; Sekins *et al.*, 1984: McMeeken and Bell, 1990b).

As the temperature of the tissue increases, the blood flow also increases and heat may be relatively rapidly and efficiently dissipated through a volume of tissue, and into other tissues as a result of conduction and convection by the circulating blood. In well-vascularized tissue such as muscle, this serves to regulate the rate of rise of temperature as well as the peak temperature, thereby protecting the tissue against overheating whilst achieving the beneficial effects from enhanced blood flow such as more rapid tissue healing.

In poorly vascularized tissues such as fat, inadequate blood supply with accompanying poor heat dissipation properties can lead to an undefended rapid rise in tissue temperature, with resulting risk of burns.

The relationship between temperature and metabolic activity is expressed by van't Hoff's law which may be expressed as for every 10°C increase in tissue temperature there is a *two-to three*-fold increase in metabolic activity. At temperatures above 45°C enzyme proteins begin to denature. At non-destructive levels, increased temperature can enhance the rate of tissue healing and infection control by increasing the metabolic activity of the phagocytic and reparative cells.

In a study investigating the effects of microwave irradiation to the forearm in 21 normal subjects, forearm temperature increased from 30.3 ± 0.2°C (average ± standard deviation) to 40.3 ± 0.5°C, and blood flow increased from 6.0 ± 0.6 to 44.9 ± 9.8 ml/100 g/min. The maximum blood flow increase to the forearm was achieved in a mean time of 15 min and hyperaemia was sustained for at least 20 min after the microwave irradiation ceased. The sustained increase in flow

appears to be due to an increase in metabolic rate in the irradiated tissues (McMeeken and Bell, 1990b).

Increased circulation from resting levels of about 3 ml/100 g/min up to about 50 ml/100 g/min could lead to several beneficial effects. These include improved nutrition to the area, enhanced removal of byproducts of injury such as prostaglandins, bradykinin and histamine which are implicated in receptor and afferent fibre sensitization, increased removal of waste products such as lactic acid, and increased destruction of foreign matter by increasing phagocytosis.

In joints covered by a thin layer of soft tissue, such as the elbow, joint structures, particularly synovium, may be selectively heated by microwave. Vigorous heating of a synovial joint should only be undertaken in the chronic stages of disease in order to improve joint range of movement by decreasing stiffness and improving extensibility of contracted soft tissues.

In the subacute stage of arthritis in superficial joints, microwave may be beneficial by improving circulation and assisting the resolution of oedema and haemorrhage. Mild heating may be used in recurring inflammatory conditions to improve blood flow, and to facilitate diffusion of oxygen and the clearance of metabolites.

The viscosity of liquids is proportional to temperature. At 44°C absolute blood viscosity is reduced by about 15%. It has been argued that reduced viscosity in tissue fluids could facilitate mobilization of joints and surrounding musculoligamentous structures, and might serve to enhance decongestion under circumstances such as infection and oedema.

Lehmann *et al.* (1983) studied the effect of 327 mm (915 MHz) microwaves on the dispersal of a haematoma created by the injection of radiolabelled blood into the thigh of six pigs. The treated side showed more rapid resolution of the haematoma and it was suggested that microwave diathermy would assist in the management of haematomata in muscle injuries. Using the same frequency, Fadilah *et al.* (1987) have shown selective heating of synovium in rabbit joints allegedly supporting the practice of using microwave for treating superficial joints.

Heat has secondary pain relieving effects when vasodilation accelerates the removal of pain-inducing metabolites or inflammatory products, and when heat reduces congestion and associated tissue tension.

Thermoreceptors and nociceptors respond to temperatures changes, hence it may be argued that microwave radiation is indicated for the relief of pain. This is distinct from any relief of pain from indirect mechanisms such as the aforementioned benefits of vasodilation and decongestion. Warmth receptors are most active in the range of 30–40°C and exhibit sustained activity at maintained skin temperatures of 30–50°C (Kenshalo, 1976). Because of the depth of heating achieved with microwave irradiation, thermal receptors located in muscle tissue could also be stimulated (Hertel *et al.*, 1976).

An increase in afferent activity from the cat muscle spindle and Golgi tendon organ has been produced by direct warming and may act in conjunction with increased activity in thermoreceptor afferents as a segmental control of pain (Mense, 1978).

Polymodal mechanothermonociceptors respond to heat with thresholds between 40 and 60°C with maximum response from 45–53°C (Yaksh and Hammond, 1982). Kanui (1985) has shown experimentally that stimulating heat receptors inhibits nociceptive impulses in rats. Thus, pain relief might be obtained directly by depressing the activity of nociceptors.

Following the pioneering work of Melzack and Wall (1965) and what was originally termed the *gate control theory of pain* (see Chapter 4), the broad principle holds true today that an interaction of relatively large (proprioception and temperature) with small (pain) afferents at multiple sites throughout the central nervous system, including the dorsal horn in the spinal cord and the brainstem reticular formation, can serve to attenuate the perception of pain. Clinical experience supports this theory; for example, heat was shown to be the preferred non-analgesic method of pain control used by 68% of cancer outpatients studied by Barbour *et al.* (1986).

Muscle guarding and pain, which occur as a result of injury to tendons and joint structures, degenerative joint disease, bursitis, sacroiliac strains and ankylosing spondylitis, may be relieved by diathermy applications to the muscles in spasm. Lehmann and de Lateur (1990) suggested this may be due to heating the secondary afferent spindle endings and the Golgi tendon organs of the affected muscles.

Heat aids local and whole body relaxation by mechanisms as yet unknown. Figure 12.7 shows the application of microwave to the upper fibres of trapezius to reduce muscle spasm using a rectangular director. This relaxation is used as a prelude to passive manipulation and active or passive exercise.

Nonthermal biological reactions may be isolated using the pulsed mode of microwave at levels where the patient does not feel warmth. Whether heat is detectable or not in pulsed mode will depend on the amount of energy absorbed. Energy absorption is dependent on the factors previously mentioned, the frequency and duration of pulses and the total power. Useful ather-

Figure 12.7   The application of microwave to the upper fibres of trapezius to reduce muscle spasm using a rectangular director.

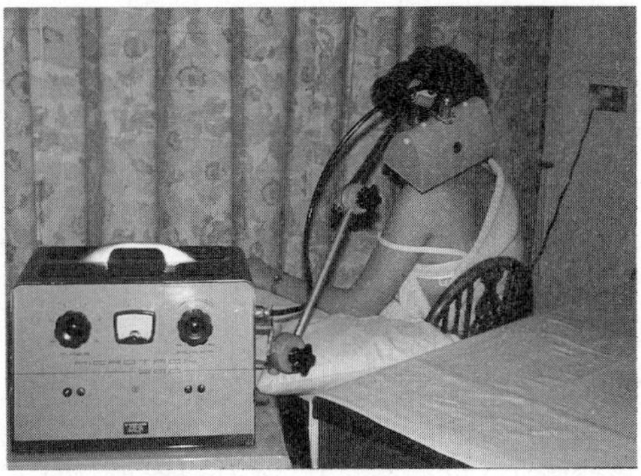

mal effects remain ill-defined. Moreover it has not been established whether a low continuous dose has the same effects as the same average dose derived from pulsed microwave.

Whilst there is some evidence of non thermal microwave effects, including the *pearl chain effect* (the alignment of molecules in the tissues) and neural excitability changes unrelated to the magnitude of heating, there is no evidence at present that these are of any physiotherapeutic relevance (Lehmann and de Lateur, 1990). Accordingly, the assumption followed below is that the consequences of microwave absorption are ultimately either a therapeutic or harmful thermal effect.

Few clinical trials have been described using microwave irradiation and those published do not describe the effects from readily available apparatus.

Weinberger *et al.* (1989) using 237 mm (915 MHz) microwave increased the intraarticular temperature to 41.3°C in patients with rheumatoid arthritis. They demonstrated reduced joint pain and increased walking time. It was further suggested by the authors that heat may have potentiated the effects of the concurrent anti-inflammatory agents.

Increased extensibility of collagenous tissue has been shown to occur with heating (Lehmann *et al.*, 1970). Joint stiffness has been found to be reduced by heating (Wright and Johns, 1961). Using direct-contact 915 MHz microwave in conjunction with stretching activities, de Lateur *et al.* (1978) demonstrated lengthening of shortened quadriceps muscle. Tissue lengthening requires stretching simultaneously or immediately following heat application whilst the relevant tissues remain pliable. Temperatures near the therapeutic limit are most effective. Stretching may be done manually or with automated mechanical devices, such as a continuous passive motion machine or functional electrical muscle stimulation devices.

Principles Underlying Application in Clinical Practice

The operating procedure of a microwave machine has been previously described and details of the control panel are provided in Figure 12.1.

Assessment of the Patient

Having assessed the patient and determined that microwave irradiation is an appropriate component of the treatment, check that all dangers and contraindications have been considered.

Treatment Preparation

Electromagnetic radiations may interact with metal objects that can act as aerials. Therefore metal plinths, chairs or tables should not be used during the application of microwave treatments. Electrical interference with other electronic equipment such as computers may also occur. Such objects should be at least 3 m away.

Patient Preparation

1 Explain the purpose of the treatment and that the treatment should never feel hot;
2 Perform a test for skin pain and temperature sensation;
3 Position the patient appropriately so that movement will not occur due to discomfort;
4 The microwave director should be positioned using as a guide the distance recommended by the manufacturer for optimum effect. If a guide is not provided commence with the director positioned a minimum of 2 cm from the part and parallel to it. If there are bony prominences separate the director 6 cm from the part. Consideration should be given to the inverse square and cosine laws;
5 Instruct the patient not to move after the unit is positioned for treatment as changes in the position may increase or decrease the amount of heat received by altering the distance or direction of the rays;
6 Increase the intensity of the current slowly, in stages, to allow the patient adequate time to become used to the sensory effects;
7 Provide the patient with the safety lead or warning device;

8 Warning the patient of the danger of overheating is mandatory;
9 No more than a minimal, mild or comfortable warmth should be experienced in the part being treated. Monitor the patient's reports of heat sensation at the inital phase of treatment and again during the treatment. When the output of the diathermy unit is adjusted, there is a delay between the time the output is changed and the time the patient becomes aware of a change in the sensation of heat. Therefore, the patient must be given sufficient time to perceive this change before further adjustments are made;
10 Set the treatment timer to the desired time;
11 Adjust the power control;
12 The physiotherapist should check with the patient regularly to ensure that all is well.

Dosage

Dosage is based on the severity, type and progress of the disorder. It is also dependent on the patient having a normal skin pain and temperature sensation. As the patient's thermal sensation is the most important indicator of dosage, this must be tested in the area to be treated before commencing treatment for the first time. The patient's ability to discriminate between warm and cool objects should be determined, and if the patient's skin temperature sensation is not normal, microwave should not be used. Under these circumstances superficial heating may be the only safe choice of electrotherapy.

When microwave treatment is indicated, subacute disorders are usually treated with a sensation of just perceptible or mild warmth for 5–15 min. Chronic disorders are usually treated with a sensation of comfortable warmth, for 10–20 min. The duration and frequency of treatment depend on the treatment goals; for example, decreased pain or increased tissue extensibility, and the status of the condition treated (subacute or chronic). However there is likely to be a treatment time below which no useful effect can be expected (5 min) and beyond which the likelihood of significant beneficial effects is slight (30 min). In this context it is wise to remember that benefits of a more prolonged heat treatment may easily be completely negated by the unwanted effects from prolonged complete immobility of, particularly, arthritic joints. Three to 8 min are required for the tissue temperature to rise to desired levels. When the temperature reaches the plateau caused by increased blood flow in 10 to 20 min, additional time addition yield no substantive gains. In contrast to the recommendation by Lehmann and de Lateur (1990) that pain may be used as a guide to indicate that the tissue temperature has reached the required level for therapeutic benefit, we suggest that temperature should not exceed a comfortable warmth.

When stretching is a major aim of treatment, positioning during the microwave treatment which elongates the tissues to be stretched, and exercising the part while the temperature is still elevated will enhance the results of the stretching techniques.

Hazards of Microwave

All electrotherapy equipment should be handled with care, and be regularly maintained and serviced. Frayed leads and improperly functioning safety leads are amongst the deficiencies that should not be tolerated. As soon as such problems are detected, the apparatus should be removed from use, appropriately labelled as faulty, and the faults repaired. Microwave units should also be tested regularly by the therapist placing a hand under the transducer and turning the intensity up to comfortable warmth and checking the power settings on the main panel. The presence and distribution of the microwave field can be tested by using an appropriate fluorescent tube. Special microwave detectors containing a fluorescent tube may also be purchased to assist in detecting reflected energy.

Contraindications

Contraindications to microwave heating are poor circulation, decreased thermal sensation, metal within 30 cm of the treatment area, moist wounds or dressings, the eyes or testis, acute inflammation, acute infection or sites of fluid under tension, recent haemorrhage, cardiac pacemakers, and if the patient has a malignancy or is pregnant.

The treating physiotherapist should not remain in the direct line of the beam or within 2 m of the director. Reflection may be from 50–75% from the patient and nearly 100% from the metal of the machine.

Hazards

The potential hazards of the use of microwaves in physiotherapy are:

1 BURNS

As with any heating devices burns are a potential risk. Burns may be due to:

a Poor technique, including overdosage and lack of communication between therapist and patient;
b Inability to dissipate heat such as poor circulation due to peripheral vascular disease or areas of poor vascularity such as the testes;

c Inability to detect heat, or decreased thermal sensation as may occur with peripheral vascular disease or neurological disturbances;

d Treatment over areas with surface or implanted metal. As may be observed in microwave ovens, metals will reflect microwaves. Within the body, the reflected radiations may overheat the adjacent tissues. Small pieces of metal may be the greatest hazard and particular care should be taken with bra clips, surgical staples, implanted stimulators and intrauterine devices. Outside the body, the radiations may reflect back to the director or to other people and objects in the environment;

e Treatment of moist open wounds, or over wet dressings as water concentrates energy. If perspiration accumulates the treatment should be interrupted and the skin dried;

f Treatment of the area near the eyes where microwave radiation could be beamed into the eyes either directly or by reflection. Due to the shape of the orbit and refraction of the microwave beam, microwaves may be focused within the eyes and damage the lens. (Lehmann and de Lateur, 1990) Precautions must be taken to ensure the eyes are not exposed. Metal goggles should not be used for eye protection as the metal of the goggles has the potential to burn adjacent skin. Due to the proximity to the eyes, it is an unacceptable risk to treat the sinuses or the temporomandibular joint with microwaves.

Areas of the body that contain a high fluid volume, such as the eye, a joint effusion, moist wound dressings or moist clothing or accumulations of excessive perspiration will focus field lines, because of the higher dielectric constant and conductivity of such body fluids compared to surrounding tissues. The same focusing effect applies to blood vessels that run through adipose tissue. The potential for overheating of the fluids particularly at the fluid–tissue interface may result in thermal necrosis of adjacent tissues.

2 EXACERBATION OF SYMPTOMS WHICH MAY BE DUE TO TREATMENT OF:

a Inflammatory conditions such as acute arthritis, tendonitis, acute nerve compressions and neuritis. An effusion in a synovial joint may pose a hazard if the temperature of the fluid is raised a few degrees. Harris and McCroskery (1974) demonstrated in vitro that an increase of 5°C produced a four-fold increase in enzymatic lysis of human cartilage by rheumatoid synovial collagenase. Feibel and Fast (1976) indicate that above-normal temperature in knees with rheumatoid arthritis may accelerate destruction of cartilage. Physiotherapists should be cautious when considering the suitability and dosage of heat for patients with an inflamed joint condition;

b Infective disorders such as tuberculosis, osteomyelitis, infective arthritis;

c Areas of increased fluid tension such as bursitis, oedema, synovial effusion;

d Haemorrhagic conditions due to acute trauma, varicose veins and ulcers and diseases such as haemophilia. Menstruation is unlikely to be affected by microwave radiation due to the limitations of penetration;

e Severe cardiac disease.

3 ELECTRIC SHOCK OR INTERFERENCE WITH CARDIAC PACEMAKERS MAY LEAD TO CARDIAC FAILURE.

4 SPREAD OF EXISTING PATHOLOGIES BY TREATMENT OF BENIGN OR MALIGNANT TUMOURS, ACTIVE TUBERCULOSIS OR ACUTE INFECTIONS.

5 HEAT HAS BEEN SHOWN TO BE
TERATOGENIC IN EARLY PREGNANCY.

Conclusion

In summary, the use of therapeutic microwave requires close attention to safety matters. Once these are addressed microwave devices provide a simple method for heating superficial muscles and joints.

References

Australian National Health and Medical Research Council (1985) *Code of Practice for the Safe Use of Microwave Diathermy Units.* Canberra.

Australian Standards Association (1992) *Australian Standard AS 3200.2.6 Particular Requirements for Safety — Microwave Therapy Equipment.* Sydney.

Barbour, LA, McGuire, DS, Kirchott, KT (1986) Non-analgesic methods of pain control used by cancer outpatients. *Oncology Nursing Forum,* 13: 56–60.

Canadian Department of Health and Welfare (1983) Shortwave diathermy guidelines for limited radio-frequency exposure, Safety Code 25. DHW, 83-EHD 98. Ottawa.

de Lateur, BJ, Lehmann, JF, Stonebridge, JB *et al.,* (1970) Muscle heating in human subjects with 915 MHz microwave contact applicator. *Archives of Physical Medicine and Rehabilitation,* 51: 147–151.

de Lateur, BJ, Stonebridge, JB, Lehmann, JF (1978) Fibrous muscular contractures: treatment with a new direct contact microwave applicator operating at 915 MHz. *Archives of Physical Medicine and Rehabilitation,* 59: 488–490.

Delpizzo, V, Joiner, KH (1987) On the safe use of microwave and shortwave diathermy units. *Australian Journal of Physiotherapy,* 33: 152–161.

Electromedical Committee of the Australian Physiotherapy Association (1990) Clinical standards for the use of electrophysical agents. *Australian Journal of Physiotherapy,* 36: 39–52.

Fadilah, R, Pinkus, J, Weinberger, A *et al.* (1987) Heating rabbit joint by microwave applicator. *Archives of Physical Medicine and Rehabilitation,* 68: 710–712.

Feibel, H, Fast, H (1976) Deep heating of joints: A reconsideration. *Archives of Physical Medicine and Rehabilitation,* 57: 513–514.

Forster, A, Palastanga, N (1985) *Clayton's Electrotherapy: Theory and Practice,* p. 138. London: Ballière Tindall.

Harris, ED, McCroskery, PA (1974) The influence of temperature and fibril stability on degradation of cartilage collagen by rheumatoid synovial collagenase. *New England Journal of Medicine,* 290: 1–6.

Hertel, HC, Howaldt, B, Mense, S (1976) Response of Group IV and Group III muscle afferents to thermal stimuli. *Brain Research,* 113: 201–205.

Ho, HS (1976) Energy absorption patterns in circular triple-layered tissue cylinders exposed to plane wave sources. *Health Physics,* 31: 97–108.

Kanui, TI (1985) Thermal inhibition of nociceptor-driven spinal cord nerves in rats. *Pain,* 21: 31–40.

Kemp, CR, Paul, WD, Hines, HM (1948) Studies concerning the effect of deep tissue heat on blood flow. *Archives Physical Medicine,* 29: 12–17.

Kenshalo, DR (1976) Correlations of temperature sensitivity in man and monkey: a first approximation. In Zotterman, Y (ed) *Sensory Functions of the Skin in Primates* with Special Reference to Man pp 305–330, Pergamon Press: Oxford.

Lehmann, JF, de Lateur, BJ (1990) Therapeutic heat in Lehmann, JF (ed) *Therapeutic Heat and Cold* 4th ed. pp. 417–581. Williams & Wilkins. Baltimore.

Lehmann, JF, Dundore, DE, Esselman, PC *et al.* (1983) Microwave diathermy: Effects on experimental muscle haematoma resolution. *Archives of Physical Medicine and Rehabilitation,* 64: 127–129.

Lehmann, JF, Masock, A, Warren, CG *et al.* (1970) Effect of therapeutic temperatures on tendon extensibility. *Archives of Physical Medicine and Rehabilitation,* 51: 481–487.

Lehmann, JF, McMillan, JA, Brunner, GD *et al.* (1962) Heating patterns produced in specimens by microwaves of the frequency of 2456 megacycles when applied with the 'A', 'B' and 'C' directors. *Archives of Physical Medicine and Rehabilitation,* 43: 538–546.

Licht, S (1982) History of therapeutic heat and cold. In Lehmann, JF (ed) *Therapeutic Heat and Cold,* 3rd edn, pp. 1–34. Williams & Wilkins, Baltimore.

Low, J, Reed, A (1990) *Electrotherapy Explained: Principles and practice.* London: Butterworth Heinemann.

McMeeken, JM, Bell, C (1990a) Effects of microwave irradiation on blood flow in the dog hindlimb. *Experimental Physiology,* 75: 367–374.

McMeeken, JM, Bell, C (1990b) Microwave irradiation of the human forearm and hand. *Physiotherapy Theory and Practice,* 6: 171–177.

Melzack, R, Wall, PD (1965) Pain mechanisms: A new theory. *Science,* 150: 971–979.

Mense, S (1978) Effects of temperature on the discharges of motor spindles and tendon organs. *Pflugers Archives,* 374: 159–166.

National Radiation Protection Board (1989) Guidance as to restrictions on exposure to time varying electromagnetic fields and the 1988 recommendations of the International Non-ionising Radiation Committee. *NRPB Report GS 11.* London: HMSO.

Richardson, AW, Imig, CJ, Feucht, BL *et al.* (1950) The relationship between deep tissue temperature and blood flow during electromagnetic irradiation. *Archives of Physical Medicine,* 31: 19–25.

Schwan, HP, Piersol, GM (1954) The absorption of electromagnetic energy in body tissues Part 1: Biological aspects. *American Journal of Physical Medicine,* 33: 371–404.

Schwan, HP, Piersol, GM (1955) The absorption of electromagnetic energy in body tissues Part 2: Physiological and clinical aspects. *American Journal of Physical Medicine,* 34: 425–448.

Scowcroft, AT, Mason, AHL, Hayne, CR (1977) Safety with microwave diathermy: A preliminary report of the CSP working party. *Physiotherapy,* 63: 359–361.

Sekins, KM, Dundore, D, Emery, AF *et al.* (1980) Muscle blood flow changes in response to 915 MHz diathermy with surface cooling as measured by Xe^{133} clearance. *Archives of Physical Medicine and Rehabilitation*, **61**: 105–113.

Sekins, KM, Lehmann, JF, Esselman, P *et al.* (1984) Local muscle blood flow and temperature responses to 915 MHz diathermy as simultaneously measured and numerically predicted. *Archives of Physical Medicine and Rehabilitation*, **65**: 1–7.

Siems, LL, Kosman, AJ, Osborne, SL (1948) A comparative study of shortwave and microwave diathermy on blood flow. *Archives of Physical Medicine and Rehabilitation*, **29**: 759.

Ward, AR (1986) *Electricity Fields and Waves in Therapy*, pp. 232–234. Marrickville: Science Press.

Weinberger, A, Fadilah, R, Lev, A *et al.* (1989) Treatment of articular effusions with local deep hyperthermia. *Clinical Rheumatology*, **8**: 461–466.

Wright, W, Johns, RJ (1961) Quantitative and qualitative analysis of joint stiffness in normal subjects and in patients with connective tissue diseases. *Annals of Rheumatic Diseases*, **20**: 30–46.

Yaksh, TL, Hammond, DL (1982) Peripheral and central substrates involved in the rostrad transmission of nociceptive information. *Pain*, **13**: 1–85.

13

Low Intensity Laser Therapy

DAVID BAXTER

Brief History

The term laser is an acronym for Light Amplification by Stimulated Emission of Radiation. Although Albert Einstein originally outlined the principles underlying the generation of such light in the early part of this century, it was not until 1960 that Theodore Maiman produced the first burst of ruby laser light at Hughes Laboratories in the USA. In the intervening decades, various laser devices based upon Maiman's original prototype have found applications ranging from laser pointers and bar code readers to military range finders and target acquisition systems.

Since their inception, lasers found immediate application in medicine and particularly in sur-gery, with ophthalmic surgeons being the first speciality to successfully use the pulsed ruby laser for the treatment of detached retina in humans. In general, most medical applications to date have relied upon the photothermal and photoablative interactions of laser with tissue; thus lasers are routinely used to cut, weld and even destroy tissue. The use of lasers as altern-atives to metal scalpels, as well as for tumour ablation and tattoo removal are all based upon such tissue reactions. In contrast, more recent interest has also focused on the potential clinical applications of the non-thermal interactions of laser light with tissue, principally based upon initial work carried out by Professor Endre Mester's group in Budapest during the late 1960s and early 1970s. Results of this work indicated the potential of relatively low intensity laser irradiation applied directly to tissue to modulate certain biological processes – in particular to photobiostimulate the wound healing process (Mester et al., 1985). Based upon Mester's work in animals and in patients, the ensuing decade saw the promotion of He–Ne laser radiation as the treatment of choice for a variety of conditions throughout the countries of the former Soviet Union, and in the far East, particularly China. Within the last ten years, the introduction of small, compact laser-emitting photodiodes has produced an increase in the use of this therapy, known as low-level or low-intensity laser therapy (LILT) in the West. Whilst the Food and Drug Administration (FDA) in the USA has still to approve laser therapy, the modality has found increasing application by physiotherapists (for human and animal use), dentists, acupuncturists, podiatrists, and indeed some physicians, for a range of conditions including the treatment of open wounds, soft tissue injuries, arthritic conditions and pain associated with various aetiologies (see Baxter et al., 1991).

Definitions and Nomenclature

Low-intensity laser therapy (see Baxter, 1994) or low- (reactive) level laser therapy (Ohshiro and Calderhead, 1988) is a generic term that defines the therapeutic application of relatively low-output (< 500 mW) lasers and monochromatic superluminous diodes for the treatment of disease and injury at dosages (usually < 35 J/cm^2) generally considered to be too low to affect any detectable heating of the irradiated tissues. Low-intensity laser therapy is thus an athermal treatment modality. For this reason, this modality has also sometimes (inappropriately) been termed 'soft' or 'cold' laser therapy to distinguish the devices and the resulting applications from high-power sources of the type used in surgery and in other medical and dental applications; however such terms are misleading and inappropriate and are therefore best avoided.

This modality is also frequently referred to as laser (photo)biostimulation, particularly in the USA, where the term is sometimes abbreviated to 'biostim'. The use of such terminology is essentially based upon the early observations of Mester's group and others which suggested the potential of such devices to selectively accelerate various wound healing processes and cellular functions. However, the term is inappropriate to define the modality for two reasons. In the first instance, the applications of the modality exceed merely the treatment of wounds. Furthermore, and more importantly, lasers also have the potential, even at therapeutic intensities, to inhibit cellular processes (i.e. laser *photobioinhibition*; see section on Arndt-Schultz Law below); thus a more accurate generic term for the biological effects of low intensity laser irradiation is laser photobiomodulation.

Physical Principles

Light Emission and Absorption and the Production of Laser Radiation

The basis of production of stimulated emission is summarized in Figure 13.1.

1 In non-laser sources, light is typically produced by *spontaneous emission of radiation* (Figure 13.1a). In such circumstances, the atoms and

Figure 13.1   Spontaneous Emission, Absorption and Stimulated Emission of Light.
(a) Spontaneous Emission: Excited electron (e) drops to lower (resting) level, emitting single photon (p);
(b) Absorption: Incident photon is absorbed by resting electron, which moves to higher level;
(c) Stimulated Emission: Incident photon interacts with already excited electron to produce two identical photons.

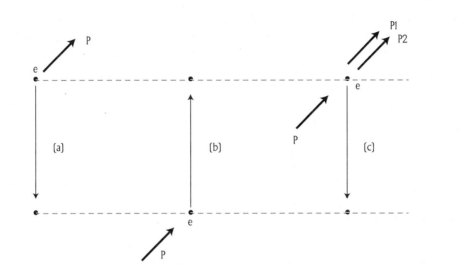

molecules comprizing the central emitter in such devices (e.g. the element/filament in a typical household light bulb) are stimulated with (electrical) energy so that the electrons shift to higher energy orbits. Once in such orbits, the electrons are inherently unstable and fall spontaneously within a short period of time to lower energy levels and in so doing release their extra energy as photons of light. The properties of the emitted photon are determined by the difference in energy levels (or valence bands) through which the excited electron 'dropped', as the difference in energy will be exactly the same as the quantal energy of the photon. As, for a given photon of light, the quantal energy (specified in electronVolts) is inversely related to the wavelength (in nm), the wavelength is effectively determined by the difference in valence bands and in turn, molecules produce typical ranges of wavelengths or emission spectra when appropriately stimulated.

2 *Absorption of radiation* occurs when a photon of light interacts with an atom or molecule in which the difference in energy of the valence bands exactly equals the energy carried by the photon (Figure 13.1b). This has two consequences: for a photon of a given quantal energy (and thus wavelength) only certain molecules will be capable of absorbing the light radiation; conversely, for a given molecule, only certain quantal energies (and thus wavelengths) can be absorbable (this is termed the *absorption spectrum* for the molecule). Thus absorption is said to be *wavelength specific*. This is an important concept in LILT applications, as this wavelength specificity of absorption effectively determines which type(s) of tissue will preferentially absorb incident radiation and (in turn) the depth of penetration of a particular treatment unit.

3 *Stimulated emission of radiation* is a unique event which occurs when an incident photon interacts with an atom which is already excited

(i.e. where the electron(s) are already in a higher energy orbit); additionally, the quantal energy of the incident photon must exactly equal the difference in energy levels between the electron's excited and resting states (see Figure 13.1c). Under these exceptional circumstances the electron, in returning to its original orbit, gives off its excess energy as a photon of light with exactly the same properties as the incident photon and completely in phase. In laser devices, the unique circumstances which give rise to stimulated emission of radiation are produced through the selection of an appropriate material or substance which, when electrically stimulated, will produce large numbers of identical photons through the rapid excitation of the medium. In order to produce such stimulated emission of radiation, laser treatment devices rely upon three essential components:

1 *A lasing medium* which is capable of being 'pumped' with energy to ultimately produce stimulated emission; for therapeutic systems, the energy source is invariably electrical, and the energy is delivered to the medium typically from the mains or (less commonly) from a battery (see below). The two media most commonly used in LILT applications are the gaseous mixture of helium and neon (He–Ne) operating at a wavelength of 632.8 nm (i.e. red light), or alternatively, gallium arsenide (Ga–As) or gallium-aluminium-arsenide (GaAlAs) semiconductors typically producing radiation at between 630–950 nm (i.e. visible red to the near infrared). While He–Ne systems were the first to be used for LILT applications, and a significant percentage of the papers published within this area are based upon such devices, their use has diminished considerably over the last decade; thus, very few He–Ne lasers currently find application in routine physiotherapeutic practice, at least in Britain or Ireland. This is due to the relative expense of such units, and the comparatively low power output associated with He–Ne systems. In addition, the relatively greater collimation (see below) of these units when applied without fibre optic applicators poses a significant hazard to the unprotected eye compared to the average semiconductor diode-based treatment unit.

2 A *resonating cavity* or chamber consisting of a structure to contain the lasing medium and incorporating a pair of parallel reflecting surfaces or mirrors. Within this chamber, photons of light produced by the medium are allowed to be reflected back and forth between the 'mirrors' to ultimately produce an intense photon resonance. As one of the reflecting surfaces (also termed the output coupler) is not a 'pure' mirror and thus does not reflect 100% of the light striking its surface, some of the radiation is allowed to pass through as the output of the device. Whilst the resonating cavity for an He–Ne unit can be relatively large and cumbersome, those for diode-based units are tiny, being the lasing medium itself, i.e. the semiconductor diode, the ends of which are carefully polished to form reflecting surfaces. This has important implications for the routine use of these units in clinical practice, as the treatment 'head' or 'probe' is usually not much larger than the size of a pen and represents another reason why diode-based units are so popular with clinicians. Furthermore, several manufacturers have incorporated a number of diodes (≤ 46 diodes) into so-called 'cluster' arrays in order to allow simultaneous treatment of larger lesions and to allow several wavelengths of radiation to be used in parallel (Figure 13.2). It should be noted that for He–

Figure 13.2   Shows a modern laser treatment unit. (Photograph courtesy of Central Medical Equipment, Nottingham).

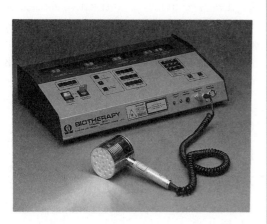

Ne-based systems, as the resonating cavity is usually more cumbersome, the laser radiation from the output coupler is usually delivered to the tissue to be treated by means of a fibre optic applicator which allows the operator to direct the radiation to the target tissue more easily.

3 A *power source* to 'pump' the lasing media to produce stimulated emission. In most cases, therapeutic devices have tended to be mains supplied and incorporate a base unit to contain the transformer and control unit (Figure 13.2). More recently, however, a number of manufacturers have produced rechargeable and battery-powered units to enhance the portability of their laser devices, e.g. for sports injuries applications.

Characteristics of Laser Radiation

The radiation generated by therapeutic laser devices differs from that produced by other sources (e.g. infrared lamps) in three respects:

MONOCHROMATICITY

The light produced by a laser is 'single coloured', with the majority of the radiation emitted by the treatment device being clustered around one single wavelength with a very narrow band width. In contrast, light generated by other sources comprises an enormous variety of wavelengths, sometimes ranging from the ultraviolet to the infrared, which result in the sensation of the colour white when the light strikes the retina of a human observer. Wavelength is a critical factor in determining the specific therapeutic effects produced by laser treatments, as this parameter determines which specific biomolecules will absorb the incident radiation and thus the basic photobiological interaction underlying any given treatment effect.

COLLIMATION

In laser light, the rays of light or photons produced by the laser device are for all practical purposes parallel, with almost no divergence of the emitted radiation over distance. This property keeps the optical power of the device bundled onto a relatively small area over considerable distances, and, to a degree, even when passing through tissue.

COHERENCE

The light emitted by laser devices is also in phase, so in conjunction with the two unique properties already outlined above, the troughs and peaks of the emitted light waves match perfectly in time (temporal coherence) and in space (spatial coherence). The biological and clinical relevance of this property is still debated, not least because of the availability of so called 'superluminous diodes' which possess all the qualities of a 'true' laser diode less the coherence, but which are a fraction of the cost of the latter; cluster treatment units incorporating some 30 or 40 diodes would be prohibitively expensive for routine clinical use if comprised of nothing other than true laser diodes and thus generally incorporate no more than several laser diodes the remainder being super-luminous diodes.

Laser–Tissue Interaction

As already indicated above, laser–tissue interaction is typically associated with the potentially destructive effects of irradiation at relatively high power and energy levels; in these circumstances, high densities of laser light from highly collimated or focused sources with output in the Watt range can easily produce photothermal reactions in tissues, including ablative or explosive effects. However, in low-intensity laser therapy the emphasis, by definition, is upon the non-thermal (or athermal) reactions of light with tissue. Light from a laser or monochromatic light therapy treatment device can interact in two ways with irradiated tissue:

1 *Scattering of incident light.* This is essentially a change in the direction of propagation of the light as it passes through the tissues, and is due to the variability in refractive indices of tissue components relative to water. Such scattering will cause a 'widening' of the beam as it passes through irradiated tissue and result in the rapid loss of coherence.

2 *Absorption of incident light by a chromophore,* i.e. a biomolecule which is capable, through its electronic or atomic configuration, of being excited by the incident photon(s). Light at the wavelengths typically employed in LILT are readily absorbed by a variety of biomolecules including melanin and haemoglobin; as a consequence, the penetration depth associated with treatment devices is limited to no more than several millimetres. It should be noted that as absorption is dependent upon the wavelength of incident light, depth of penetration is similarly wavelength dependent.

Of these two modes of interaction, absorption may be regarded as the most important in terms of the photobiological basis of laser therapy, as without absorption, no photobiological, and thus clinical, effects would be possible.

Conceptual Basis of Laser Photobiomodulation: Arndt-Schultz Law

The photobiological effects of laser or monochromatic light upon tissue are many and complex, and to a large degree still poorly understood, particularly in terms of the variable stimulative/inhibitory reactions which may be affected by such irradiation. In providing a theoretical basis for the observed biological and clinical effects of this modality, the Arndt-Schultz Law has been proposed as a suitable model; the main tenets of this Law are illustrated in Figure 13.3. It should be stressed that while this model can account for such phenomena as the 'inverse' dosage dependency reported in some papers (e.g. Lower *et al.,*

Figure 13.3 The Arndt-Schultz Law.
(a) Pre-threshold: no biological activation (resting);
(b) Biostimulation: activation of biological processes;
(c) Bioinhibition: inhibition of biological processes.

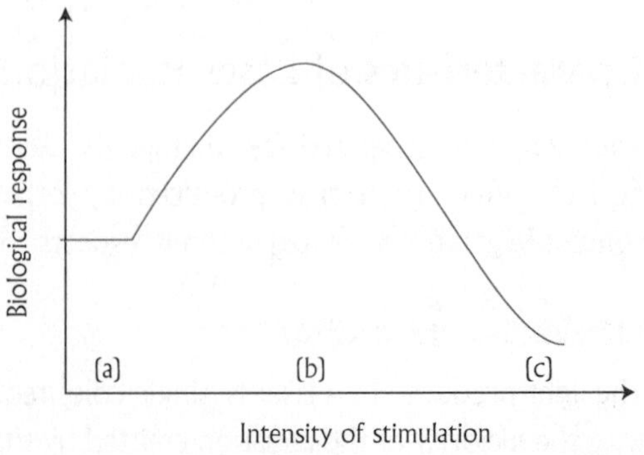

1994), it essentially applies to radiant exposure (or energy density — see below); the putative relevance of manipulation of other irradiation parameters such as pulse repetition rate or power output remains, at least for the time being, unclear.

Biological and Physiological Effects

Investigations of the biological and physiological effects of low-intensity laser radiation can usefully be considered under three main areas: cellular studies involving the use of well-established cell-lines and explanted cells, studies in various species of animals (*in vivo* and *in vitro*), and finally research in healthy human volunteers.

Whilst the following provides an overview of the findings to date in these areas, a full and comprehensive review of the literature on the biological and physiological effects of low-intensity laser radiation is beyond the scope of this book; for further detail the reader is directed to the reviews of Basford (1986, 1989), King (1990), Kitchen and Partridge (1991), Shields and O'Kane (1994) and Baxter (1994).

Cellular Research

A range of studies have examined the effects of low-intensity laser irradiation in a variety of cell lines and explanted cells to establish the photo-biological basis of the clinical use of this modality, especially for the promotion of wound healing. In these studies a number of possible indicators have been used to assess the photobiomodulatory effects of laser irradiation, including cell proliferation (Boulton and Marshall, 1986; Hallman *et al.*, 1988), collagen production (Castro *et al.*, 1983; Lam *et al.*, 1986) and ultrastructural changes

(Bosatra *et al.*, 1984). Because of their importance in wound repair, the cells most commonly used to date have been fibroblasts and macrophages (e.g. Lam *et al.*, 1986; O'Kane *et al.*, 1994). However it should be stressed that while findings from such studies are generally positive, results are not exclusively favourable nor straightforward; results in some cell types have tended to be more variable; e.g. research on lymphocytes has typically shown inhibitory effects upon cellular proliferation as a result of laser irradiation (Ohta *et al.*, 1987), while other groups have failed to find any significant laser-mediated effect (Hallman *et al.*, 1988).

Cellular studies such as those outlined above are important in two respects; in the first instance for providing a scientific basis for the clinical application of low-intensity lasers for the management of wounds, through demonstration of the photo-biological mechanisms underlying such treatments. Second, by using such well-controlled laboratory research techniques, systematic investigations by some groups have demonstrated the importance of laser irradiation parameters such as wavelength, dosage, and pulse repetition rate to the observed effects (e.g. van Breugel *et al.*, 1993; O'Kane *et al.*, 1994; Rajaratnam *et al.*, 1994).

This notwithstanding, the extrapolation of findings from this type of study to the clinical setting is difficult, as the precise relevance of the reported observations to clinical treatments are not always entirely clear. For example, where photobiostimulatory effects are reported at a radiant exposure of 1.5 J/cm^2 in a laboratory study involving the direct irradiation of artificially maintained murine macrophage-like cell lines, what direct relevance has this for dosage selection in the laser treatment of a venous ulcer in a 67-year-old patient? Given such problems, particularly the vast difference between the cell lines and the highly complicated micro-environment of the clinical wound, a number of groups have employed animal studies and experimental studies on healthy human volunteers to assume further the biological and physiological effects of this modality in the laboratory.

Animal Studies

To date, animal studies have concentrated on two main areas of research: the photobiostimulative effects of laser irradiation upon wound healing and tissue repair in experimentally induced lesions, and the neurophysiological and in particular the antinociceptive effects of such irradiation. For the former studies, small loose-skinned animals such as rats and mice have been most commonly used (e.g. Mester et al., 1985; Lyons et al., 1987); in these species, a range of experimental wounds have been employed including muscle injuries (Mester et al., 1975), burns (Rochkind et al., 1989), tendon injuries (Enwemeka et al., 1990) and open skin wounds of various types (Haina et al., 1982; Mester et al., 1985; Abergel et al., 1987). While these studies have typically reported positive effects of laser irradiation (in terms of increased rates of healing, wound closure, enhanced granulation tissue formation etc.) the experimental lesions in these animals are considered to represent a poor model for wounds in humans because of the species differences in tegument compared to humans (e.g. Basford, 1989; King, 1990). As a consequence, some investigators have preferred to use porcine wound healing as a more appropriate experimental assay to study the potential benefits of laser irradiation for management of wounds in humans, with more variable findings (Hunter et al., 1984; Abergel et al., 1987); thus while findings from animal research has generally demonstrated biostimulative effects upon wound healing, particu-

larly in rodents, findings are not exclusively positive (see Shields and O'Kane, 1994 for detailed review).

Perhaps the most interesting aspect of this type of animal work has been reports, principally by Rochkind's group, of the potential of laser irradiation to accelerate regeneration of nerves, together with associated electrophysiological and functional recovery, after various types of experimental lesions (e.g. Rochkind et al., 1989; Khullar et al., 1994). If such effects are also possible in humans, the implications for future applications of this modality would be enormous; interestingly, Rochkind's group has already conducted some limited clinical work in humans using relatively high dosages (> 100 J/cm^2) with encouraging early results in both peripheral and central nerve lesions (Rochkind et al., 1994a,b).

Neurophysiological and antinociceptive effects of laser irradiation have also been investigated in a variety of species. In particular, withdrawal and avoidance behaviours such as the tail-flick and hot plate tests have been used to assess hypoalgesic effects of laser irradiation, its mechanism of action and dependence upon the pulse repetition rate used (e.g. Wu, 1983; Ponnudurai et al., 1987, 1988). These studies consistently demonstrated a significant hypoalgesic effect of laser irradiation, in terms of increased latency to tail flick or paw lick, which was found to be most pronounced at the lower pulse repetition rates (4 Hz; Ponnudurai et al., 1987); furthermore the hypoalgesia was found not to be reversible when the opiate antagonist naloxone was administered, thus suggesting that the observed pain relief was not mediated by endogenous opiates (Ponnudurai et al., 1988). However, the hypoalgesic effects of laser irradiation, at least in animals, are not straightforward, as one group has also reported laser-mediated *hyper*algesic effects in experimental mice using a hot plate paradigm to assess pain relief (Zarkovic *et al.*, 1989).

It can thus be seen that animal studies have provided some evidence of beneficial effects of laser irradiation upon experimental wounds and pain. While studies in animals such as those outlined above do go some way towards bridging the gap between cellular work and clinical practice, some of the problems in extrapolating and applying results from animal studies to clinical practice in humans remain. As a consequence, several groups have used controlled studies in healthy human volunteers as a useful means of investigation without recourse to patients and the considerable problems inherent in undertaking controlled clinical research.

Controlled Studies in Humans

Studies in this area have focused principally on the physiological and hypoalgesic effects of laser radiation. This approach has been particularly useful in investigating the effects of laser upon peripheral nerves; while early studies provided contradictory findings (e.g. Walker and Akhanjee, 1985; Wu *et al.*, 1987; Greathouse *et al.*, 1986; Snyder-Mackler and Bork, 1989), more recent studies have demonstrated significant effects upon peripheral nerve conduction in the median and superficial radial nerves which would appear to be critically-dependent upon the dosage and pulse repetition rate of the laser source (Walsh, 1993; Basford *et al.*, 1993; Baxter *et al.*, 1994; Lowe *et al.*, 1994). Although these papers typically report changes in nerve conduction latencies or velocities in response to laser irradiation applied to the skin overlying the course of the nerve, the precise relevance of such observations to the clinical applications of this modality are debatable. Of more direct relevance to clinical prac-

tice, a number of studies have assessed the effects of laser upon various types of experimentally-induced pain in humans. These studies have essentially relied upon two main types of pain induction: thermal pain threshold and the submaximal effort tourniquet technique. Noxious heat stimulation has been used by several groups to assess the efficacy of single-diode laser application, applied directly to the site of noxious stimulation or to appropriate acupuncture points, with variable findings (e.g. Seibert and Gould, 1984; Brockhaus and Elger, 1990); in particular the latter study found the hypoalgesic effects of needle acupuncture to be significantly superior to laser acupuncture. Variable findings have also been obtained with experimentally-induced ischaemic pain; significant hypoalgesic effects upon this model of pain have been reported with combined phototherapy/low intensity laser therapy using a multiwavelength, multisource 'cluster' array at radiant exposures of over 30 J/cm^2 (e.g. Mokhtar *et al.*, 1992), but not with low-intensity laser applied using a single (830 nm) diode (Lowe *et al.*, 1995).

Clinical Studies

While a vast number of clinical studies have been completed and published in this area, in the main with positive results, reviewers have consistently noted the following problems with the literature:

1 Most studies have been published in foreign language journals, often without English abstracts, making the work inaccessible to the anglophone;
2 The studies reported in the literature (regardless of language) are often poorly controlled with only very limited bending; indeed a

significant proportion of the studies are merely anecdotal in nature;

3 The irradiation parameters and treatment protocols used are frequently inadequately specified, thus limiting comparison of results and rendering replication and application in the clinical setting impossible. Even where irradiation parameters are specified, the bewildering number of possible permutations and combinations of wavelength, irradiance, pulse repetition rate etc. will often mean that precise replication is problematic.

This notwithstanding, it is important to stress that the published database of clinical studies on low-intensity laser therapy represents a significant body of anecdotal evidence in favour of the modality; while the constraints of the current text precludes an exhaustive review of this literature, the following at least provides an overview of some of the most relevant papers to date.

Wound Healing

The popularity of laser therapy among physiotherapists for the treatment of various types of wounds is witnessed by the results of a recent survey on current clinical practice in this field (Baxter et al., 1991). Treatment of various types of chronic ulceration was the first application for low-intensity laser to be trialled in humans during the late 1960s and early 1970s (see Mester and Mester, 1989), using He–Ne sources and dosages of up to 4 J/cm^2; it was based upon the reported success of these early studies in terms of enhanced rates of wound healing and pain reduction that the modality quickly achieved popularity in this application. In the ensuing decades, laser therapy has been assessed in the treatment of a variety of wounds and ulcerated lesions with positive results generally, especially when applied

in more chronic, intractable cases (e.g. Karu, 1985; Sugrue et al., 1990; Robinson and Walters, 1991). However, given that many of the reports to date are poorly controlled and based upon relatively small numbers, and furthermore that results are not exclusively positive (e.g. Santioanni et al., 1984), additional studies are warranted to definitively establish the benefit of this modality for the promotion of wound healing, and particularly the relevance of irradiation parameters to such effects.

Arthritic Conditions

The potential benefit of laser therapy in the management of such conditions as rheumatoid arthritis, osteoarthritis and arthrogenic pain has been assessed by a number of groups with varying degrees of success reported. While several papers have reported decreased joint pain and inflammation coupled with increased functional status in rheumatoid joints after treatment with a low output Nd:YAG laser (Goldman et al., 1980; Vidovich and Olson, 1987), it is important to stress that such units, which are typically used at higher output levels for surgical applications, are not suitable for routine use in physiotherapeutic laser therapy. Using more commonly available He–Ne and diode-based units, a number of groups have reported significant decreases in pain with concomitant improvements in function as a result of laser treatment of these patients (Lonauer, 1986; Walker et al., 1987; Palmgren et al., 1989; Trelles et al., 1991); equally, several groups have failed to find any significant benefit of laser treatment in well-controlled and reported trials (Bliddal et al., 1987; Basford et al., 1987; Jensen et al., 1987). While the precise reasons for such discrepancies are not entirely clear, it may be due in part to the differences in laser parameters employed in these studies and in particular the relatively low-power output units used in some of the latter studies (< 1 mW). For the time being at least, this is another area in which further research would appear to be indicated.

Musculoskeletal Disorders

Given the evidence on the potential biostimulative effects of laser irradiation at the cellular and clinical level, it is not surprising that a number of groups have assessed the efficacy of these devices in the management of a range of musculoskeletal disorders. Laser therapy for tendinopathies have been investigated by several groups with both positive (England et al., 1989) and negative (Siebert et al., 1987) findings being reported. However, the disparate findings between these two studies may in part be explained by the irradiation techniques used in that the investigators in the latter study inappropriately employed a non-contact technique (see below), using the laser source at a distance of some 10 cm from the target tissue; this would have significantly reduced the intensity of radiation on the tissue (i.e. irradiance) and thus the effectiveness of the applied laser treatment in this trial. Similarly, the use of inappropriately-low dosage levels may in part explain the non-significant results reported by some groups in the laser treatment of other musculoskeletal conditions such as myofascial pain (Waylonis et al., 1988) and lateral epicondylitis (Lundeberg et al., 1987), compared to the typically positive findings at other centres (Choi et al., 1986; Glykofridis and Diamantopoulos, 1987; Li, 1990). However, it should be stressed that while the former studies may be criticized on the basis of their use of inappropriate irradiation parameters, these studies were in the main better designed and controlled than many of the case-series type of paper typically published in this area.

Pain

Early observations of concomitant reductions in reported pain in wound patients treated with laser led to attempts at exploitation and investigation of the analgesic effects of this modality. Apart from decreases in pain associated with the laser-mediated treatment effects documented in those studies already indicated above, a number of groups have also reported analgesic effects of laser irradiation in various types of chronic pain as well as in neuropathic and neurogenic pain syndromes (Walker, 1983; Lukashevich, 1985; Moore et al., 1988; Shiroto et al., 1989; Amoils and Kues, 1991). However, and despite such positive reports, the treatment of pain remains one of the most contentious areas of laser application, particularly in terms of the management of chronic pain syndromes; while the reasons for scepticism are essentially those already identified, the lack of an obvious mechanism of action further confounds acceptance of the pain relieving effects of this modality (see Devor, 1990). This notwithstanding, the modality has become a popular treatment method with physiotherapists for the relief of pain, and one which is highly rated against alternative electrotherapeutic modalities (Baxter et al., 1991).

Principles of Clinical Application

INDICATIONS

While laser therapy finds a variety of applications in routine clinical practice, these can be usefully summarized under the following headings:

1 Stimulation of wound healing in various types of open wounds;
2 Treatment of various arthritic conditions;

3 Treatment of soft tissue injuries; and,
4 Relief of pain.

These are considered in outline below, after an overview of the principles underlying effective laser treatment. As a basis for subsequent sections and to aid the reader in more critical review of the work published in this area, the method of calculating dosage and the importance of other irradiation parameters is presented below.

Dosage and Irradiation Parameters

Apart from wavelength, which is determined by the lasing medium used in the device, the other irradiation parameters that appear to be important in laser treatments are:

POWER OUTPUT

The power output of a unit is usually expressed in milliwatts (mW) or thousandths of a watt. While usually fixed and invariable, some machines allow operator selection of the percentage of the total power output (e.g. 10%, 25% etc.); in addition, where pulsing of the output is provided as an option by the manufacturer, this can have profound effects upon the power output of the unit. Over the last decade, the trend in commercially available units has been towards higher output devices (~ 30–200 mW), rather than the once popular 1–10 mW devices, not least because higher output units can deliver a specified treatment in a much shorter period of time.

IRRADIANCE (POWER DENSITY)

The power per unit area (mW/cm^2) is an important irradiation parameter, which is usually kept as high as possible for a given unit by so called 'in contact' treatment technique and applying a firm pressure through the treatment head during treatment. It should be noted that, even with

the small degrees of divergence associated with laser treatment devices, treatment out of contact from the target tissue will significantly reduce the effectiveness of treatment as the irradiance falls due the inverse square law and because of increased reflection from the skin or tissue interface. For in-contact treatments, the irradiance is simply calculated by dividing the power output (or average power output for a pulsed unit) by the spot size of the treatment head; typical values for the latter are 0.1–0.125 cm^2.

ENERGY

This is given in joules (J) and is usually specified per point irradiated, or sometimes for the total treatment where a number of points are treated. It is calculated by multiplying the power output in *Watts* by the time of irradiation or application in seconds. Thus a 30 mW (i.e. 0.03 W) device applied for 1 minute (i.e. 60 s) will deliver 1.8 J of energy.

RADIANT EXPOSURE (ENERGY DENSITY)

This is generally considered to be the best means of specifiying dosage, and is given in joules per unit area (i.e. J/cm^2); typical values for routine treatments may range from less than 1 to over 30 J/cm^2, however 1–12 J/cm^2 would be most commonly used (see below). Energy density is usually calculated by dividing the energy delivered (in Joules) by the spot size of the treatment unit (in cm).

PULSE REPETITION RATE

While a large percentage of the laser units routinely used in clinical practice are continuous wave (CW) output (i.e. the output power is essentially invariable over time), most units currently available in the UK allow some form of pulsing of their output. For pulsed units, the pulse repetition rate is expressed in hertz (Hz, pulses per second). Typical values for pulse repetition rate can vary from 2 to tens of thousands of Hz. Although the potential biological and clinical relevance of pulse repetition rate is still far from being universally accepted, recent research would suggest that this parameter is critical to at least some of the biological effects of this modality (e.g. Rajaratnam *et al.*, 1994).

Importance of the Use of Contact Technique

(See Figure 13.4)

While the method of application may vary depending on what specific condition the operator is treating, in general and wherever possible the treatment head or probe should be applied with a firm pressure to the area of tissue to be treated. In the first instance, this makes the laser treatment inherently safer by reducing the poten-

tial for accidental intrabeam viewing, as already indicated above. However, the primary reason for using so-called contact technique is to maximize the irradiance or power density on the tissue surface and thus the light flux within the target tissue, which are important in ensuring the effectiveness of laser treatment. Where the treatment head is used out of contact, light flux within the tissue is reduced due to several factors; most importantly, the inverse square law applies to such non-contact applications, leading to reduced incident irradiance on surface of the irradiated tissue. Furthermore, more reflection of incident photons will occur where the probe is not maintained directly in contact with the tissue (Figure 13.4).

Apart from producing the highest levels of light flux within the tissue, application of contact technique will also allow the operator to press the treatment probe into the tissues to treat deeper seated lesions more effectively. Apart from compensating for the relatively limited penetration of therapeutic laser devices by

Figure 13.4   Contact versus non-contact technique.
(a) Non-contact technique;
(b) Contact technique.

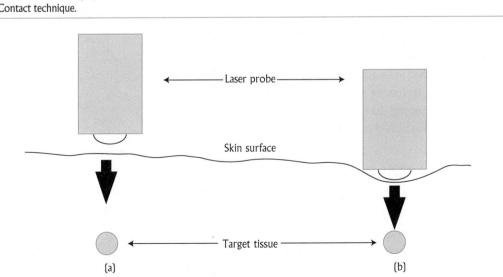

approximating the treatment probe with the target tissue, the deep pressure will drive red blood cells from the area of tissue directly under the probe head and thus reduce the attenuation of light due to such cells.

Application of the laser treatment probe also affords the opportunity of applying pressure treatments to key points (e.g. trigger or acupoints) and thus effectively combines laser with acupressure-type treatments. Despite the above, there are situations where laser treatment cannot be applied using contact technique; principally these are where such application would be too painful or aseptic technique is required e.g. in cases of open wounds. Less commonly, the contours of the tissue to be treated may not allow use of a so-called 'cluster' head in full contact, thus non-contact technique must be used. Where this is the case, the treatment head should not be held more than 0.5–1 cm from the surface of the target tissue.

Treatment of Open Wounds and Ulcers

The treatment of open wounds and ulcers represents the cardinal application for low-intensity laser devices and combined phototherapy / low-intensity laser therapy units (Figure 13.5). For comprehensive treatment of such conditions, irradiation is applied in two stages: the first using standard contact technique around the edges of the wounds, the second during which the wound bed is treated using non-contact technique.

TREATMENT OF WOUND MARGINS

For this a single-diode probe is the ideal unit to apply treatment around the circumference of wound at approximately 1–2 cm from its edges. Points of application should be no more than 2–3 cm apart, and the treatment unit should be

Figure 13.5   Laser treatment of wounds. Wound margin is treated with single probe using contact technique (~1 cm from wound; 2 cm intervals); Wound bed is treated using non-contact technique, using either gridding or scanning technique (single diode probe) or multidiode 'cluster' unit.

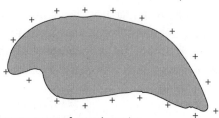

Spot treatment of wound margins

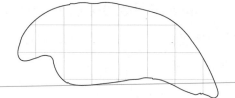

Gridding technique for wound bed

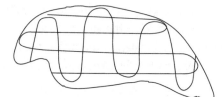

Treatment of wound margins and bed with 'cluster' array

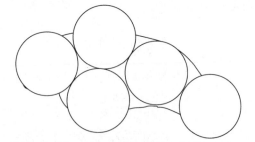

Treatment of wound margins and bed with 'cluster' array

applied with a firm pressure to the intact skin within the patient's tolerances.

For such treatments of the wound margins, dosages applied should be no more than 1 J per point, or approximately 10 J/cm^2.

Figure 13.6 Laser treatment of wounds. Wound margin is treated with single probe using contact technique (~ 1 cm from wound; 2 cm intervals); Wound bed is treated using non-contact technique, using either gridding or scanning technique (single diode probe) or multidiode 'cluster' unit.

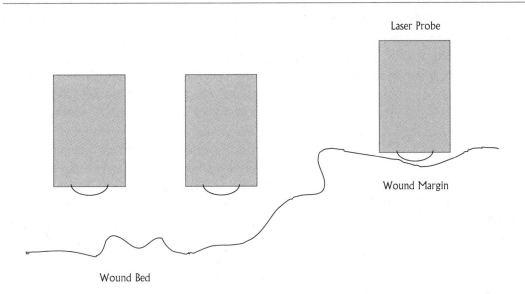

Laser Probe

Wound Margin

Wound Bed

TREATMENT OF THE WOUND BED

As already indicated above, treatment of the wound bed will invariably be completed using non-contact technique. As the wound lacks the usual protective layer of dermis, the dosages applied during treatment will be much lower than during application over intact skin, and typically cited radiant exposures are somewhere in the range of 1–10 J/cm², with 4 J/cm² being most commonly recommended as the 'Mester protocol' based upon the pioneering work of Professor Endre Mester's group.

However, the problem of applying such a dosage in a standardized fashion across the surface of an open wound is obvious and has led to several means of application being recommended in these conditions. At the simplest level, where only a single probe or fibre optic applicator is available, the wound may be 'mapped' with a hypothetical grid of equal sized squares (typically 1–2 cm square), each of which may be

regarded as an individual area of target tissue and treatment applied accordingly at the recommended dosage. In order to standardize the 'grid', some therapists have employed acetate sheets marked with the grid, upon which the outline of the wound can also be traced at regular intervals as a method of recording the progress of the patient's lesion to treatment. Alternatively, a clear plastic sheet with holes drilled in a regular grid has also been successfully used in some units as a means of standardizing wound treatments; in such cases, the size of the holes correspond to the circumference of the tip of the laser treatment probe, which is applied in sequence to each of the holes overlying the wound, for the time required to deliver the prescribed dosage.

Apart from such gridding, some therapists have also employed some variant of scanning technique to treat the wound bed where single-diode or fibre-optic applicators are used. In these cases, the probe is moved slowly over the area of the lesion using a non-contact technique while taking care to deliver a standardized radiant exposure to all areas and maintain the head at a distance of no more than 1 cm from the wound bed. Perhaps not surprisingly, most therapists find this technique difficult to perform, and thus it is increasingly rare to find units where manual scanning treatments are performed.

SPECIAL DEVICES FOR TREATMENT OF WOUNDS

Given the problems inherent in performing effective standardized laser irradiation of wound beds, a number of special devices have been produced and marketed in an attempt to simplify and improve the efficacy of such treatments. In the first instance, several manufacturers have produced scanning devices that may be used in conjunction with their treatment units; these scanners mechanically direct the output of the device over an area defined by the operator by means of controls on the scanning unit. While such devices have been popular in some circles in offering a 'hands off' approach to providing a well-standardized treatment across the whole wound area, particularly in cases of more extensive wounds (e.g. burns) the relatively high cost and potentially greater hazards associated with these units have prevented them becoming as popular as they perhaps might otherwise be.

As an alternative to scanners, a number of manufacturers now provide the option of so-called 'cluster' units, typically incorporating an array of diodes in a single hand-held unit. The number of diodes provided in these clusters varies between 3 and over 50, but it is generally true that the larger units incorporate a mixture of superluminous (monochromatic) diodes as well as (true) laser sources in their arrays, due to the prohibitive cost of the latter. Such cluster units allow simul-taneous treatment of an area of tissue, the extent of which is decided by the number and configuration of the diodes included in the array. Furthermore, at least several manufacturers have incorporated diodes operating at a variety of wavelengths (i.e. multisource/multiwavelength arrays) in their cluster units, claiming enhanced clinical effects through parallel (and possibly synergistic) wavelength-specific effects. In routine clinical practice, the relative difficulty in treating extensive ulceration with single diode units has led to cluster units being frequently cited as the most popular units by therapists (see Baxter *et al.*, 1991). In treating wound beds, cluster units can be used in isolation or in conjunction with single probes to access deeper or recessed areas, and in either case present a more time efficient means of treatment than single probes units used in isolation.

Treatment of Other Conditions

As already indicated, when treatment is applied to intact skin, contact technique is the application of choice. For such treatment of general musculoskeletal conditions, laser therapy can usefully be applied in a number of ways.

DIRECT TREATMENT OF THE LESION

In such cases, the laser probe is applied directly to the lesion (area of bruising, site of pain etc.) using a firm pressure within the patient's tolerance. Where extensive bruising/haematoma is present, an 'in contact' version of wound treatment as already summarized above is applied; for these cases, dosages applied are correspondingly higher than those used for the treatment of open wounds, given the presence of the skin as a barrier to laser irradiation.

TREATMENT OF ACUPUNCTURE AND TRIGGER POINTS

In China and Japan, the main method of laser application is as an alternative to needles for acupuncture. While the comparative efficacy of such application with respect to needles or other non-invasive alternatives (e.g. TENS, acupressure etc.) is still to be definitively determined and a matter for intense debate, there are many reports in the literature of successful application of laser in this area (see Baxter, 1989; Ellis, 1994). Taut muscles with associated, well localized areas of pain upon palpation (i.e. trigger points; Baldry, 1989) may also be treated with laser irradiation; while no definitive recommendations can be made on dosage for such trigger point therapy, in the author's experience the best results are achieved when a relatively high power unit (i.e. 50–200 mW) is employed to deliver initial dosages of at least 10 J/cm^2.

IRRADIATION OVER NERVE ROOTS, TRUNKS ETC.

In the laser treatment of pain syndromes, or in cases where pain represents a major feature of the clinical presentation of the condition to be treated, irradiation may usefully be applied to the skin overlying the appropriate nerve root, plexus or trunk. For example, in treating upper limb pain, laser therapy might be applied over the relevant cervical nerve roots, the brachial plexus by irradiation over Erb's Point as well as to points where the nerves in the arm are relatively superficial such as the radial, median or ulnar nerves at the elbow or wrist.

Key Points on Laser Treatment of Some Selected Conditions

SOFT TISSUE INJURIES

In such conditions, treatment should be initiated as early as is practically possible within the acute stage, using relatively low dosages in the region of 1.5–4 J/cm^2 applied directly to the site of injury and any areas of palpable pain. Within the first 72–96 hours post-injury, such treatment may be applied up to three times daily with no risk of overtreatment provided that dosages are kept low. It is important to reiterate that low-intensity laser treatment is by definition athermal and thus eminently suitable for treatment in these situations. As the condition resolves, the frequency of laser treatment may be reduced and dosage correspondingly increased, up to a maximum of 30 J/cm^2. Where pulsed systems are available, early treatments should be initiated with relatively low pulse repetition rates (< 100 Hz) and increased into the megahertz range as treatment progresses. Where haematoma or bruising is present, it should be treated using the general principles already outlined for the treatment of open wounds, although in this case a firm contact technique should be used within the patient's tolerance, particularly where the lesion is relatively deep.

Recommended initial dosages should be in the region of 4–8 J/cm^2 around the margins of the lesion, and with an average of 6–8 J/cm^2 using a grid technique or a multisource array applied over the centre of the bruise. In the treatment of muscle tears and injuries, laser therapy can be highly effective in accelerating the repair process and thus the return to normal function. This, coupled with its ability to be applied early in the acute stage – in some cases immediately after injury — makes it a popular modality in the treatment of sports injuries.

NEUROPATHIC AND NEUROGENIC PAIN

Where the patient presents with chronic neurogenic pain, laser irradiation is typically applied in a systematic fashion to all relevant nerve roots, plexus and trunks, using a middle range dosage ($\sim$ 10–12 J/cm^2) to initiate treatment. Where trigger or tender points are identified, these are also treated, using a initial dosage of at least 10–12 J/cm^2, which is increased to achieve desensitization of the point upon repalpation. Irradiation is also applied directly to any areas of referred pain, and to the affected dermatome etc.

ARTHROGENIC PAIN

Arthralgia of various aetiologies may be effectively managed with laser treatment applied in a comprehensive manner to the affected joints; for this care should be taken (especially with regard to patient positioning), to ensure that all aspects of the joint are systematically treated.

Hazards

Classification of Lasers and Ocular Hazard

Under a classification system internationally agreed which grades laser devices on a scale from 1–4 according to the associated dangers to the unprotected skin and eye, the units typically used in LILT are classed as Class 3B lasers, although much lower output Class 1 and 2 devices have also been used in the past. This essentially means, for the majority of systems used in physiotherapy applications (i.e. Class 3B units), that although

the laser's output may be considered harmless when directed onto the unprotected skin, it poses a *potential* hazard to the eye if viewed along the axis of the beam (i.e. intrabeam viewing), due to the high degree of collimation of the laser light.

For this reason, the use of protective goggles, which must be appropriate for the wavelength(s) used, are recommended for operator and patient. Care is also recommended in ensuring that the beam is never directed towards the unprotected eye; the patient should be specifically warned about the ocular hazard associated with the device and asked not to stare directly at the treatment site during application. Furthermore, the laser treatment unit should ideally be used only in an area specifically designated for this purpose; outside this area, the appropriate laser warning symbols should be clearly displayed. Having outlined these fundamental safety rules, it is important to stress that the ocular hazard associated with therapeutic units is (for all practical purposes) negligible, especially where the treatment head or probe is used with the recommended 'in contact' technique (see *Principles of Application*).

Contraindications (see C.S.P. Safety of Electrotherapy Working Group, 1991)

Apart from direct treatment of the eye (for whatever reason), the use of low-intensity laser therapy is also contraindicated in the following cases:

1 *In patients with active or suspected carcinoma.* Studies at the cellular level testify to the potential photobiostimulatory effects of laser radiation; given this, it is possible that therapeutic laser application could accelerate carcinogenesis in patients where carcinoma is present.

Despite this potential danger, it should be stressed that laboratory studies in normal cells have consistently failed to demonstrate any carcinogenic effects of laser radiation; indeed, recent results would suggest that laser irradiation might affect DNA repair mechanisms (Logan et al., 1994).

2 *Direct irradiation over the pregnant uterus.* In the absence of hard evidence to show no associated hazard to foetus or mother, no direct treatment over the pregnant uterus represents a prudent and standard contraindication which applies to all forms of electrotherapy.

3 *Areas of haemorrhage.* This represents an absolute contraindication to laser treatment due to the possibility of laser induced vasodilatation, which would exacerbate the condition.

Other Safety Considerations

Whilst the above are usually regarded as the cardinal contraindications to treatment with low-intensity laser therapy, the Chartered Society of Physiotherapy's Safety of Electrotherapy Equipment Working Group also recommended the exercise of caution in a number of other situations.

Principally these included:

1 *Treatment of infected tissue (e.g. infected open wounds).* As laser light has the potential to stimulate the bacteria *Escherichia coli* in culture (vide Shields and O'Kane, 1994), it would seem only prudent to recommend caution in the application of laser therapy to infected tissue, and especially infected open wounds. However, the situation is far from clear as there is evidence to suggest that clinicians have successfully treated such conditions with laser therapy, and in some cases regard the presence of infection as an *indication* for such treatment (Baxter et al., 1991).

2 *Treatment over the sympathetic ganglia, vagus nerves and cardiac region in patients with heart disease.* In such cases, the possibility of laser-mediated alterations in neural activity resulting in adverse effects upon cardiac function can represent an unacceptable risk for these patients.

3 *Treatment over photosensitive areas.* Patients with a history of photosensitivity (e.g. adverse reactions to sunlight) should be treated with care, and in such cases the use of a test dose is recommended. In addition, the current use of photosensitizing drugs should also be excluded.

References

Abergel, RP, Lyons, RF, Castel, JC (1987) Biostimulation of wound healing by lasers; experimental approaches in animal models and fibroblast cultures. *Journal of Dermatological Surgery Oncology,* 13: 127–133.

Amoils, S, Kues, J (1991) The effect of low level laser therapy on acute headache syndromes. *Laser Therapy,* 3: 155–157.

Baldry, P (1989) *Acupuncture, trigger points and musculoskeletal pain.* Churchill Livingstone: Edinburgh.

Basford, JR (1986) Low energy laser treatment of pain and wounds: hype, hope or hokum? *Mayo Clinic Proceedings,* 61: 671–675.

Basford, JR (1989) Low-energy laser therapy: controversies and new research findings. *Lasers Surgery Medicine,* 9: 1–5.

Basford, JR, Hallman, JO, Matsumoto, JY et al. (1993) Effects of 830 nm laser diode irradiation on median nerve function in normal subjects. *Lasers Surgery Medicine,* 13: 597–604.

Basford, JR, Sheffield, CG, Mair, SD et al. (1987) Low energy helium-neon laser treatment of thumb osteoarthritis. *Archives Physical Medicine Rehabilitation,* 68: 794–797.

Baxter, GD (1989) Laser acupuncture analgesia: an overview. *Acupuncture in Medicine,* 6: 57–60.

Baxter, GD (1994) *Therapeutic Lasers: Theory and Practice.* Edinburgh: Churchill Livingstone.

Baxter, GD, Bell, AJ, Ravey, J et al. (1991) Low level laser therapy: current clinical practice in Northern Ireland. *Physiotherapy,* 77: 171–178.

Baxter, GD, Walsh, DM, Lowe, AS et al. (1994) Effects of low intensity infrared laser irradiation upon conduction in the human median nerve in vivo. *Experimental Physiology,* 79: 227–234.

Bliddal, H, Hellesen, C, Ditlevsen, P et al. (1987) Soft laser therapy of rheumatoid arthritis. *Scandinavian Journal Rheumatology,* 16: 225–228.

Bosatra, M, Jucci, A, Olliano, P et al. (1984) In vitro fibroblast and dermis fibroblast activation by laser irradiation at low energy. *Dermatologica*, **168**: 157–162.

Boulton, M, Marshall, J (1986) He–Ne laser stimulation of human fibroblast proliferation and attachment in vitro. *Lasers in Life Sciences*, **1**: 125–134.

Brockhaus, A, Elger, CE (1990) Hypoalgesic efficacy of acupuncture on experimental pain in man. Comparison of laser acupuncture and needle acupuncture. *Pain*, **43**: 181–186.

Castro, DJ, Abergel, P, Meeker, C et al. (1983) Effects of Nd-Yag laser on DNA synthesis and collagen production in human skin fibroblast cultures. *Annals Plastic Surgery*, **11**: 214–222.

Chartered Society of Physiotherapy (1991) Guidelines for the safe use of lasers in physiotherapy. *Physiotherapy*, **77**: 169–170.

Choi, JJ, Srikantha, K, Wu, W-H (1986) A comparison of electroacupuncture, transcutaneous electrical nerve stimulation and laser photobiostimulation on pain relief and glucocorticoid excretion. *International Jnl Acupuncture Electrotherapeutics Research*, **11**: 45–51.

Devor, M (1990) What's in a beam for pain therapy? *Pain*, **43**: 139.

Ellis, N (1994) *Acupuncture in clinical practice: a guide for health professionals.* London: Chapman and Hall.

England, S, Farrell, AJ, Coppock, JS et al. (1989) Low power laser therapy of shoulder tendonitis. *Scandinavian Journal Rheumatology*, **18**: 427–431.

Enwemeka, CS, Rodriquez, O, Gall, NG et al. (1990) Correlative ultrastructural and biomechanical changes induced in regenerating tendons exposed to laser photostimulation. *Lasers Surgery Medicine*, Suppl. 2: 12.

Glykofridis, S, Diamantopoulos, C (1987) Comparison between laser acupuncture and physiotherapy. *Acupuncture in Medicine*, **4**: 6–9.

Goldman, JA, Chiapella, J, Casey, H et al. (1980) Laser therapy of rheumatoid arthritis. *Lasers Surgery Medicine*, **1**: 93–101.

Greathouse, DG, Currier, DP, Gilmore, RL (1985) Effects of clinical infrared laser on superficial radial nerve conduction. *Physical Therapy*, **65**: 1184–1187.

Haina, D, Brunner, R, Landthaler, M et al. (1982) Animal experiments in light induced wound healing. *Laser Basic Biomedical Research*, **22**: 1.

Hallman, HO, Basford, JR, O'Brien, JF et al. (1988) Does low energy He–Ne laser irradiation alter in vitro replication of human fibroblasts? *Lasers Surgery Medicine*, **8**: 125–129.

Hunter, JG, Leonard, LG, Snider, GR et al. (1984) Effects of low energy laser on wound healing in a porcine model. *Lasers Surgery Medicine*, **3**: 328.

Jensen, H, Harreby, M, Kjer, J (1987) Is infrared laser effective in painful arthrosis of the knee? *Ugeskr Laeger*, **149**: 3104–3106.

Karu, TI (1985) Biological action of low intensity visible monochromatic light and some of its medical applications. In *International Congress on Lasers in Medicine & Surgery*, June 26–28, Bologna, pp. 25–29. Monduzzi Editore: Bologna.

Khullar, SM, Brodin, P, Hanaes, HR (1994) The effects of low level laser therapy (LLLT) on function and neurophysiological activity in the injured rat sciatic nerve. *Laser Therapy*, **6**: 19.

King, PR (1990) Low level laser therapy: a review. *Physiotherapy Theory and Practice*, **6**: 127–138.

Kitchen, SS, Partridge, CJ (1991) A review of low level laser therapy. *Physiotherapy*, **77**: 161–167.

Lam, T, Abergel, P, Meeker, C et al. (1986) Low energy lasers selectively enhance collagen synthesis. *Lasers Life Sciences* **1**: 61–77.

Li, XH (1990) Laser in the department of traumatology. With a report of 60 cases of soft tissue injury. *Laser Therapy*, **2**: 119–122.

Logan, ID, Craig, HE, Barnett, Y (1994) Low intensity laser irradiation induces DNA repair in X-Ray damaged friend erythroleukaemia and HL-60 cells. *Laser Therapy*, **6**: 30.

Lonauer, G (1986) Controlled double blind study on the efficacy of He–Ne laser beams versus He–Ne plus infrared laser beams in the therapy of activated osteoarthritis of finger joints. *Lasers Surgery Medicine*, **6**: 172.

Lowe, AS, Baxter, GD, Walsh, DM et al. (1994) The effect of low intensity laser (830 nm) irradiation upon skin temperature and antidromic conduction latencies in the human median nerve: relevance of radiant exposure. *Lasers Surgery Medicine*, **14**: 40–46.

Lowe, AS, McDowell, BC, Walsh, DM et al. (1994) Failure to demonstrate any hypoalgesic effect of low intensity laser irradiation of Erb's Point upon experimental ischaemic pain in humans. *Lasers Surgery Medicine*, (in press).

Lukashevich, IG (1985) Use of a helium-neon laser in facial pains. *Stomatologiia*, **64**: 29–31.

Lundeberg, T, Haker, E, Thomas, M (1987) Effects of laser versus placebo in tennis elbow. *Scandinavian Journal Rehabilitation Medicine*, **19**: 135–138.

Lyons, RF, Abergel, RP, White, RA et al. (1987) Biostimulation of wound healing in vivo by a helium neon laser. *Annals Plastic Surgery*, **18**: 47–50.

Mester, AF, Mester, A (1989) Wound healing. *Laser Therapy*, **1**: 7–15.

Mester, E, Korenyi-Both, A, Spiry, T et al. (1975) The effect of laser irradiation on the regeneration of muscle fibers. *Zeitschrift Experimentelle Chirurgie*, **8**: 258–262.

Mester, E, Mester, AF, Mester, A (1985) The biomedical effects of laser application. *Lasers Surgery Medicine*, **5**: 31–39.

Mokhtar, B, Walker, D, Baxter, GD et al. (1992) A double blind placebo controlled investigation of the hypoalgesic effects of low intensity laser irradiation of the cervical nerve roots using experimental ischaemic pain. In *Proceedings, Second Meeting, International Laser Therapy Association*, 61.

Moore, KC, Hira, N, Kumar, PS et al. (1988) A double blind crossover trial of low level laser therapy in the treatment of post herpetic neuralgia. *Laser Therapy*, Pilot Issue, 7–9.

Oshiro, T, Calderhead, RG (1988) *Low Level Laser Therapy: A Practical Introduction.* Chichester: Wiley.

Ohta, A, Abergel, RP, Vitto, J et al. (1987) Laser modulation of human immune system: Inhibition of lymphocyte proliferation by Gallium-Arsenide laser at low energy. *Lasers Surgery Medicine*, **7**: 199–201.

O'Kane, S, Shields, TD, Gilmore, WS et al. (1994) Low intensity laser irradiation inhibits tritiated thymidine incorporation in the haemopoietic cell lines HL-60 and U-937. *Lasers Surgery Medicine*, **14**: 34–39.

Palmgren, N, Jensen, GF, Kaae, K et al. (1989) Low power laser in rheumatoid arthritis. *Lasers Medical Science*, **4**: 193–196.

Ponnudurai, RN, Zbuzek, VK, Niu, H-L et al. (1988) Laser photobiostimulation-induced hypoalgesia in rats is not naloxone reversible. *International Jnl. Acupuncture Electrother. Res.*, **13**: 109–117.

Ponnudurai, RN, Zbuzek, VK, Wu, W (1987) Hypoalgesic effect of laser photobiostimulation shown by rat tail flick test. *International Jnl. Acupuncture Electrotherapeutics Research*, **12**: 93–100.

Rajaratnam, S, Bolton, P, Dyson, M (1994) Macrophage responsiveness to laser therapy with varying pulsing frequencies. *Laser Therapy*, **6**: 107–112.

Robinson, B, Walters, J (1991) The use of low level laser therapy in diabetic and other ulcerations. *Journal British Podiatric Medicine*, **46**: 10.

Rochkind, S, Rousso, M, Nissan, M et al. (1989) Systemic effects of low power laser irradiation on the peripheral and central nervous system, cutaneous wounds and burns. *Lasers Surgery Medicine*, **9**: 174–182.

Rochkind, S, Alon, M, Dekel, S et al. (1994a) Peripheral nerve and brachial plexus injuries: results of surgery and/or low level laser therapy. *Laser Therapy*, **6**: 53.

Rochkind, S, Alon, M, Sosnov, Y et al. (1994b) Severe spinal cord or cauda equina injuries: results of low level laser therapy *Laser Therapy*. **6**: 55.

Santionnai, P, Monfrecola, G, Martellotta, D et al. (1984) Inadequate effect of Helium-Neon laser on venous leg ulcers. *Photodermatology*, **1**: 245–249.

Seibert, DD, Gould, WR (1984) The effect of laser stimulation on burning pain threshold. *Physical Therapy*, **64**: 746.

Shields, D, O'Kane, S (1994) Laser photobiomodulation of wound healing. In Baxter, GD (ed) *Therapeutic Lasers: Theory and Practice.* Edinburgh: Churchill Livingstone.

Shiroto, C, Ono, K, Onshiro, T (1989) Retrospective study of diode laser therapy for pain attenuation in 3635 patients: detailed analysis by questionnaire. *Laser Therapy*, **1**: 41–48.

Siebert, W, Siechert, N, Siebert, B et al. (1987) What is the efficacy of 'soft' and 'mid' lasers in therapy of tendinopathies? *Archives Orthopaedic and Traumatic Surgery*, **106**: 358–363.

Snyder-Mackler, L, Bork, CE (1988) Effect of Helium-Neon laser irradiation on peripheral sensory nerve latency. *Physical Therapy*, **68**: 223–225.

Sugrue, ME, Carolan, J, Leen, EJ et al. (1990) The use of infra-red laser therapy in the treatment of venous ulcerations. *Annals Vascular Surgery*, **4**: 179–181.

Trelles, MA, Rigau, J, Sala, P et al. (1991) Infrared diode laser in low reactive-level laser therapy (LLLT) for knee osteoarthrosis. *Laser Therapy*, **3**: 149–153.

van Breugel, HHF, Engels, C, Bar PR (1993) Mechanisms of action in laser-induced photo-biomodulation depend on the wavelength of the laser. *Lasers Surgery Medicine*, Suppl. **5**: 9.

Vidovich, D, Olson, DR (1987) Neodymium YAG laser stimulation as a treatment modality in acute and chronic pain syndromes and in rheumatoid arthritis. *Lasers Surgery Medicine*, **7**: 79.

Walker, J (1983) Relief from chronic pain by low power laser irradiation. *Neuroscience Letters*, **43**: 339–344.

Walker, J, Akhanjee, LK (1985) Laser-induced somatosensory evoked potential: evidence of photosensitivity in peripheral nerves. *Brain Research*, **344**: 281–285.

Walker, J, Akhanjee, LK, Cooney, MM et al. (1987) Laser therapy for pain of rheumatoid arthritis. *Clinical Journal Pain*, **3**: 54–59.

Walsh, DM (1993) *Investigations of the neurophysiological and hypoalgesic effects of low intensity laser therapy and transcutaneous electrical nerve stimulation.* DPhil Thesis: University of Ulster.

Waylonis, GW, Wilkie, S, O'Toole, D et al. (1988) Chronic myofascial pain: management by low output helium-neon laser therapy. *Archives Physical Medicine Rehabilitation*, **69**: 1017–1020.

Wu, W (1983) Recent advances in laserpuncture. In Atsumi, K (ed) *New Frontiers in Laser Medicine and Surgery.* Amsterdam: Elsevier.

Wu, W-H, Ponnudurai, R, Katz, J et al. (1987) Failure to confirm report of light-evoked response of peripheral nerve to low power Helium-Neon laser light stimulus. *Brain Research*, **401**: 407–408.

Zarkovic, N, Manev, H, Pericic, D et al. (1989) Effect of semiconductor GaAs laser irradiation on pain perception in mice. *Lasers Surgery Medicine*, **9**: 63–66.

14

Ultraviolet Therapy

BRIAN DIFFEY AND PETER FARR

Introduction

The foundation of modern-day ultraviolet (UV) phototherapy began with the work of the Danish physician Niels Finsen, who is best remembered for his successful treatment of cutaneous tuberculosis, and who, in 1903, was awarded the Nobel Prize for Medicine in recognition of this work. Following the pioneering work of Finsen, the early part of the twentieth century saw the rapid expansion of heliotherapy (using the sun as the source of radiation) and actinotherapy (using lamps as the source) throughout Europe and the USA for the treatment of many skin diseases. The practice of actinotherapy continued to expand through the middle part of the twentieth cen-

tury and was accompanied by an enormous literature on the subject during the 1920s and 1930s. This rapid growth is reflected by the many revisions of the handbook *Actinotherapy Technique*, which was first published by the Sollux Publishing Company in 1933 and was reprinted for the ninth time (7th edition) in 1949. Most of the irradiation protocols for the countless number of diseases described in this book are now of historical interest only. The advent of effective antibiotics and the realization that the successes claimed in many of these diseases were little more than anecdotal have resulted today in a much reduced role of ultraviolet radiation in clinical medicine. This applies also to the treatment of conditions such as leg ulcers and pressure sores which, although still treated by UV radiation in some physiotherapy departments, are more effectively managed by techniques such as modern drug therapy and skilled nursing practice. For this reason, the water-cooled Kromayer lamp, familiar to many physiotherapists, will not be covered in this chapter.

On the other hand, one of the major contributions to dermatological practice in the past 20 years has been the introduction of a treatment for several skin diseases, including psoriasis, known as photochemotherapy; the combination of ultraviolet radiation (UVR) and photoactive drugs producing a beneficial effect in the skin.

The first sources of artificial ultraviolet radiation were carbon arc lamps of the type developed by Finsen at around the turn of the century. These lamps were unpopular in clinical practice because of their noise, odour and sparks, and were superseded by the development of mercury arc lamps. Fluorescent lamps were developed in the late 1940s and, since then, a variety of phosphor and envelope materials have been used to produce lamps with different emissions in the ultraviolet region, such that today there exists a wide range of lamps which are used for the phototherapy of skin diseases.

The Nature of Ultraviolet Radiation

Ultraviolet radiation covers a small part of the electromagnetic spectrum. Other regions of this spectrum include radiowaves, microwaves, infrared radiation (heat), visible light, x-rays and gamma radiation. The feature that characterizes the properties of any particular region of the spectrum is the wavelength of the radiation.

Ultraviolet radiation spans the wavelength region from 400–100 nm. Even in the ultraviolet por-

tion of the spectrum the biological effects of the radiation vary enormously with wavelength and, for this reason, the ultraviolet spectrum is further subdivided into three regions:

1 UVA: 400–320 nm;
2 UVB: 320–290 nm;
3 UVC: 290–200 nm.

The divisions between the different wavebands are not rigidly fixed, and 315 nm is sometimes taken as the boundary between UVA and UVB, and 280 nm as that between UVB and UVC.

It has been common practice in physiotherapy to talk of *ultraviolet light* or *UVL*. This is incorrect; the term *light* should be reserved for those wavelengths of radiation (approximately 400–700 nm) which reach the retina and result in a sensation of vision. The correct term is *ultraviolet radiation* or *UVR*.

Production of Ultraviolet Radiation

Ultraviolet radiation is produced artificially by the passage of an electric current through a gas, usually vaporized mercury. The mercury atoms become excited by collisions with the electrons flowing between the lamp's electrodes. These excited electrons return to particular electronic states in the mercury atom and in doing so release some of the energy they have absorbed in the form of radiation, that is, ultraviolet, visible and infrared radiation.

The spectrum of the radiation emitted consists of a limited number of discrete wavelengths (so-called 'spectral lines') corresponding to electron transitions which are characteristic of the mercury atom; the relative intensity of the different wavelengths in the spectrum depends upon the pressure of the mercury vapour. For lamps containing mercury vapour at about atmospheric pressure (medium-pressure mercury arc lamps), radiation is emitted with several different wavelengths in the UVC, UVB, UVA, visible and near infrared (IR-A) regions. By adding traces of metal halides, such as lead iodide or iron iodide, to mercury vapour lamps, both the power and the composition of the spectrum emitted, particularly in the UVA and visible regions, may be enhanced.

The other common way of producing ultraviolet radiation is by fluorescent lamps, or tubes. A fluorescent lamp is a low-pressure mercury vapour lamp which has a phosphor coating applied to the inside of the glass tube (sometimes referred to as the *envelope*). At low pressures in mercury vapour there is a predominant spectral line at a wavelength of 253.7 nm, and radiation of this wavelength is efficiently absorbed by the phosphor. This results in the re-emission of radiation of longer wavelengths by the phenomenon of fluorescence. The wavelength range of the fluorescent radiation will be a property of the chemical nature of the phosphor material. Phosphors are available which produce

Figure 14.1   The spectral power distribution of ultraviolet radiation from a medium-pressure mercury arc lamp of the type used in an Alpine Sunlamp. The graph shows the intensity of the radiation emitted at each wavelength. The specific wavelengths are characteristic of mercury and are the same irrespective of the manufacturer of the mercury lamp, although the intensity at the different wavelengths may differ. The prominent wavelengths (*spectral lines*) in the ultraviolet region from a mercury lamp are at 254, 265, 280, 297, 302, 313, 334 and 365 nm. There are also spectral lines in the visible spectrum (not shown on the graph) which occur at 405 (violet), 436 (blue), 546 (green), and 578 (yellow) nm, which combine to give these lamps a bright white light.

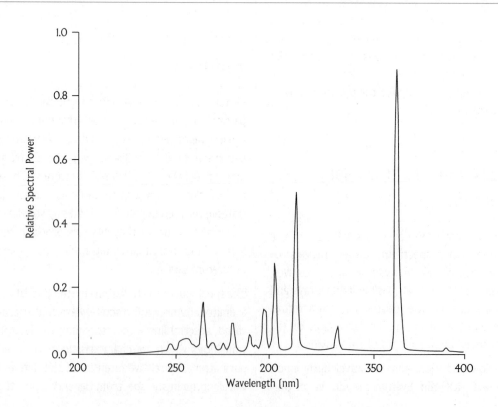

their fluorescence radiation mainly in the visible region (for artificial lighting purposes), the UVA, or the UVB regions.

Spectral Power Distribution

It is common practice to talk loosely of 'UVA lamps' or 'UVB lamps'. However, such a label does not characterize ultraviolet lamps adequately since nearly all phototherapy lamps will emit UVA and UVB, and even UVC, visible light, and infrared radiation. The only correct way to specify the nature of the emitted radiation is by reference to the spectral power distribution. This is a graph (or table) which indicates the radiated power as a function of wavelength. Figure 14.1 shows the spectral power distribution of ultraviolet radiation emitted by a medium-pressure mercury arc lamp (commonly called a 'hot quartz' lamp in the USA). This type of lamp has been used for many years for the phototherapy of skin diseases in apparatus such as the Alpine Sunlamp. The exact shape of the spectrum, particularly at wavelengths of less than 300 nm, depends on factors including the lamp envelope material and the vapour pressure of the mercury. The spectrum of several other lamps used for phototherapy can be found in Diffey (1990a).

Stability of Radiation Output

The radiation output from ultraviolet lamps will fluctuate with factors such as the voltage of the mains supply and operating temperature. Medium- and high-pressure lamps take several minutes to reach a stable output since, shortly after striking these lamps, there is an excess of liquid mercury which vaporizes during the heating process. Also, since these lamps cannot be struck again until they have cooled down, it is not feasible to switch them on and off between patients unless there is a gap of about 30 minutes or more. Fluorescent lamps, on the other hand, reach their full output within 1 minute of switching on, and yield maximum radiation output when the lamp is running in free air at an ambient temperature of about 25°C. As the temperature increases, the output decreases, and this can be a problem in irradiation units which incorporate large numbers of fluorescent lamps packed closely together (unless adequate, forced-air cooling is incorporated into the unit).

Some medium- and high-pressure lamps will be located behind optical glass filters in order to remove unwanted components of the emission spectrum. The problem here is that glass filters will change their transmission spectrum as they heat up and this can result in an appreciable change in both the quality (or spectrum) and quantity (or dose) of UVR received during irradiation if patients are treated shortly after switching on the lamps. The solution is to run the lamp for 20 minutes or so before exposing patients to allow the glass filters to reach thermal equilibrium.

The output from ultraviolet lamps deteriorates with time. There is a 'running-in' time with all lamps during which period the rate of fall in radiation output is considerably greater than for later times. For fluorescent lamps, the running-in period is about 100 hours, but is only about 20 hours for medium- and high-pressure lamps. The useful lifetime of most ultraviolet lamps is between 500 and 1000 hours. After this period, the output will have fallen to around 80% of the value at the end of the running-in period.

The UV output of medium- and high-pressure lamps deteriorates more rapidly than the visible light output. With fluorescent lamps, however, the relative decrease in radiation output with usage is more or less independent of wavelength — in other words, the spectrum of the radiation

Brian Diffey and Peter Farr

remains approximately constant even though the absolute radiation output decreases.

Biological Effects of Ultraviolet Radiation

Effects on Skin

ERYTHEMA

Erythema, or redness of the skin due to dilatation of superficial dermal blood vessels, is one of the commonest and most obvious effects of ultraviolet exposure ('sunburn'). The potential for development of erythema is the major factor which limits the exposure that may be given during phototherapy. Erythema is usually encountered only when UVB treatment is used as, without psoralen sensitization (see the section *Psoralen Photochemotherapy* below), the skin is between 100 and 1000 times less sensitive to UVA than to UVB.

The mechanism of erythema production following ultraviolet exposure is understood poorly. It is known that erythema from UVB is mediated, at least in part, by the release from the epidermis of pharmacologically active compounds, such as prostaglandins, which diffuse to act on dermal blood vessels. The erythemal response may also be related to the DNA-damaging effects of UVR, as patients with the rare condition of xeroderma pigmentosum, in which there are defective mechanisms to repair UVR-induced DNA damage, also have abnormal erythemal responses to UVR. Further details of this and other light-related disorders can be found in Magnus (1976).

Following UVR exposure, there is usually a latent period of 2–4 hours before erythema develops, although after sufficient exposure to UVA some immediate erythema may occur. Ultraviolet-induced erythema reaches maximum intensity between 8 and 24 hours after exposure, but may take several days to resolve completely. If a high enough exposure has occurred, the skin will also become painful and oedematous, and blistering may result.

The smallest dose of UVR to result in erythema that is just detectable by eye at between 8 and 24 hours after exposure is termed the *minimal erythema dose* (MED). The MED is measured normally by exposing small areas of normal skin, usually on the back, to different doses of UVR. Ideally, a series of doses increasing geometrically is used (e.g. successive doses increasing by 40%). This is a widely used indicator of an individual's sensitivity to UVR, and is a useful clinical measure of exposure as the goal of many phototherapy regimens is to achieve a mild degree of erythema. The MED shows a wide variation between individuals: even within Caucasians, a 4–6-fold difference in MED will occur between those who burn easily in sunlight and those who rarely burn. At doses higher than the MED, the intensity of erythema increases rapidly, e.g. an exposure of twice the MED (2MED) would result in erythema of moderate intensity, but 3 MED might cause a severe and painful response. The characteristics of erythema induced in psoralen-sensitized skin during PUVA therapy are different in a number of important respects (see the section *Psoralen Photochemotherapy* p. 231).

TANNING

Another consequence of exposure to UVR (which at present still seems to be socially desirable) is the delayed pigmentation of the skin known as *tanning*, or melanin pigmentation. Melanin pigmentation of skin is of two types: constitutive (the colour of the skin seen in different races and determined by genetic factors only), and facultative (the reversible increase in tanning in response to UVR and other external stimuli).

Individuals may be classified according to their self-reported erythemal and pigmentary response to natural sunlight exposure. This skin type system is used widely to choose a starting dose of UVR at the beginning of a course of phototherapy. However, wide variation in MED values occur both within each skin-type category and between categories, limiting its clinical usefulness. The four categories of ths skin type system are as follows:

- Group I – always burns, never tans;
- Group II – always burns, sometimes tans;
- Group III – sometimes burns, always tans;
- Group IV – never burns, always tans.

HYPERPLASIA

In addition to tanning, the skin is capable of another, perhaps even more important adaptive response, which limits damage from further ultraviolet exposure – epidermal thickening or hyperplasia. This begins to occur around 72 hours after exposure, is a result of an increased rate of division of basal epidermal cells, and results eventually in thickening of both epidermis and stratum corneum which persist for several weeks (for further details see Johnson, 1984). This adaptive process, unlike tanning, occurs with all skin types, and is the major factor which protects those who tan poorly in sunlight (skin types I and II). That epidermal hyperplasia occurs mainly following UVB exposure, rather than UVA, is shown by the poor sunburn protection achieved with a UVA only-induced tan (e.g. from a sunbed) compared with an equivalent tan achieved from natural sunlight exposure (UVA and UVB).

The adaptive processes of tanning and epidermal hyperplasia that occur during a course of phototherapy treatment mean that, in order to maintain an effective dose of UVR at the key target site in the skin (considered for most disorders to be around the basal layer of the epidermis), the exposure dose to the skin surface needs to be gradually increased (see the sections on treatment regimens in *Phototherapy* and *Psoralen Photochemotherapy* below).

PRODUCTION OF VITAMIN D

The skin absorbs UVB radiation in sunlight and converts sterol precursors in the skin, such as 7-dehydrocholesterol, to vitamin D_3. Vitamin D_3 is further transformed by the liver and kidneys to biologically active metabolites such as 25-hydroxyvitamin D; these metabolites then act on the intestinal mucosa to facilitate calcium absorption, and on bone to facilitate calcium exchange.

AGEING OF THE SKIN

Chronic exposure to sunlight can result in an appearance of the skin often referred to as premature ageing or actinic damage. The clinical changes associated with skin ageing include a dry, coarse, leathery appearance, laxity with wrinkling, and various pigmentary changes. These changes are believed to be due mainly to exposure to the ultraviolet component of sunlight.

SKIN CANCER

The three common forms of skin cancer, listed in order of seriousness, are: basal-cell carcinoma, squamous-cell carcinoma and malignant melanoma. Exposure to UVR is considered to be a major aetiological factor for all three forms of cancer. For basal-cell carcinoma and malignant melanoma, neither the wavelengths involved nor the exposure pattern that results in risk have been established with certainty; whereas for squamous-cell carcinoma, both UVB and UVA are implicated, and the major risk factors seem to be cumulative lifetime exposure to UVR and a poor tanning response (e.g. skin types I and II). The development of squamous-cell carcinoma is a significant risk for patients treated for long periods with psoralen photochemotherapy (see the section *Psoralen Photochemotherapy* below).

Effects on Eyes

PHOTOKERATITIS AND CONJUNCTIVITIS

The acute effects of exposure to UVC and UVB radiation are primarily those of conjunctivitis and photokeratitis.

Conjunctivitis is an inflammation of the membrane which lines the insides of the eyelids and covers the cornea; it may often be accompanied by an erythema of the skin around the eyelids. There is the sensation of 'gritty eyes' and also varying degrees of photophobia (aversion to light), lacrimation (tears), and blepharospasm (spasm of the eyelid muscles) may be present.

Photokeratitis is an inflammation of the cornea that can result in severe pain. Ordinary clinical photokeratitis is characterized by a period of latency that tends to vary inversely with the severity of UV exposure. The latent period may be as short as 30 minutes or as long as 24 hours, but it is typically 6–12 hours. The acute symptoms of visual incapacitation usually lasts from 6–24 hours. Almost all discomfort usually disappears within 2 days and rarely does exposure result in permanent damage. Unlike the skin, the ocular system does not develop tolerance to repeated exposure to UVR. Many cases of photokeratitis have been reported following exposure to UVR produced by welding arcs and by the reflection of solar radiation from snow and sand. For this reason, the condition is sometimes referred to as 'welders flash', or 'arc eye', or 'snow blindness'.

CATARACT

A cataract is a partial or complete loss of transparency of the lens or its capsule. The mechanism of formation of cataracts probably involves several factors but, from epidemiological studies, there is some evidence that sunlight, particularly the UVB component, plays a role.

In PUVA therapy (see the section *Psoralen Photochemotherapy* below) patients are administered photosensitizing drugs called psoralens which are deposited in the lens. Evidence from animal studies shows that subsequent UVA irradiation can lead to cataract formation and, for this reason, adequate eye protection should always be worn for 12 hours or so following the ingestion of psoralens.

Phototherapy

Treatment of skin disease by exposure to UVR is termed *phototherapy*, and is often used in combination with agents applied topically (for example, dithranol plus UVB phototherapy for psoriasis). When treatment with UVR is combined with a photosensitizing agent (for example psoralen plus UVA exposure), the term *photochemotherapy* is used.

Diseases which are Treated by Ultraviolet Phototherapy

Diseases that are treated with ultraviolet phototherapy are:

- Psoriasis;
- Eczema;
- Acne;
- Pityriasis lichenoides;
- Polymorphic light eruption (and other photo-sensitive disorders);
- Pruritus (particularly related to renal disease).

The vast majority of patients treated with ultraviolet phototherapy will have psoriasis, eczema (particularly atopic eczema) or acne. UVB phototherapy is also used to treat a number of photosensitive skin disorders, only one of which (polymorphic light eruption) is at all common. Increased tolerance to sun exposure is achieved by tanning and skin thickening and, probably of equal importance, by immunological and pharmacological actions (see, for example, Farr and Diffey, 1988).

Spectrum of Therapeutic Response

The erythemal or 'sunburn' sensitivity of the skin varies greatly with the wavelength of ultraviolet radiation; UVB being 100–1000 more potent at inducing erythema than UVA. The variation in erythemal sensitivity may be depicted graphically as an action spectrum (Figure 14.2); other effects of ultraviolet exposure can be described in a similar way, e.g. the relative effectiveness of

Figure 14.2   A plot of effectiveness of radiation against wavelength (action spectrum) for erythema (dashed line) and for the clearance of psoriasis with daily phototherapy (solid line). The two curves diverge at wavelengths shorter than 290 nm where even doses greater than 10-times the MED fail to result in clearance of psoriasis. A logarithmic scale has been used for the vertical axis in order to allow the large change in response of the skin with wave length to be visible, together with relatively small but biologically-important differences between the two curves. (Figure modified form Parrish JA, Jaenicke KF (1981) Action spectrum for phototherapy of psoriasis. *J Invest Dermatol* 76: 359–362).

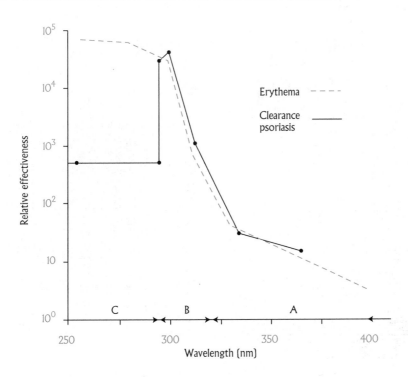

different wavelengths at healing skin disease. Unfortunately, at present, only the action spectrum for the clearance of psoriasis with ultraviolet phototherapy is established with any degree of certainty (Parrish and Jaenicke, 1981). Figure 14.2 shows that for wavelengths shorter than 290 nm, even when doses are used that are considerably in excess of the MED, no healing of psoriasis occurs. With wavelengths longer than 290 nm, the action spectrum for clearance of psoriasis is very similar to that for the development of erythema. This has important implications for the selection of ultraviolet lamps to treat psoriasis: lamps with a large

component of UVC will produce erythema easily but will not clear psoriasis. Based on this therapeutic action spectrum, lamps have been designed specifically to treat psoriasis (such as the Philips TL01), and have been shown to be more effective than conventional UVB lamps. It is to be hoped that more efficient treatment will become available for the other diseases in which ultraviolet phototherapy is used once further disease-specific action spectra have been determined.

Ultraviolet Lamps for Phototherapy

Ultraviolet sources for phototherapy are either arc lamps or fluorescent lamps. The arc lamp that is most widely used in physiotherapy departments is the single, medium-pressure mercury arc lamp (Figure 14.3) typified by the Alpine Sunlamp and

Figure 14.3   The Alpine Sunlamp (Hanovia Ltd, Slough, England). This unit incorporates a 220-watt medium-pressure mercury arc lamp mounted at the focus of a parabolic reflector.

Figure 14.4   Three columns, each incorporating 5 high pressure metal halide lamps (courtesy of Uvalight Technology Ltd, Birmingham, England).

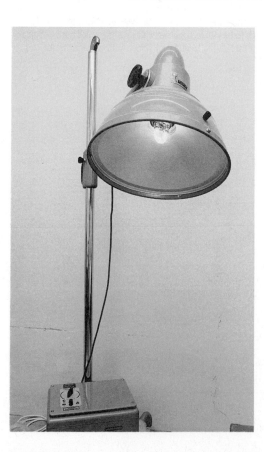

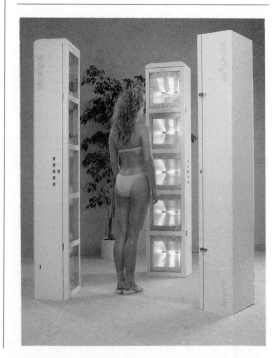

Hohensonne lamp. This type of lamp emits a broad spectrum of ultraviolet radiation (Figure 14.1) with significant quantities at wavelengths shorter than 290 nm which, although ineffective in clearing psoriasis, contributes appreciably to skin reddening (see section *Spectrum of Therapeutic response* above).

Mercury arc lamps can be made more efficient by adding a metal halide to the lamp to enhance the radiation spectrum, and housing the lamp behind a glass filter which absorbs radiation at wavelengths below about 290 nm but transmits at longer wavelengths. Stacking lamps in a vertical column and using 2 or more columns simultaneously improves the uniformity of irradiation and reduces treatment times. An example of a unit of this type is shown in Figure 14.4.

A survey of the practice of phototherapy in the UK carried out in 1993 (Dootson *et al.*, 1994) showed that 70% of treatment machines for whole-body irradiation incorporate fluorescent lamps, rather than arc lamps. In this survey, the machine used most frequently was the Theraktin ultraviolet bath or tunnel. This is a semicylindrical frame containing four 120 cm-long fluorescent lamps with an ultraviolet spectrum extending from 270–400 nm, peaking at 310 nm. The frame is normally suspended from a ceiling. This unit has several drawbacks, which include low irradiance and uneven skin exposure, often with relative sparing of the lower legs and sides of trunk. It has no place in a modern phototherapy service. More efficient units are either:

- Semicylindrical or cylindrical cubicles incorporating up to 48 fluorescent lamps, extending for 2 m in length, and mounted vertically around the inner circumference;

Figure 14.5   A bed and canopy incorporating a total of 28 Helarium (UVB) fluorescent lamps (courtesy of Sun Health Services Ltd, Crowborough, England).

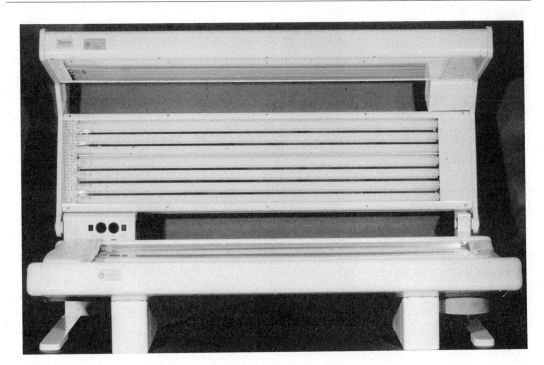

Figure 14.6 A whole-body cubicle incorporating 27 UVA lamps (shown illuminated) and 13 UVB fluorescent lamps (not illuminated) which can be used for either UVB or PUVA therapy (model 7001K, Waldmann GmbH, Schwenningen, Germany).

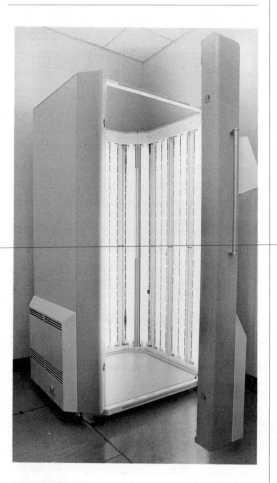

- A bed and canopy incorporating up to 28 fluorescent lamps for simultaneous anterior and posterior irradiation with patients lying supine (Figure 14.5).

Some cylindrical cubicles incorporate a mixture of UVB and UVA fluorescent lamps (Figure 14.6). The advantage of such a cubicle is that the one machine can be used for phototherapy (when the UVB lamps are switched on) or PUVA therapy (when the UVA lamps are switched on). The disadvantage is that both UVB and UVA irradiances are lower than can be obtained from a unit incorporating just one type of lamp. Consequently, longer treatment times are necessary, but this may not be a problem in a department with a low throughput of patients.

There are several types of UVB fluorescent lamps with varying spectral emissions, as indicated in Table 14.1.

Irradiation with lamps such as the Sylvania UV21 and Philips TL12 requires shorter exposure times than with lamps such as the Sylvania UV6, Wolff Helarium or Philips TL01 in which the spectrum is shifted to longer wavelengths and considerably less UVC is present. However, for a given degree of erythema the latter three lamps will be more effective because they emit much less erythemally effective, but therapeutically ineffective, radiation

Table 14.1
Spectral properties of different UVB fluorescent lamps used in phototherapy

| Type of UVB fluorescent lamp | Wavelength range and spectral peak (% of total ultraviolet) | | | | |
	Range (nm)	Peak (nm)	UVA	UVB	UVC
Philips TL12	276–380	313	34	60	6
Sylvania UV21	276–380	313	34	60	6
Sylvania UV6	286–370	313	40	59	< 1
Wolff Helarium	295–400	340	92	8	0
Philips TL01	300–320	311	10	90	0

at wavelengths shorter than 290 nm. An appraisal of the different lamps used for phototherapy has been given by Diffey and Farr (1987).

TREATMENT TIMES

Treatment times depend not only upon the spectrum of the radiation, but also upon factors such as electrical power, number of lamps, lamp-to-skin distance and differences in patient susceptibility to UVR. Initial treatment times with most phototherapy lamps are about 0.5–3 minutes. Treatment times need to be increased throughout a course of phototherapy in order to maintain an erythema on increasingly acclimatized skin (see section on treatment regimens in *Phototherapy*).

UNIFORMITY OF IRRADIATION

Single lamps, such as the Alpine Sunlamp (Figure 14.3), limit radiation to regions such as the chest or back. In order to achieve whole-body irradiation, the lamp-to-patient distance is so great that the treatment times become unacceptably long. Most modern phototherapy units incorporate several lamps and are designed for partial- or whole-body irradiation. Studies have shown that the vertical distribution of ultraviolet radiation in phototherapy cabinets is non-uniform when fluorescent lamps are used, with a reduction in intensity of between 20 and 50% near the ends of the tubes compared with the middle, resulting in significantly lower radiation doses at the extremities. In contrast, when columns incorporating five or six high-pressure metal halide lamps are, used as shown in Figure 14.4, the vertical variation of radiation intensity is normally no more than 10% (Chue *et al.*, 1988).

Phototherapy lamps of the type shown in Figure 14.4 have the advantage that not all of the lamps need to be switched on, so that partial-body irradiation is possible. This is not the case with fluorescent lamp systems, although fluorescent lamps are available in a variety of lengths ranging from 30 cm to 2 m so that units designed for treating small areas, such as the hands or feet, are available.

In addition to geometrical problems associated with the lamps, variation in irradiance over a patient's skin will depend also on the topology and self-shielding of the patient's body. Measurements of the ultraviolet dose received at different body sites have shown that a large fraction of the body surface area receives more than 70% of the maximum dose which occurs on the trunk, while areas such as the groin and axillae receive a smaller fraction, as expected (Diffey *et al.*, 1978).

INSTALLATION REQUIREMENTS

Single lamps require no special electrical supply or room modification. With whole-body systems, however, it may be necessary to install a high-current mains electrical supply. Consideration should also be given to maintaining a satisfactory environmental temperature by installing air conditioning units.

In the UK there are no specific guidelines published on the installation of phototherapy machines. This type of apparatus falls under the umbrella of Medical Electrical Equipment and as such it should be installed in compliance with the British Standard BS5724. Standards in other countries should be consulted as appropriate.

SERVICING

There is very little required in the way of servicing phototherapy units. Lamp surfaces should be cleaned regularly to remove dust and skin, both of which will attenuate the radiation. Lamps should be replaced when the irradiance has dropped sufficiently low that treatment times become unacceptably long. When this point occurs depends very much on local circumstances and workload. Changing lamps, both high-pressure and fluorescent, is a tedious but straightforward process and could be carried out by electronics technicians from either the Medical Physics or Works Departments within a hospital. Maintenance contracts on phototherapy equipment which are offered by some suppliers are probably unnecessary and uneconomical if competent support is available locally.

UVB Dosimetry

Dosimetry is the science of radiation measurement. There are two principal reasons why ultraviolet radiation should be measured:

1 To allow consistent radiation exposure of patients over many months and years within a local department;
2 To allow the results of irradiations made in different departments to be published and compared.

It is important to distinguish between these two objectives. The first requires *precision*, or reproducibility. The dosemeter is used as a monitor to give a reference measurement and so needs to be stable. *Accuracy*, that is, absolute calibration against some accepted standard, is not essential. The second objective requires both precision *and* accuracy. Here the dosemeter must not only be stable from one day to the next, but also the display (in milliwatts per square centimetre, mW/cm^2) must be traceable to absolute standards.

Ultraviolet radiation exposure of patients in most centres is prescribed in units of time. Where exposure is prescribed in radiometric units (J/cm^2) it is generally limited to the newer whole-body machines which often incorporate internal dosimetry systems. The problem with attempting to make absolute measurements of irradiance and dose in UVB phototherapy is that it can lead easily to misunderstanding. The erythemal sensitivity of skin changes very rapidly with wavelength in the UVB waveband; at 300 nm the skin is 100 times more sensitive than at 320 nm. Thus, the dose of UVB radiation from a particular lamp necessary to result in a given degree of erythema depends strongly on the spectral emission of the lamp. For example, about 50 mJ/cm^2 of UVB from the TL12 lamps used in a Theraktin unit would produce minimal erythema 8–24 hours later in unacclimatized white skin. The UVB doses required to produce the same degree of erythema from an Alpine Sunlamp or a phototherapy unit containing either UV21, UV6 or TL01 fluorescent lamps (all of which are referred to as *UVB lamps*) are 20, 50, 100, and 300 mJ/cm^2, respectively.

Treatment Regimens

PSORIASIS

For psoriasis, UVB phototherapy is given usually on a daily basis, although less frequent exposures may also be effective. Ideally, the initial exposure dose will be based on the minimal erythema dose established for each patient (e.g., 70% of the MED). If this is not possible or practical, the first exposure time should be selected according to the skin type of the patient and the degree of any pre-existing melanin pigmentation. The operator should have established the approximate range of times required to achieve erythema in the local population with a particular type of lamp. One successful approach is to use fairly large dose increments for the first few days of treatment (e.g. dose increments of 50–100%) *until* a degree of erythema is noted or reported by the patient. Once erythema has developed, exposure times should be increased more cautiously (for example, by 10–20%) to maintain an effective treatment dose as the skin adapts. If severe or symptomatic erythema is present, further exposure should be avoided until the skin returns to normal.

Treatment is continued until the desired clinical response is obtained, or until no further improvement is occurring. Complete clearance of psoriasis may take several weeks of phototherapy.

OTHER DISORDERS

Protocols for the treatment of other skin disorders should be agreed with the referring physician. Erythema and skin irritation from phototherapy may be a significant problem for patients with atopic eczema and photosensitivity disorders, such as polymorphic light eruption.

ADJUNCTIVE AGENTS

Both tar and emollients are used topically in an attempt to improve the effectiveness of phototherapy for psoriasis. Tar preparations used alone for psoriasis do have a limited effect, but there is little evidence that responses to phototherapy are improved over those achieved with an emollient alone. Emollients are used in an attempt to improve optical transmission of UVB through the scaly surface of psoriasis. Oily preparations, such as arachis oil or coconut oil, may be applied to the skin some minutes before phototherapy. Several ointment preparations (e.g. emulsifying ointment, white soft paraffin and yellow soft paraffin) and products containing the keratolytic agent salicylic acid, have a sunscreening action and may reduce the effectiveness of phototherapy (Hudson-Peacock et al., 1994).

In the UK, hospital-based treatment of psoriasis is usually with daily topical treatment with dithranol (a synthetic derivative of chrysarobin, a tree bark extract). This is applied each day in an ointment or paste formulation to lesions of psoriasis and left in contact with the skin surface for 15–60 minutes (short-contact therapy) or for nearly 24 hours (Ingram regime). Clearance of psoriasis is achieved with around 14–21 days of treatment. Ultraviolet phototherapy is often used in addition to dithranol treatment and, when given optimally, can reduce by around one third the number of days of treatment required for clearance (Farr et al., 1987).

Side-effects

The main side-effect of UVB phototherapy is the development of erythema or, in more severe cases, blistering and subsequent peeling of the skin. Severe erythema can usually be avoided providing further exposure is not given if the patient has any residual erythema from the previous day's treatment. Once symptomatic erythema has developed, treatment with emollients may provide some relief and topical corticosteroids are often prescribed.

Although sun exposure is the major risk factor for the development of skin carcinoma, particularly squamous carcinoma, no additional risk from UVB phototherapy has been reported and, on theoretical grounds, any risk is likely to be minimal (Studniberg and Weller, 1993).

Psoralen Photochemotherapy (PUVA)

Psoralen photochemotherapy is the combined treatment of skin disorders with a photosensitising drug (psoralen) and ultraviolet A radiation.

Psoralens are naturally occurring plant compounds and their therapeutic potential for the treatment of vitiligo has been recognized for many thousands of years. Photochemotherapy of psoriasis, using synthetic psoralen compounds such as 8-methoxypsoralen (8-MOP) or 5-methoxypsoralen (5-MOP), was introduced in the 1970s and is now widely used as a second-line form of treatment, being available in around 100 dermatology units in the UK (Farr and Diffey, 1991).

Diseases that Respond to PUVA

Although used principally to treat psoriasis, many disorders show partial or complete response to PUVA:

- Psoriasis;
- Vitiligo;
- Eczema;
- Lichen planus;
- Graft-versus-host disease;
- Pityriasis lichenoides chronica;
- Cutaneous T-cell lymphoma (mycosis fungoides);
- Urticaria pigmentosa;
- Photosensitive disorders (polymorphic light eruption, actinic prurigo, chronic actinic dermatitis).

Further details on the role of PUVA in the treatment of these diseases can be found in the guidelines prepared by the British Photodermatology Group (Norris et al., 1994).

Pharmacology and Mechanism of Action

Psoralen is usually given orally using a dose system based on body weight or surface area (0.6 mg/kg or 25 mg/m^2 for the crystalline form of 8-MOP; 1.2 mg/kg or 50 mg/m^2 for 5-MOP). Absorption and resulting plasma concentrations show considerable variation between subjects, but UVA exposure is given usually 2 hours after ingestion at the average time of peak plasma concentration (Stevenson et al., 1981). PUVA may also be given using topical psoralen, either painted onto the skin surface or, more frequently, using a bath delivery system in which the patient soaks for 15 minutes in a weak psoralen solution (e.g. 3.75 mg/l of 8-MOP), followed immediately by UVA exposure. Significant concentrations of psoralen in plasma are not achieved with topical psoralen.

Psoralen molecules, when activated by UVA radiation form cross-links between adjacent strands of DNA, thus interfering with DNA and cellular replication. Although it has been assumed that this is the mechanism of action of PUVA in disorders associated with increased cell division (such as psoriasis), PUVA also has other important actions on the skin, including induction of pigmentation and epidermal hyperplasia, suppression of certain components of the immune system and release of reactive oxygen and free radicals which damage cell membranes and cytoplasmic structures.

Unlike ultraviolet phototherapy, the therapeutic wavelength response (or action spectrum for clearance of psoriasis) for PUVA has not yet been fully established. However, there is some evidence that lamps which emit shorter wavelengths (around 320–330 nm) may be more effective than conventional lamps (Farr et al., 1991).

Psoralen Erythema

Following oral administration of 8-MOP, the cutaneous photosensitivity to UVA parallels the plasma psoralen concentration – maximally sensitive after around 2 hours and gradually returning to normal by 8–12 hours. The photosensitivity from topical psoralen lasts for a much shorter period (<4 hours). Unlike UVB erythema (or UVA erythema without psoralen), PUVA erythema has a delayed onset, being first noticeable 24–48 hours after irradiation, and does not reach maximum intensity until 72 hours. The smallest dose of UVA required to achieve erythema in psoralen-sensitized skin is referred

Figure 14.7   The spectral power distribution of the ultraviolet radiation emitted by two different types of lamp used for PUVA therapy. Upper curve – UVA fluorescent lamps; note that the spectrum lies almost entirely between 320 and 400 nm (the UVA waveband) and peaks at 350 nm. Lower curve – optically-filtered high-pressure metal-halide lamps; note that most of the radiation is emitted at wavelengths longer than 360 nm.

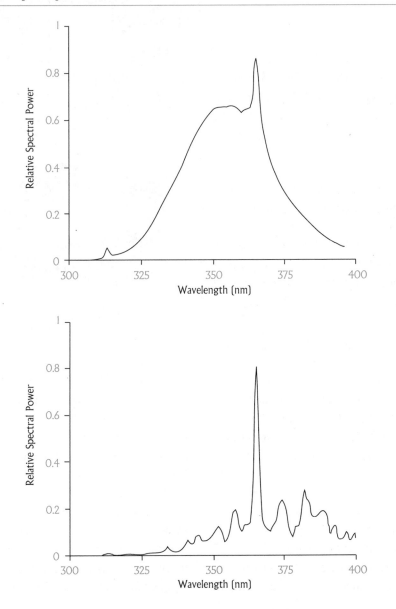

to usually as the *minimal phototoxic dose* (MPD), the term phototoxic indicating that an external agent has been used to increase the sensitivity of the skin. Unlike UVB erythema, where doses above the MED cause severe burning easily, 2 or 3 times the MPD results only in mild or moderate erythema when psoralen has been given orally. Burning may happen more easily with topical psoralen however.

Treatment Apparatus

Photoirradiation systems designed for PUVA therapy of psoriasis and other skin diseases normally incorporate UVA fluorescent lamps (e.g. Philips TLO9, Sylvania FR90T12/PUVA) emitting a continuous distribution from about 315–400 nm and peaking at around 352 nm. The spectrum from this lamp is shown in the upper half of Figure 14.7. Although it would seem that the true peak is at 365 nm (one of the characteristic spectral lines of mercury vapour), there is actually very little energy present in this spectral line. A variety of treatment units are available, ranging from small area (Figure 14.8) to whole-body cabinets (Figure 14.6).

Some centres use high-pressure metal halide lamps behind glass filters to remove the UVB and UVC components of the radiation and allow UVA to be transmitted, similar to the unit shown in Figure 14.4. The UVA irradiance from this arrangement at typical treatment distances can be 2–3 times higher than can be achieved in conventional UVA fluorescent lamp units and might be thought to be a positive feature in favour of this type of unit. However, high-pressure metal halide lamps behind glass filters emit a spectrum as shown in the lower half of Figure 14.7. Whereas the spectrum from UVA fluorescent lamps peaks at around 350 nm, the optically

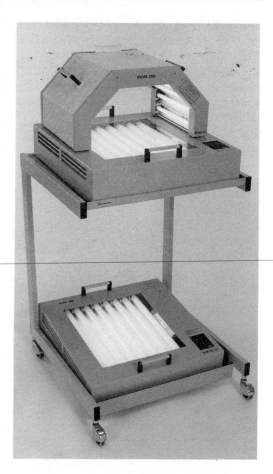

Figure 14.8 Small area PUVA units used for treating hands and feet (courtesy of Athrodax Surgical Ltd, Ross-on-Wye, England).

filtered metal halide lamps used in the high-power units emit much of their ultraviolet radiation in the band between 360 and 380 nm. The action spectrum for the clearance of psoriasis by psoralen photochemotherapy is such that shorter UVA wavelengths are more effective than radiation at the long-wavelength end of the UVA spectrum (see section on *Pharmacology and Mechanism of Action* above). The apparent advantage of higher UVA irradiances from high-pressure lamp systems may be more than offset by the relative lack of radiation in the shorter wavelength interval (320–340 nm) of the UVA spectrum compared with the commonly used UVA fluorescent lamps.

UVA Dosimetry

Accurate UVA dosimetry in PUVA therapy is important for two reasons:

1 To ensure that patients receive the correct prescribed dose of UVA – thus allowing treatment regimens to be optimally effective;
2 To maintain accurate records of patients' lifetime UVA exposure received during PUVA treatment – important when the risk of PUVA-related malignancy is considered.

There are several makes of UVA dosemeter that are used in PUVA therapy. The dosemeter consists of two parts: a *sensor* incorporating an ultraviolet-sensitive detector; and a *meter* which displays the intensity (more strictly called the *irradiance*) in units of milliwatts per square centimetre (mW/cm^2). A simple calculation allows an exposure time to be determined for a prescribed UVA dose in joules per square centimetre (J/cm^2):

Exposure Time (minutes) =

$$\frac{1000 \times \text{Prescribed dose } (J/cm^2)}{60 \times \text{Measured irradiance } (mW/cm^2)}$$

The UVA irradiance in whole body PUVA cubicles can range from 4–16 mW/cm^2 depending upon the number of installed lamps and their age.

Many PUVA machines have a built-in sensor which controls patient exposure. Yet there can be dangers with this approach:

1 The sensor inside the PUVA cabin may 'see' only a small fraction of the lamps, and the output from these may not be representative;
2 The patient may shield the sensor either inadvertently or deliberately;

3 The sensor may accumulate dust and skin with the consequence that it gives a false low measurement of irradiance which results in patients receiving an overdose of radiation;
4 Prolonged exposure to radiation inside the PUVA cabin will cause the sensitivity of the sensor to change with time.

Ideally, therefore, a hand-held UVA dosemeter should be available so that regular checks can be made on the integrity of built-in sensors. It is a sound policy to have the dosemeter recalibrated annually.

Treatment Regimens

For psoriasis, PUVA treatment regimens are now well established. Protocols for treatment of other disorders, however, remain to be developed.

Treatment for psoriasis in the UK has been given usually three times per week. However, as PUVA erythema does not reach a maximum until around 72 hours after exposure, treatment on a Monday, Wednesday and Friday, leaving only 48 hours between some exposures, considerably increases the risk of burning. Consequently, many dermatology units in the UK are changing to twice-weekly treatment. This has been shown to be effective for psoriasis (Sakuntabhai et al., 1993), is considerably more convenient for patients than 3-times-weekly treatment, and allows greater efficiency of operation of a PUVA unit.

Starting doses of UVA are often based on the skin type of the patient, such as:

- Skin type I: 0.5 J/cm^2
- Skin type II: 1.0 J/cm^2
- Skin type III: 1.5 J/cm^2
- Skin type IV: 2.0 J/cm^2

However, the additional factor of variable skin photosensitivity due to differences between patients in psoralen pharmacokinetics, means that skin typing is even less useful as a method of prediction of erythemal sensitivity for PUVA compared with UVB phototherapy. Measurement of each patient's minimal phototoxic dose (MPD) at the start of a course of treatment allows high-dose treatment regimens to be used without increased risk of burning, and results in faster clearance of psoriasis. The MPD may be measured by exposing small areas of normal skin (e.g. 1 cm diameter sites) on the forearm or back to increasing doses of UVA (e.g. 1, 2, 4 and 8 J/cm^2 for oral 8-MOP treatment), and then observing which, if any, of the sites become erythematous at 72 hours (Diffey et al., 1993). Whole-body treatment is given using between 40 and 70% of the MPD. Doses are increased usually weekly by between 10 and 40% to maintain the response to treatment as the skin adapts by pigmentation and epidermal thickening. Using a twice weekly protocol with MPD measurement to choose the starting dose, it is typically possible to clear psoriasis with 12 exposures and a cumulative UVA dose of around 50 J/cm^2. The response to treatment is quite variable, however, and some patients will clear faster than this, whilst others show a slower response. For topical (bath) PUVA, smaller UVA doses are used as the skin is more photosensitive than with oral PUVA. Typical starting doses are 0.2–0.5 J/cm^2.

Once clearance of psoriasis has been achieved, it was common practice to continue with PUVA for a variable period to maintain remission. With the long-term side-effects of PUVA now well defined, many dermatologists prefer to avoid maintenance treatment wherever possible.

Adjunctive Agents

Vitamin A derivatives (retinoids), given orally, are sometimes used in conjunction with PUVA ther-apy for psoriasis. They may reduce the cumulative UVA dose required for clearance, particularly in patients who are poor or slow responders to PUVA.

Side effects

The main short-term side-effects of PUVA are erythema and nausea. PUVA erythema has a delayed onset compared with UVB erythema, can persist for a week or more, and may be associated with severe itching, blistering and local skin pain. The risk of burning is minimized if care is taken not to treat patients who have any residual erythema from the previous treatment. Once symptomatic erythema has developed, emollients and topical corticosteroids may aid resolution. Severe erythema may be followed by the development of new lesions of psoriasis arising within areas of damaged skin.

Nausea is quite common with oral 8-methoxypsoralen, lasting 1–4 hours after ingestion. In some patients, this problem can be overcome if the drug is taken with a light meal. For the 5% of patients in whom nausea prevents the use of 8-methoxypsoralen, 5-methoxypsoralen may be substituted, although this drug may be less effective at clearing psoriasis.

Many patients who have received PUVA in high doses over long periods will have some signs of skin damage. Multiple, small hyperpigmented lesions, termed PUVA freckles (or PUVA lentigines) are seen in up to 70% of high-dose patients. They have not been shown to have malignant potential, but may be perceived by some patients as a cosmetic problem. More worrying is the development of warty, keratotic lesions (PUVA keratoses), usually up to 1 cm in diameter, which may show premalignant features on histological examination. It is now clearly established that long-term PUVA treatment results in an increased risk of cutaneous squamous-cell carcinoma. This risk has shown to be dose-dependent: a cumulative UVA dose received through PUVA of <500 J/cm^2 is unlikely to result in significant risk; above 1000 J/cm^2 is associated with definite risk, and around 50% of patients who have received >2000 J/cm^2 will have PUVA keratoses or squamous carcinoma (Lever and Farr, 1994). In some centres, malignant tumours have occurred on the male genitalia and it is now recommended that this area should be protected by clothing whenever possible during a course of treatment. The very real risk of serious skin damage through PUVA emphasizes the importance of accurate dosimetry, careful selection of patients for PUVA treatment, and frequent medical assessment of patients during the course.

Safety

Considerations of safety relate to both patients and staff (Diffey, 1990b).

Patient Safety

It goes without saying that there must be adequate protection against electrical hazards. Patients (and physiotherapists) should not be able to touch any live electrical parts, and all metal components, such as handrails and safety grids, must satisfy national electrical safety standards and codes of practice.

Ideally, patients should not be able to come in contact with bare lamps. In high-pressure units this is achieved by interposing a glass filter(s) between the patient and lamps. However, in whole-body phototherapy units incorporating large numbers of fluorescent lamps, it is normally possible for patients to touch the lamps. The main risk is that from flying glass if a fluorescent lamp implodes. Although the occurrence is rare, it does happen.

Other features that relate to patients' safety include hand rails to support patients during treatment, a cord within the cabinet that can be pulled by the patient to summon help, doors that can be opened easily by the patient from inside the irradiation cabinet, non-skid flooring in the cabinet, and adequate air flow to maintain patient comfort during the irradiation period.

Finally, there is one potential hazard associated with high-pressure lamp phototherapy units which incorporate optical filters to allow either UVA or UVA plus UVB irradiation. If only UVA irradiation is intended but the operator fails to ensure that the correct filter is in place, the patient may be exposed to high doses of UVB (depending on the treatment times) which can lead to severe, painful erythema. A similar hazard exists with combination units incorporating both UVA and UVB fluorescent lamps.

Because psoralens are deposited in the lens of the eye there is the possibility of cataract induction if the eyes are exposed to UVA irradiation in the 12 hours or so following the ingestion of the drug. Consequently, patients should be avoid unnecessary exposure to sunlight for the remainder of the day after taking the psoralens, and should be instructed to wear UVA-opaque spectacles or sunglasses for the following 12 hours. (Some dermatology units recommend wearing eye protection for 24 hours). The effectiveness of spectacles in blocking UVA should ideally be measured in a spectrophotometer (a laboratory instrument for measuring light transmission on a wavelength-by-wavelength basis) but, failing this, staff can check spectacles by using the radiation from a PUVA unit and a hand-held UVA dose-meter. Spectacles are only acceptable if there is a zero or near-zero reading on the dosemeter.

Staff Safety

Exposure to ultraviolet radiation can produce harmful effects in the eyes and the skin, and measurements have shown that an ultraviolet exposure hazard exists in the vicinity of many lamps used for phototherapy, e.g. at 1 m from an Alpine Sunlamp, the maximum permissible exposure for 8-hour working periods recommended by national regulatory authorities can be exceeded in less than 2 minutes. For this reason, operators should always keep away from the primary beam as much as is practicable when working with unenclosed lamps. Measures which can be taken to minimize the unnecessary exposure of staff to ultraviolet radiation include: proper engineering design of ultraviolet apparatus; wearing appropriate goggles or face shields, accompanied, if necessary, by suitable UVR-opaque clothing; limiting access to the area to persons directly concerned with the work; and ensuring that staff are aware of the potential hazards associated with exposure to ultraviolet radiation sources.

Patients undergoing UV irradiation are often given green tinted, occlusive goggles (e.g. Portia Actinotherapy Goggles, Solport Ltd), whereas staff may prefer to wear clear spectacles with side shields which have negligible transmission of UVR (e.g. Blak-Ray Contrast Control Spectacles Model No UVC-303, Ultraviolet Products Ltd, Cambridge).

It is not acceptable for staff to experience either skin erythema or photokeratitis. If this does occur, working practices should be examined and steps taken to ensure that overexposure is unlikely in the future (Diffey, 1989).

Hazards from Ozone

Ozone is a colourless, toxic, irritant gas formed by a photochemical reaction between short-wavelength UVR and the oxygen present in the air. It is possible to find ozone near ultraviolet lamps, especially those where radiation of wavelengths shorter than about 250 nm is transmitted through the envelope of the lamp. Most modern phototherapy lamps are so-called 'ozone-free', that is, the lamp envelope is opaque to wavelengths below about 260 nm, thus preventing shorter-wavelength UVR from forming ozone in the air. If ozone is suspected, either by measurement or smell, the gas should be removed by adequate ventilation.

References

Chue, B, Borok, M, Lowe, NJ (1988) Phototherapy units: comparison of fluorescent ultraviolet B and ultraviolet A units with a high-pressure mercury system. *Journal of the American Academy of Dermatology* 18: 641–645

Diffey, BL (1990a) Ultraviolet Radiation Lamps for the Phototherapy and Photochemotherapy of Skin Diseases, in Champion, RH, Pye, RJ (eds) *Recent Advances in Dermatology* (8th edition), pp. 21–40. Churchill Livingstone, Edinburgh.

Diffey, BL (1990b) Ultraviolet Radiation Safety, in Pal, SB (ed) *Handbook of Laboratory Health and Safety Measures* (2nd edition), pp. 349–396. Kluwer Academic Publishers, London.

Diffey, BL, Harrington, TR, Challoner, AVJ (1978) A comparison of the anatomical uniformity of irradiation in two different photochemotherapy units. *British Journal of Dermatology* 99: 361–363.

Diffey, BL, Farr, PM (1987) An appraisal of ultraviolet radiation lamps used in the phototherapy of psoriasis. *British Journal of Dermatology* 117: 49–56.

Diffey, BL (1989) Ultraviolet radiation and skin cancer: are physiotherapists at risk? *Physiotherapy* 75: 615–616.

Diffey, BL, de Berker, DAR, Saunders, PJ, Farr, PM (1993) A device for phototesting patients before PUVA therapy. *British Journal of Dermatology* 129: 700–703.

Dootson, G, Norris, PG, Gibson, CJ, Diffey, BL (1994) The practice of UVB phototherapy in the United Kingdom. *British Journal of Dermatology* 131: 873–877.

Farr, PM, Diffey, BL, Marks, JM (1987) Phototherapy and anthralin treatment of psoriasis: new lamps for old. *British Medical Journal* **294**: 205–207.

Farr, PM, Diffey, BL (1991) PUVA treatment of psoriasis in the United Kingdom. *British Journal of Dermatology* **124**: 365–367.

Farr, PM, Diffey, BL, Higgins, EM, Matthews, JNS (1991) The action spectrum between 320 and 400 nm for clearance of psoriasis by psoralen photochemotherapy. *British Journal of Dermatology* **124**: 443–448.

Hudson-Peacock, MJ, Diffey, BL, Farr, PM (1994) Photoprotective action of emollients in ultraviolet therapy of psoriasis. *British Journal of Dermatology* **130**: 361–365.

Johnson, BE (1984) The Photobiology of the Skin, in Jarrett A (ed) *The Physiology and Pathophysiology of the Skin*, pp. 2434–2437. Academic Press, London.

Lever, LR, Farr, PM (1994) Skin cancers or premalignant lesions occur in half of high-dose PUVA patients. *British Journal of Dermatology* **131**: 215–219.

Magnus, IA (1976) *Dermatological Photobiology.* Blackwell Scientific Publications, Oxford.

Norris, PG, Hawk, JLM, Baker, C *et al.* (1994) British Photodermatology Group guidelines for PUVA. *British Journal of Dermatology* **130**: 246–255.

Parrish, JA, Jaenicke, KF (1981) Action spectrum for phototherapy of psoriasis. *Journal of Investigations in Dermatology* **76**: 359–362.

Sakuntabhai, A, Sharpe, GR, Farr, PM (1993) Response of psoriasis to twice weekly PUVA. *British Journal of Dermatology* **128**: 166–171.

Stevenson, IH, Kenicer, KJA, Johnson, BE, Frain-Bell W (1981) Plasma 8-methoxypsoralen concentrations in photochemotherapy of psoriasis. *British Journal of Dermatology* **104**: 47–51.

Studniberg, HM, Weller, P (1993) PUVA, UVB, psoriasis, and non-melanoma skin cancer. *Journal of the American Academy of Dermatology* **29**: 1013–1022.

E

Ultrasound

15

Ultrasound Therapy

STEVE YOUNG

Introduction
•
Physical Effects of Ultrasound
•
Wound Repair
•
Ultrasound Application
•
Wound Assessment
•
Summary

Introduction

The aim of this chapter is to provide a detailed source of reference about ultrasound and its mechanisms of action on tissues, in both the physical and biological sense. Once clinicians know how a modality works they are then in a position to predict with a high degree of accuracy what the correct treatment regime should be for a particular injury, without having to rely solely on clinical experience (which every clinician may not have) and heresay. This chapter could be written in the form of a recipe book, with no thinking to be done: just follow the guidlines – for injury X apply modality Y for 5 minutes at an intensity of . . . and so on. This is not desirable for a number of reasons. There is no general agreement in the clinical and laboratory research literature on how best to treat each individual type of injury. Many clinicians, like all good chefs, each have their own ideas how best to tackle the job presented to them. Also, no two injuries are identical. What may work for one venous leg ulcer, for example, may not work for another. It is vital that the clinician has as much knowledge as possible about the biology of wound healing and how electrotherapies interact with it. Armed with this knowledge, the clinician is in a strong position to work out why a particular wound is not responding to therapy and how best to alter the treatment regime to provide the much-needed repair stimulus. It must be understood that some wounds will not repair irrespective of which electrotherapy modality is applied, because of the presence of some underlying deficiency in the wound environment.

Bearing this in mind, one of the first steps to be taken by the clinician before embarking on a course of therapy is to make sure that they have a full patient history so that any underlying complications are known, e.g. diabetes, venous insufficiency. These complications should be addressed before a course of therapy is undertaken. Failure to do this means that both clinician and patient waste time and money, and, most importantly, there is a likelihood of compounding the problem and putting the patient at further risk.

This leads onto another problem: once therapy has begun, how does the clinician then assess wound healing. It is important to have sensitive, quantitative diagnostic techniques which are easy to use and to interpret, and by which changes in a wound in response to therapy can be assessed. The more sensitive the technique is, the earlier the clinician will detect whether the therapy being used is working. In an age of cost-guided medical care where the term 'clinical audit' is the buzz word (DOH, 1989) it is vital that the time a patient is under care is cut to the absolute minimum. To save even a few days by changing more rapidly to a more appropriate therapy could, nationally, account for an enormous saving in health-care costs. The government white paper defines audit as 'The systematic critical analysis of the quality of care, including the procedures used for diagnosis and treatment, the use of resources and the resulting outcome and quality of life for the patient'. As an example of how current resources are being stretched, consider the cost of pressure sore care in the UK. Estimates of the prevalence of pressure sores in hospitals and nursing homes is approximately 10% of the all patients (Goode *et*

al., 1992; Allman, 1989); the hospital population in the UK in 1992 was approximately 300 000 (HMSO, 1994) and, therefore, 30 000 patients in hospital suffer from pressure sores. In the UK, there are approximately 225 000 nursing home beds. Based on these figures, the total number of patients with pressure sores in the nursing home community is approximately 22 500 (Potter, 1994; David, 1983). This brings the total number of patients suffering from pressure sores in hospitals and nursing homes to 52 500. In terms of cost of treatment of pressure sores, the most frequently quoted figure is £150 million per year (Collier, 1990; Morison, 1992; Young, 1990; Watson, 1989; Hibbs, 1989; Livesey and Simpson, 1989; Scales *et al.*, 1982). One estimate of the cost of treatment for a single patient with a pressure sore is £25 905 (Hibbs, 1988), which represented a 12-week period of treatment in hospital.

Therefore, it can be seen that the costs for just one particular type of wound is enormous; adding the costs of all the other wounds (e.g. venous leg ulcers, diabetic ulcers, acute surgical wounds), the total cost becomes astronomical. For this reason, techniques for assessing the effectiveness of your therapy will be discussed in this chapter.

To say that ultrasound is a frequently used therapeutic modality in physiotherapy practice is a gross understatement. The results of a survey carried out in Britain in 1985 (ter Haar *et al.*, 1985) showed that 20% of all physiotherapy treatments in NHS departments and 54% of all private treatments involved therapeutic ultrasound. It is obvious that if a modality is used so widely then it is vital that we understand fully its biological effects and mechanisms of action so that it can be used effectively and, more important, safely. In this survey, physiotherapists were asked to complete a questionnaire covering a range of topics including: technical details of their ultrasound machine, intensities and frequencies most commonly used, calibration procedures, contraindications — leaving out for using ultrasound. The survey revealed that there existed large inconsistencies in the use of ultrasound and, therefore, signalled an urgent need for further education in the use of this modality. In summary, the survey highlighted the following:

1 Intensities used varied by a factor of 300, from 0.1–3.0 W/cm^2;
2 Confusion existed in the choice of pulsed- or continuous-exposure mode;
3 Some of the inclusions in the list of contraindications were based on little or no scientific evidence;
4 Calibration was carried out, at best, once every 3–6 months in NHS departments and on average once a year in private practice. The availability of calibration equipment to physiotherapists was low, with only 20% of NHS and 6% of those in private practice having access to radiation balances.

Problems also appear to exist when it comes to making a choice of which type of electrotherapy to use when presented with the wide range of injuries that arrive at the clinic daily. A recent national survey (Kitchen, 1995) highlighted this uncertainty. The work pointed out that knowledge about electrotherapy's biological effects, clinical efficacy and safety are limited, and this compounds the decision-making process.

The purpose of this chapter is to present the relevant quantitative, clinical and laboratory data about therapeutic ultrasound. This should provide the clinician with the capacity to choose when and when not to use the modality and how to use it effectively and safely.

Physical Effects of Ultrasound

When ultrasound enters the body it can exert an effect on the cells and tissues via two physical mechanisms: thermal and nonthermal. It is important that we understand these mechanisms fully as some are stimulatory in their effect on the wound healing process, whereas others are potentially dangerous. For further details of the physical principles that underlie the behaviour of ultrasound, see Chapter 1.

Thermal Effects

When ultrasound travels through tissues a percentage of it is absorbed, and this leads to the generation of heat within that tissue. The amount of absorption depends upon the nature of the tissue, its degree of vascularization, and the frequency of the ultrasound. Tissues with a high protein content absorb more readily than those with a higher fat content, and the higher the frequency the greater the absorption. A biologically significant thermal effect can be achieved if the temperature of the tissue is raised to between 40–45 °C for at least 5 minutes. Controlled heating can produce desirable effects (Lehmann and De Lateur, 1982) which include pain relief, decrease in joint stiffness, and increased blood flow.

The advantage of using ultrasound to deliver this heating effect is that the therapist has control over the depth at which the heating occurs. To do this, it is important that the therapist has knowledge of half-value depth measurements (i.e. the depth of penetration of the ultrasound energy at which its intensity has decreased by a half) and of the selective heating of tissues. For example, the half-value depth for soft, irregular connective tissue is approximately 4 mm at 3 MHz, but is about 11 mm at 1 MHz. Structures which will be heated preferentially include periosteum, superficial cortical bone, joint menisci, fibrotic muscle, tendon sheaths and major nerve roots (Lehmann and Guy, 1972), and intermuscular interfaces (ter Haar and Hopewell, 1982). It is therefore important that the therapist has knowledge of the structures which lie between the ultrasound source and the injured tissue, and also beyond it.

Once delivered, the heat is then dissipated by both thermal diffusion and local blood flow, which can present a problem when treating injuries where the blood supply has been restricted by either the nature of the injury or the relatively avascular nature of the tissue itself (e.g. tendon). Another complication can occur when the ultrasound beam hits bone or a metal prosthesis. Because of the great acoustic impedance difference between these structures and the surrounding soft tissues there will be a reflection of about 30% of the incident energy back through the soft tissue. This means that further energy is deposited as heat during the beam's return journey. Therefore, heat rise in soft tissue will be higher when it is situated in front of a reflector. To further complicate matters, an interaction termed *mode conversion* also occurs at the interface of the soft tissue and the reflector (e.g. bone or metal prosthesis). During mode conversion, a percentage of the reflected incident energy is converted from a longitudinal waveform into a transverse or shear waveform which cannot propagate on the soft tissue side of the interface and is therefore absorbed rapidly, causing heat rise (and frequently pain) at the bone–soft tissue interface (periosteum).

Nonthermal Effects

There are many situations where ultrasound produces bioeffects and yet significant temperature is not involved (e.g. low spatial-average temporal-average [SATA] intensity). Evidence exists as to where nonthermal mechanisms are thought to play a primary role in producing a therapeutically significant effect: stimulation of tissue regeneration (Dyson et al., 1968), soft tissue repair (Dyson, Franks and Suckling, 1976; Paul et al., 1960), blood flow in chronically ischaemic tissues (Hogan, Burke and Franklin, 1982), protein synthesis (Webster et al., 1978), and bone repair (Dyson and Brookes, 1983).

The physical mechanisms thought to be involved in producing these nonthermal effects are one or more of the following: cavitation, acoustic streaming, and standing waves.

CAVITATION

Ultrasound can cause the formation of micron-sized bubbles or cavities in gas-containing fluids. Depending upon the pressure amplitude of the energy, the resultant bubbles can be either useful or dangerous. Low pressure amplitudes result in the formation of bubbles which vibrate to a degree where reversible permeability changes are produced in cell membranes near to the cavitational event (Mortimer and Dyson, 1988). Changes in cell permeability to various ions such as calcium can have a profound effect upon the activity of the cell (Sutherland and Rall, 1968). High pressure amplitudes can result in a more violent cavitational event (often called transient or collapse cavitation). During this event, the bubbles collapse during the positive pressure part of the cycle with such a ferocity that pressures in excess of 1000 MPa and temperatures in excess of 10 000 K are generated. This violent behaviour can lead to the formation of highly reactive free radicals. Although free radicals are produced by cells naturally, e.g. during cellular respiration, they are removed by free-radical scavengers. Production in excess of the natural free-radical scavenger system could, however, be damaging. Avoidance of a standing-wave field and use of low intensities during therapy makes it unlikely that transient cavitation will occur.

ACOUSTIC STREAMING

This refers to the unidirectional movement of a fluid in an ultrasound field. High velocity gradients develop next to boundaries between fluids and structures such as cells, bubbles and tissue fibres. Acoustic streaming can stimulate cell activity if it occurs at the boundary of the cell membrane and the surrounding fluid. The resultant viscous stress on the membrane, providing it is not too severe, can alter the membrane's permeability and second messenger activity (Dyson, 1982, 1985). This could result in therapeutically advantageous changes such as increased protein synthesis (Webster *et al.*, 1978), increased secretion from mast cells (Fyfe and Chahl, 1982), fibroblast mobility changes (Mummery, 1978), increased uptake of the second messenger calcium (Mummery, 1978; Mortimer and Dyson, 1988), and increased production of growth factors by macrophages (Young and Dyson, 1990a). All these effects could account for the acceleration of repair following ultrasound therapy.

STANDING WAVES

When an ultrasound wave hits the interface between two tissues of different acoustic impedances, e.g. bone and muscle, reflection of a percentage of the wave will occur. The reflected waves can interact with oncoming incident waves to form a standing-wave field in which the peaks of intensity (*antinodes*) of the waves are stationary and are separated by half a wavelength. Because the standing wave consists of two superimposed waves in addition to a traveling component, the peak intensities and pressures are higher than the normal incident wave. Between the antinodes, which are points of maximum and minimum pressure, there are *nodes* which are points of fixed pressure. Gas bubbles collect at the antinodes, and cells (if in suspension) collect at the nodes (NCRP Report No. 74, 1983). Fixed cells, such as endothelial cells which line the blood vessels, can be damaged by microstreaming forces around bubbles if they are situated at the pressure antinodes. Erythrocytes can be lysed if they are swept through the arrays of bubbles situated at the pressure antinodes. Reversible blood cell stasis has been demonstrated, the cells forming bands, half a wavelength apart, centred on the pressure nodes (Dyson *et al.*, 1974). The increased pressure produced in standing-wave fields can cause transient cavitation and consequently free radical formation (Nyborg, 1977). It is therefore important that therapists move the applicator continuously throughout treatment, and also use the lowest intensity required to cause an effect, to minimize the hazards involved in standing-wave field production (Dyson *et al.* 1974).

Having covered how ultrasound imparts its energy to the tissue we will now look at how this energy is utilized by cells and tissues in the wound healing process.

Wound Repair

Following injury, a number of cellular and chemical events occur in soft tissues. Although these events are explained in detail in an earlier section of this book (Chapter 3), it is worth summarizing them here in the context of ultrasound therapy.

The major cellular components of the repair process include platelets, mast cells, polymorphonuclear leucocytes (PMNLs), macrophages, T lymphocytes, fibroblasts and endothelial cells. These cells migrate as a module into the injury site in a well-defined sequence which is controlled by numerous soluble wound factors. These wound factors originate from a number of sources such as inflammatory cells (e.g. macrophages and PMNLs), inflammatory cascade systems (e.g. coagulation and compliment), or from the products of damaged tissue breakdown.

The whole repair process, for convenience, can be divided into three phases (Clark, 1990), although it must be stated that these phases overlap considerably, lacking any distinct border between each other. The three phases are:

1 Inflammation;
2 Proliferation/granulation tissue formation;
3 Remodelling.

There is now overwhelming evidence showing that the effectiveness of therapeutic ultrasound is dependent upon the phase of repair in which it is used. This will be discussed in more detail later in this chapter.

Inflammation

This early, dynamic phase of repair is characterized initially by clot formation. The blood platelet is a major constituent of the blood clot and, in addition to its activities associated with clotting, platelets also contain numerous biologically active substances, including prostaglandins, serotonin, platelet-derived growth factor (PDGF). These substances have a profound effect upon the local environment of the wound and its subsequent repair (Clark, 1990). Mast cells present another source of biologically active substances, or wound factors, which help orchestrate the early repair sequences.

Neutrophils are the first PMNLs to enter the wound bed, attracted by an array of wound factors present at the wound site. The neutrophils function is to clear the wound site of foreign particles such as bacteria and damaged tissue debris.

Macrophages enter the wound bed soon after the neutrophils, where they phagocytose bacteria and wound tissue debris. They also produce wound factors which direct granulation tissue formation (Leibovich and Ross, 1975).

Evidence will be presented later in this chapter which shows that, when used at the right time during wound repair and at the right levels of output, ultrasound can influence the release of these wound factors from the cells in and around the wound bed.

Proliferation/granulation Tissue Formation

During normal acute injury repair, the inflammatory phase is followed within several days by granulation tissue formation. This stage is often referred to as the proliferative phase. During this phase the wound void is filled with cells (mainly macrophages and fibroblasts), numerous blood vessels (angiogenesis), and a connective tissue matrix (composed of fibronectin, hyaluronic acid and collagen types I and III).

A new epidermis also forms during this phase of repair. The new epidermal cells migrate from the edge of the wound (and also from around hair follicles within the injury site in the case of partial-thickness wounds) towards the centre of the wound.

Wound contraction occurs during this phase of repair and can be defined as the process by which the size of a wound decreases by the centripetal movement of the whole thickness of surrounding skin (Peacock, 1984). In man, skin is relatively immobile due to its attachment to underlying structures. Therefore, in some instances where wounds occur over joints, any wound contraction may lead to immobilization due to the tension developed through attachment of the skin to underlying structures. Thus excessive contraction is often seen as a serious complication to healing.

The stimulus controlling all of these events comes from numerous sources, with the macrophage being a main one. The release of active factors from macrophages is thought to be controlled, in part, by the relatively hypoxic environment of the wound (Knighton et al., 1983). The effect of ultrasound on the macrophage will be discussed in detail later.

Remodelling

Remodelling can continue for many months or years after the proliferative phase of repair. During remodelling, granulation tissue is gradually replaced by a scar which is a relatively acellular and avascular tissue. As the wound matures, the composition of the extracellular matrix changes. Initially, the extracellular matrix is composed of hyaluronic acid, fibronectin, collagens types I, III and V. The ratio of type I to III then changes during remodelling until type I is the dominant collagen. Scar tissue is a poor substitute for unwounded skin. The rate at which wounds gain tensile strength is slow (Levenson et al., 1965), gaining only between 20 and 25% of their maximum strength three weeks after injury. The increase in wound strength depends upon two main factors: the rate of collagen deposition, remodelling and alignment, with the gradual formation of larger collagen bundles (Kischer and

Shetlar, 1974), and an alteration of intermolecular cross-links (Bailey et al., 1975). It will be shown later that, if used at the correct time after injury, ultrasound can improve both the cosmetic appearance and the mechanical properties of the resulting scar tissue.

The Effect of Ultrasound on the Inflammatory Phase of Repair

As indicated previously, the inflammatory phase is extremely dynamic and, during it, numerous cell types (e.g., platelets, mast cells, macrophages, neutrophils) enter and leave the wound site. There is evidence to show that therapeutic ultrasound can interact with the above cells, influencing their activity and leading to the acceleration of repair.

Acoustic streaming forces have been shown to produce changes in platelet membrane permeability leading to the release of serotonin (Williams, 1974, 1976). In addition to serotonin, platelets contain wound factors essential for successful repair (Ginsberg, 1981). If streaming can stimulate the release of serotonin, it may also influence the release of these other factors.

One of the major chemicals that modifies the wound environment at this time after injury is histamine. The mast cell is the major source of this factor, which is normally released by a process known as mast cell degranulation. In this process, the membrane of the cell, in response to increased levels of intracellular calcium (Yurt, 1981), ruptures, releasing histamine and other products into the wound site. It has been shown that a single treatment of therapeutic ultrasound if given soon after injury, i.e. during the early inflammatory phase, can stimulate mast cells to degranulate, thereby releasing histamine into the surrounding tissues (Fyfe and Chahl, 1982;

Hashish, 1986). It is possible that ultrasound is stimulating the mast cell to degranulate by increasing its permeability to calcium. Increased calcium ion permeability has been demonstrated by a number of researchers. Calcium ions can act as intracellular messengers; when their distribution and concentration changes in response to environmental modifications of the plasma membrane they act as an intracellular signal for the appropriate metabolic response. There is much evidence that ultrasound can produce membrane changes in a number of cell types. These range from gross destructive changes to the more subtle reversible changes. Gross changes can be achieved if levels of ultrasound are high enough. Even when using therapeutic levels of ultrasound it is possible to achieve the necessary conditions for destruction if a standing-wave field is allowed to form due to bad clinical practice, i.e. in failing to keep the applicator head moving. Dyson *et al.* (1974) demonstrated that if this phenomena occurs in the region of fine blood vessels it is possible to damage the endothelial cells lining the luminal side of the vessels.

Reversible membrane permeability changes to calcium have been demonstrated using therapeutic levels of ultrasound (Mummery, 1978; Mortimer and Dyson, 1988; Dinno *et al.*, 1989). The fact that this effect can be suppressed by irradiation under pressure suggests that cavitation is the physical mechanism responsible. Changes in permeability to other ions such as potassium have also been demonstrated (Chapman *et al.*, 1979). Work by Dinno *et al.* (1989) demonstrated, in a frog-skin model, that ultrasound can modify the electrophysiological properties of the tissue. The work reported an ultrasound-induced reduction in the sodium–potassium ATPase pump activity. A decrease in pump activity, if it occurs in neuronal plasma membranes, may inhibit the trans-

duction of noxious stimuli and subsequent neural transmission, which may account, in part, for the pain relief which is often experienced following clinical exposure to therapeutic ultrasound. It should be noted, however, that the mechanism of pain relief is still not understood fully, and much of it can be attributed to placebo effects.

As discussed above, the evidence is clear: therapeutic ultrasound can alter membrane permeability to various ions. The ability to affect calcium transport through cell membranes is of considerable clinical significance since calcium, in its role as intracellular or second messenger, can have a profound effect on cell activity, e.g. increasing synthesis and secretion of wound factors by cells involved in the healing process. This has been shown to occur in macrophages in response to therapeutic levels of ultrasound (Young and Dyson, 1990a) which, as discussed earlier, is one of the key cells in the wound healing system, being a source of numerous wound factors. This *in vitro* study demonstrated that the ultrasound-induced change in wound factor secretion is frequency dependent. Ultrasound at an intensity of 0.5 W/cm^2 (SATA) and a frequency of 0.75 MHz appeared to be most effective in encouraging the immediate release of factors already present in the cell cytoplasm, whereas the higher frequency 3.0 MHz appeared to be most effective in stimulating the production of new factors which were then released some time later by the cells normal secretory processes. Therefore, there appeared to be a delayed effect when treating with the higher frequency; however, the resulting liberated factors when compared to those liberated using 0.75 MHz, were more potent in their effect on the stimulation of fibroblast population growth. One possible reason why these two frequencies induce different effects is due to the physical mechanisms involved. At both frequencies the peak pressures generated by the ultrasound was that necessary for cavitation to occur (Williams, 1987). Cavitation is more likely to occur at the lower frequency, whereas heating is more likely to occur at the higher one. Therefore, the differing proportions of nonthermal to thermal mechanisms present in each of the two treatments may explain the difference seen in the resulting biological effects.

Hart (1993) also found that following the *in vitro* exposure of macrophages, a wound factor was released into the surrounding medium which was mitogenic for fibroblasts.

It was often thought that ultrasound was an anti-inflammatory agent (Reid, 1981; Snow and Johnson, 1988). When viewed from a clinical standpoint, i.e. rapid resolution of oedema (El Hag *et al.*, 1985), this conclusion is understandable. However, research has shown that ultrasound is not anti-inflammatory in its action (Goddard *et al.*, 1983); rather, it encourages oedema formation to occur more rapidly (Fyfe and Chahl, 1985; Hustler *et al.*, 1978) and then to subside more rapidly than control sham-irradiated groups, so accelerating the whole event and driving the wound into the proliferative phase of repair sooner.

Further confirmation of this has been shown experimentally in acute surgical wounds (Young and Dyson, 1990b). In this study, full-thickness excised skin lesions in rats were exposed to therapeutic ultrasound (0.1 W/cm^2 SATA, 0.75 MHz or 3.0 MHz) daily for seven days (5 minutes per day per wound). By five days after injury, the ultrasound-treated groups had significantly fewer inflammatory cells in the wound bed and more extensive granulation tissue than the sham-irradiated controls. Also, the alignment of the fibroblasts – parallel to the wound surface – in the wound beds of the ultrasound-treated groups

was indicative of a more advanced tissue than the random alignment of fibroblasts seen in the sham-irradiated control wounds. The results obtained suggest that there had been an acceleration of the wounds through the inflammatory phase repair in response to ultrasound therapy. It was also noted that there were no abnormalities such as hypertrophy of the wound tissue seen in response to ultrasound therapy. Therefore, ultrasound therapy appears to accelerate the process without the risk of interfering with the control mechanisms which limit the development of granulation.

The Effect of Ultrasound on the Proliferative Phase of Repair

The main events occurring during this phase of repair include cell infiltration into the wound bed, angiogenesis, matrix deposition, wound contraction and re-epithelialization.

Cells such as fibroblasts and endothelial cells are recruited to the wound site by a combination of migration and proliferation. Mummery (1978) showed *in vitro* that fibroblast motility could be increased when they were exposed to therapeutic levels of ultrasound. With regard to cell proliferation, there is little evidence in the literature to suggest that ultrasound has a direct stimulatory effect on fibroblast stimulation. Most of the *in vitro* studies report either no effect or even an inhibitory effect on cell proliferation when exposed to therapeutic levels of ultrasound (Loch *et al.*, 1971; Kaufman *et al.*, 1977). However, the literature shows that when tissues are exposed to ultrasound *in vivo*, a marked increase in wound bed cell number can be demonstrated (Young and Dyson, 1990b; Dyson *et al.*, 1970). This anomaly may be explained if we examine the cellular interactions which occur during healing.

It was illustrated earlier that during wound repair much of the stimulus which controls the cellular events is derived from the macrophage. Therefore, it is highly likely that any increase in, for example, fibroblast proliferation, may be due in part to an indirect effect of ultrasound via the macrophage. Work by Young and Dyson (1990a) showed that if one exposes macrophages to therapeutic levels of ultrasound *in vitro*, then remove the surrounding culture medium and place it on fibroblast cultures, there is a large stimulatory effect on the proliferation of the fibroblasts. It therefore appears that the macrophage is sensitive to ultrasound and, in response to therapeutic levels of it ($0.5W/cm^2$ SAPA), they release a factor or factors which stimulate fibroblasts to proliferate.

Ultrasound can also effect the rate of angiogenesis. Hogan *et al.* (1982) showed that capillaries develop more rapidly in chronically ischaemic muscle when is exposed to ultrasound. Other work has shown that the exposure of skin lesions to ultrasound can stimulate the growth of blood capillaries into the wound site (Hosseinpour, 1988; Young and Dyson, 1990c).

When fibroblasts are exposed to ultrasound *in vitro* a marked stimulation in collagen secretion can be detected (Harvey *et al.*, 1975). It should be added that the degree of response was intensity dependent. When the fibroblasts were exposed to continuous ultrasound ($0.5W/cm^2$ SA), a 20% increase in collagen secretion was recorded; however, when the ultrasound was pulsed ($0.5 W/cm^2$ SATA), a 30% increase was recorded. Webster *et al.* (1978) demonstrated an increase in protein-synthesis when fibroblasts were exposed to ultrasound.

Wound contraction can be accelerated with ultrasound. Work by Dyson and Smalley (1983) showed that pulsed ultrasound (3 MHz, 0.5 W/cm^2 SATA) could stimulate the contraction of cryo-surgical lesions. More recently, Hart (1993) showed that exposure of full-thickness excised skin lesions to low levels of pulsed ultrasound stimulated contraction, leading to a significantly smaller scar. Interestingly, he found that the degree of contraction he induced using an intensity of 0.5 W/cm^2 (SATA) could also be achieved using the much lower intensity of 0.1 W/cm^2 (SATA). This is a significant finding which implies that clinicians can reduce their ultrasound treatment intensities by a significant degree and still achieve the desired results, via nonthermal effects. It is vital that when treating tissues which have a compromised blood system, and hence no effective mechanism of dispersing excess heat, the lowest possible ultrasound intensity is used.

In humans, wound closure is due mainly to granulation tissue formation and re-epithelialization, whereas in animals, where the skin is more loosely connected to the underlying tissues, wound closure is due mainly to contraction. Dyson *et al.* (1976) found that ultrasound therapy (3 MHz, pulsed, 0.2 W/cm^2 SAPA), accelerated the reduction in varicose ulcer area significantly (Figure 15.1). Similar findings were reported by Roche and West (1984).

Figure 15.1 Ultrasound treatment to the edge of a varicose ulcer using a sterile gel medium.

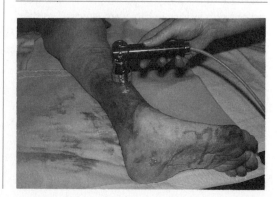

Callam *et al.* (1987) studied the effect of weekly ultrasound therapy (1 MHz, pulsed, 0.5 W/cm² SAPA) on the healing of chronic leg ulcers. They found that there was a 20% increase in the healing rate of the ultrasound-treated ulcers. There have been negative reports as to the use of ultrasound treatment on these chronic conditions. Lundeberg *et al.* (1990) did not demonstrate any statistically significant difference between ultrasound-treated and sham-treated venous ulcers. However, a trend was noted by the investigators that suggested ultrasound was more effective than placebo treatment. Interestingly, they stated that their experimental design, particularly their sample size (n = 44), was such that an improvement of less than 30% could not be detected.

Accelerated wound closure has also been recorded in other chronic wounds such as pressure sores (Paul *et al.*, 1960; McDiarmid *et al.*, 1985). McDiarmid *et al.* also reported an interesting finding that microbiologically infected sores were more responsive to ultrasound therapy than uninfected sores. It is likely that the low-grade infection had in some way primed or further activated the healing system (e.g. recruiting more macrophages to the area), which in turn would produce an amplified signal to herald an early start to the other phases of repair.

The Effect of Ultrasound on the Remodelling Phase of Repair

During remodelling the wound becomes relatively acellular and avascular, collagen content increases, and the tensile strength of the wound increases. The remodelling phase can last from months to years, depending upon the tissue involved and the nature of the injury. The mechanical properties of the scar are related to both the amount of collagen present and also the arrangement or alignment of the collagen fibres within the wound bed.

The effect of ultrasound on the properties of the scar depend very much upon the time at which the therapy was first instigated. By far the most effective regimes are those that are started soon after injury, i.e. during the inflammatory phase of repair. Webster *et al.* (1980) found that when wounds were treated three times per week for two weeks after injury (0.1 W/cm² SATA) the resulting tensile strength and elasticity of the scar was significantly higher than that of the control group. Byl *et al.* (1992, 1993), demonstrated an increase in tensile strength and collagen content in incised lesions whose treatment was commenced during the inflammatory phase. They also compared different ultrasound intensities and found that the lower intensity (1 MHz, pulsed, 0.5 W/cm² SATA) was the most effective. Treatment with ultrasound during the inflammatory phase of repair not only increases the amount of collagen deposited in the wound but also encourages the deposition of that collagen in a pattern whose three-dimensional architecture more resembles that of uninjured skin than the untreated controls (Dyson, 1981). Jackson *et al.* (1991) showed that the mechanical properties of injured tendon can be improved with ultrasound if treatment starts early enough, however, the levels used were relatively high, at 1.5 W/cm². Enwemaka *et al.* (1990) reported that increased tensile strength and elasticity can be achieved in injured tendons using much lower intensities (0.5 W/cm² SA). Figure 15.2 shows application of ultrasound to the elbow to treat tennis elbow.

The Effect of Ultrasound on Bone Repair

Bone repairs in much the same way as soft tissues. Both repair processes consist of three

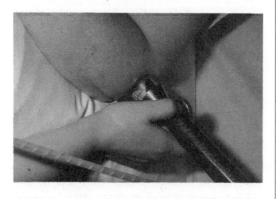

Figure 15.2   Ultrasound treatment for tennis elbow using gel as the transfer medium.

overlapping phases: inflammation, proliferation and remodelling. However, in bone repair, the proliferative phase is subdivided into soft and hard callus formation. The soft callus is an equivalent to granulation tissue in soft tissue injuries, and it is within this tissue that new bone regenerates to form the hard callus. Much work has been carried out investigating the effects of ultrasound therapy on this process. Dyson and Brookes (1983) showed that it was possible to accelerate the repair of fibular fractures using therapeutic levels of ultrasound (1.5 or 3 MHz, pulsed, 0.5 W/cm² SATP). The treatments were for five minutes, four times per week. Treatments were carried out at different combinations of weeks after injury, e.g. during the first two weeks only, or during the third and fourth week only. The most effective treatments were found to be those which were carried out during the first two weeks of repair, i.e. during the inflammatory phase of repair. It was found that if treatment was delayed (i.e. started on weeks 3 or 4 after injury) the ultrasound appeared to stimulate cartilage growth, postponing bony union. Of the two frequencies used, 1.5 MHz was the more effective.

There have been many other reports of the effectiveness of ultrasound in the treatment of bone fractures. Pilla et al. (1990) showed that low-intensity ultrasound (1.5 or 3MHz, pulsed, 0.3 W/cm²) could stimulate fracture repair to such a degree that maximum strength was gained in the treated limbs by 17 days after injury, compared to 28 days in the controls. Tsai et al. (1992a) demonstrated an increase in femoral fracture repair when using low intensities of ultrasound (1.5 MHz, pulsed, 0.5 W/cm²); however, when they tried 1.5 W/cm² they found that treatments inhibited repair. The same team (Tsai et al., 1992b) found that in the most effective output levels for stimulating repair, the production of endogenous PGE2 was highest. They suggested that bone healing stimulated by ultrasound may be mediated via the production of PGE2. More recent work (Heckman et al., 1994) investigated the effectiveness of low-intensity ultrasound on the healing of tibial fractures. The fractures were examined in a prospective, randomized, double-blind evaluation of low-intensity ultrasound. The treated group showed a significant decrease in the time to healing (86 days) when compared to the control group (114 days).

As with soft tissue repair, the evidence suggests that the best results are achieved when treatment is started as soon after injury as possible.

Ultrasound Application

A number of factors must be considered before using ultrasound:

1 Choice of ultrasound machine;
2 Calibration;
3 Choice of coupling medium;
4 Frequency;
5 Intensity;
6 Pulsed or continuous mode;
7 Treatment intervals;

8 Duration of treatment;

9 Potential hazards to both therapist and patient.

CHOICE OF ULTRASOUND MACHINE

Most ultrasound machines have the same basic design, consisting of an ultrasound generator which may be mains or battery-powered (or have dual capability). The generator comprises an oscillator circuit, transformer and microcomputer, and is linked via a coaxial cable to the treatment applicator. The applicator houses the transducer which produces ultrasound when stimulated by the oscillating voltage from the generator. Machines generally come with a number of treatment applicators, each capable of producing a different output frequency. Intensity can be varied, and also the choice of output can be varied from pulsed mode (a range of pulses is usually available) to continuous mode.

The choice of machine purchase should be made using the following guidelines:

1 Safety: use only machines that carry the British Standard mark BS 5724:part 1. This guarantees that the machines design has been checked for electrical safety.

2 Beam non-uniformity ratio (BNR): use machines that have transducers with low BNRs (5–6). This means that the ultrasound field is relatively uniform across the transducer face and lacks high-intensity hotspots.

3 Frequency: depth of penetration and the choice of desired physical mechanism (thermal or nonthermal) are frequency dependent; it makes sense to buy a machine that offers the greatest variety of frequencies e.g. 0.75–3.0 MHz, thereby giving you greater flexibility in your therapy range.

4 Digital controls/displays: these controls are easy to use and are more precise than the dated analogue meters and manual dials.

5 Self diagnostics: many machines now have inbuilt diagnostic circuits which check the generator output each time the machine is turned on. If a fault occurs in the machine this system ensures rapid diagnosis of the fault and allows maintenance to be carried out more effectively.

6 Automatic timer: preset treatment times reduces the risk of over exposure to ultrasound.

CALIBRATION

The machine must be calibrated on a regular basis, ideally once a week. The constant heavy usage that this type of equipment gets and the busy environment of the typical physiotherapy clinic (where items of equipment are sometimes dropped), mean it is likely that settings which corresponded to $1\,W/cm^2$ last month may not give that output this month. It is very important to note that the reading on the machine power-output meter is not an accurate guide as to what is actually coming out of the treatment head; the machine must be calibrated against a dedicated calibration device such as a radiation balance. Such a device is inexpensive, accurate, and simple to use, taking only minutes to carry out the calibration.

CHOICE OF COUPLING MEDIUM

By the very nature of ultrasound it cannot travel through air and so, without an adequate exit path, the sound generated by the transducer would reflect back from the interface between the air and the applicator treatment surface which could damage the delicate transducer. In order to provide the generated ultrasound with an 'escape route' from the treatment head into the body, some form of coupling agent needs to be placed between the applicator face and the body. The best coupling agent in terms of acoustic properties is water. The difference in acoustic impedance

Steve Young

between water and soft tissue is small, which means that there is approximately only 0.2% reflection at the interface between the two.

The ideal coupling agent would have not only the acoustic properties of water, but would also satisfy the following (Dyson, 1990):

1 No gas bubbles or other reflective objects;
2 Gel-like viscosity, allowing ease of use;
3 Sterile;
4 Hypoallergenic;
5 Chemically inert;
6 Perform also as a wound dressing;
7 Transparent;
8 Inexpensive.

Unfortunately, the ideal agent does not exist. However, there are a number of agents that are adequate and, as long as the user is aware of each agent's limitations, we can make the necessary allowances for them during the treatment session.

Degassed Water Freedom from gas bubbles and other inclusions, together with the close acoustic impedance match of water with soft connective tissues when compared to air (water – 1.52×10^6; fat – 1.35×10^6; muscle – 1.65–1.74×10^6; air – 429) make water the ideal agent, acoustically. However, the very nature of water, in terms of its viscosity, limits its use and it can therefore be used only if it is containerized; this does not present a problem when treating the extremities of the body such as the hand, wrist, ankle and foot, where they can be easily placed in a bowl of water (Figure 15.3).

The ideal treatment bowl should be lined with ultrasound-absorbing material to prevent unwanted reflections from the side of the dish. The therapist can adapt a regular washing-up bowl easily by lining its entire submerged surface with the type of dimpled rubber matting used in cars as foot mats. The degassed water (distilled water will

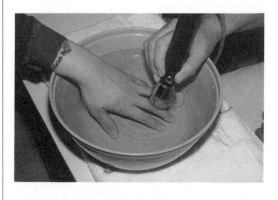

Figure 15.3   Ultrasound to the middle phalanges using degassed water as the transfer medium.

suffice) should be maintained at 37°C sterile if an open wound is being treated. The injured area and treatment head are then submerged in the bowl. It is not necessary to make contact between the treatment head and the injury because of the good transmission of ultrasound through water. If there is any risk of the operators hand being submerged in the water during treatment, a rubber surgical glove over a thin cotton glove should be worn on the hand (Figure 15.4); this reduces the possibility of ultrasound reflections being absorbed by the operator (the air trapped by the surgical glove makes a good reflective layer between the glove and the skin of the operator) and also reduces the possibility of cross infection in the case of open wounds.

This form of ultrasound application has the advantages that the treatment head does not need to touch painful injury sites, and that irregular areas such as the finger can be treated easily.

As with all ultrasound treatments, the treatment head must be kept moving at all times in a circular motion to avoid standing-wave formation.

Aqueous Gels, Oils and Emulsions These materials have similar acoustic properties to water with the advantage that their higher viscosities make them more user friendly. Examples of gels used

Figure 15.4   The incorrect and correct way to apply ultrasound therapy using the water immersion methods (P — ultrasound probe, S — surgical rubber glove, W — degassed water).

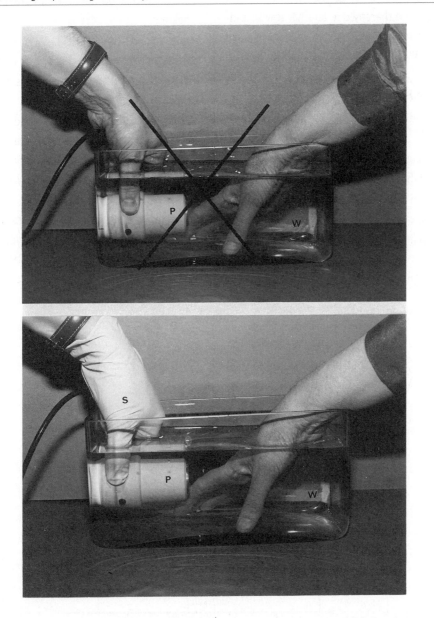

commonly used gels are Sonogel (Enraf-Nonius) and Camcare (Electro-Medical Supplies Ltd). They can be applied directly to the skin, but care should be taken to ensure that no air bubbles become trapped in them. If used on broken skin then sterile materials only should be used; if these are not available then treatment should be limited to the surrounding intact skin. This can still be an effective form of treatment as many of the reparative cells originate in this surrounding area and ultrasound will still have have a stimulatory effect on their activity.

Wound Dressings There are now a number of wound dressings that can be used in conjunction with ultrasound therapy due to their low sound-attenuation properties (Pringle, 1993). They fall into two main categories:

1 Polyurethane film dressings (e.g. OpSite, Smith and Nephew);
2 Polyacrylamide agar gel dressings (e.g. Geli-perm, Geistlich Pharmaceuticals).

Both dressing types attenuate little of the ultrasound energy (less than 5%). The dressings are used in the following way (Figure 15.5):

1 If there is a wound cavity it must be filled with sterile saline until the surface of the saline is continuous with the surface of the surrounding edge of the wound.

2 The dressing is then placed over the wound site, ensuring that no air becomes trapped underneath it.
3 Ultrasound coupling gel is then placed on the dressing surface, covering the wound site.
4 The ultrasound treatment head is then placed on the gel and treatment started.
5 After treatment, the excess gel can be wiped off the dressing and the dressing left in place to confer all the benefits of a moist environment to the healing wound (Dyson *et al.*, 1989).

This form of treatment allows therapists whose treatment has been restricted previously to the edge of the wound to treat directly over the wound bed. This area is a rich source of new cells

Figure 15.5 The correct procedure for applying ultrasound therapy to a cavity wound.

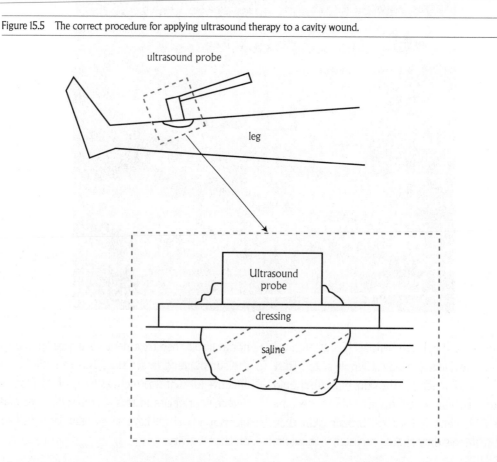

and tissue, thus making ultrasound therapy even more effective.

FREQUENCY

Having control over the frequency of the ultrasound output gives the therapist control over the depth at which the energy can be targeted, and also over which physical mechanism is active. The basic rule is that the higher the frequency, the more superficial the depth of penetration leading to rapid attenuation of the ultrasound causing a biological effect mainly via thermal mechanisms (cavitation is more likely to occur at lower frequencies). It must also be noted that the amount of attenuation is also dependent upon the nature of the tissue through which the ultrasound travels. Tissues with high protein content absorb energy more readily than those with a high fat or water content. Table 15.1 shows a guide to tissue absorption properties based upon half value-depth data. Putting this information into practice, the therapist confronted with a superficial skin lesion would choose a 3 MHz applicator; a deeper muscular injury would require a 1 MHz applicator.

INTENSITY

Once the choice of frequency has been made so that the required depth of penetration can be achieved, the therapist has to make the decision as to what intensity level to use, i.e. the damaged area can be reached, so now, how much ultrasound do we apply?

There is no quantitative scientific or clinical data that indicates we must use high levels of ultrasound, i.e. greater than $1 \, W/cm^2$ (SATA), to cause a significant biological effect in injured tissues. On the contrary, the data presented earlier in this chapter supported the use of intensities of 0.5 W/cm^2 (SATA) and less to achieve maximum healing rates in tissues such as skin, tendons and bone. The evidence also showed that levels of ultrasound in excess of 1.5 W/cm^2 (SATA) have an adverse effect on healing tissues. Significant thermal effects can be achieved using intensities of between 0.5 and $1 \, W/cm^2$ (SATA). Treat below 0.5 W/cm^2 (SATA) to invoke primarily non-thermal mechanisms.

Fortunately, there has been a trend over recent years towards the use of lower-intensity treatments. The advice to the therapist is **always use the lowest intensity that produces the required therapeutic effect, since higher intensities may be damaging** (Dyson, 1990). Generally, with acute conditions, the intensity used should be no higher than 0.5 W/cm^2 (SATA), and for chronic conditions levels should be no higher than $1 \, W/cm^2$ (SATA).

Table 15.1

The half value depth for 1 MHz ultrasound in a range of different media*

Medium	1 MHz (mm)	3 MHz (mm)
Water	11 500.0	3833.0
Adipose tissue	50.0	16.5
Skeletal muscle (fibres parallel to sound beam)	24.6	8.0
Tendon	6.2	2.0
Skin	11.1	4.0
Skeletal muscle (fibres at right angles to sound beam)	9.0	3.0
Cartilage	6.0	2.0
Air	2.5	0.8
Compact bone	2.1	–

* from Hoogland, 1986

PULSED OR CONTINUOUS MODE ?

Pulsing ultrasound has a major effect on reducing the amount of heat generated in the tissues. A controversy exists as to what the major mechanisms are by which ultrasound stimulates injuries to heal. It is unlikely that a specific bioeffect occurs as a result of the exclusive action of either thermal or nonthermal mechanisms; it is more likely to be as a mixture of both. Therefore, the area is rather a gray one. However, based on the literature available, the the flow diagram in Figure 15.6 gives an indication as to how the decision may be made.

Thermal effects are not desirable where the injury site has a compromised or low blood supply, e.g. tendon. In this case, healing should be achieved using nonthermal mechanisms, i.e. pulse the ultrasound to reduce the temporal average (reduced heating) whilst maintaining the pulse average at a level high enough to achieve a biological effect.

TREATMENT INTERVALS

The interval between successive treatments depends upon the nature of the injury.

ACUTE

The weight of the evidence with regards to the effectiveness of ultrasound therapy indicates that the earlier it is used after injury, the more effective it is, i.e. it is best applied during the early inflammatory phase of repair (Oakley, 1978; Patrick, 1978). During the inflammatory phase of repair, macrophages and mast cells occupy the wound site and it has been shown that these cells are responsive to therapeutic ultrasound (Fyfe and Chahl, 1985; Young and Dyson, 1990a). This action of therapeutic ultrasound accelerates the inflammatory phase of repair, resulting in a more rapid entry into the proliferative phase (Dyson, 1990; Young and Dyson, 1990). During the inflammatory phase of repair, treatments should be once a day for approximately a week, or until swelling and pain have subsided. Treatments through the subsequent proliferative phase of repair can then be reduced to three times per week (McDiarmid and Burns, 1987). This should be maintained until the condition is resolved.

CHRONIC

The literature with regards to the treatment of chronic wounds is sparse, and also mixed in

---

Figure 15.6   Flow diagram showing some criteria on which the decision to use pulsed or continuous ultrasound can be based.

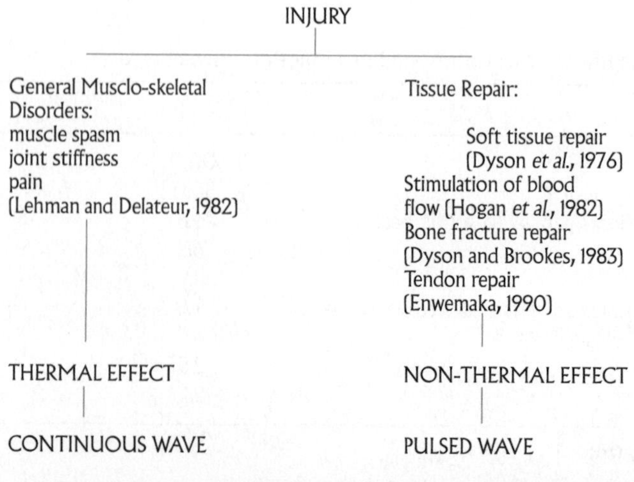

INJURY

General Musclo-skeletal Disorders:
muscle spasm
joint stiffness
pain
(Lehman and Delateur, 1982)

Tissue Repair:

Soft tissue repair
(Dyson et al., 1976)
Stimulation of blood
flow (Hogan et al., 1982)
Bone fracture repair
(Dyson and Brookes, 1983)
Tendon repair
(Enwemaka, 1990)

THERMAL EFFECT

NON-THERMAL EFFECT

CONTINUOUS WAVE

PULSED WAVE

respect to the efficacy of ultrasound treatments and also about the treatment intervals. In the case of venous leg ulcers, the positive reviews state a treatment regime of once per week (Callam, 1987), and three times per week (Dyson *et al.*, 1976). It is advisable to maintain treatment of chronic wounds beyond the inflammatory phase of repair into the proliferative phase as it has been shown that ultrasound can effect many of the processes that occur during this time, e.g. angiogenesis (Young and Dyson, 1990c), fibroblast activity (Webster, 1980; Dyson, 1987), and wound contraction (Hart, 1993). These effects have been achieved using low intensity (maximum of $0.5W/cm^7$), which utilizes primarily non-thermal mechanisms.

DURATION OF TREATMENT

The duration of treatment depends upon the area of the injury. Typically, the area should be divided into zones which are approximately 1.5 times the area of the ultrasound treatment head, and then treat for 1 or 2 minutes per zone (Oakley, 1978). Subsequent treatment times should then be increased by 30 seconds per zone up to a maximum of 3 minutes (Oakley, 1978). Hoogland (1986) recommends that a total maximal treatment time of 15 minutes and that at least 1 minute should be spent in treating an area of 1 cm.

POTENTIAL HAZARDS

Ultrasound can be an effective therapy or a potential hazard depending upon how it is applied. There exists a number of extensive lists of contraindications and precautions (Reid, 1981; Hoogland, 1986; Dyson, 1988). These include irradiation of:

- Uterus during pregnancy;
- Gonads;
- Malignancies and precancerous lesions;
- Tissues previously treated by deep x-ray or other radiation;
- Vascular abnormalities, e.g. deep vein thrombosis, emboli, severe atherosclerosis;
- Acute infections;
- Cardiac area in advanced heart disease;
- Eye;
- Stellate ganglion;
- Haemophiliacs not covered by factor replacement;
- Areas over subcutaneous bony prominences;
- Epiphyseal plates;
- Spinal cord after laminectomy;
- Subcutaneous major nerves;
- Cranium;
- Anaesthetic areas.

Many of these contraindications have been included in the list even though they are not based on any hard scientific evidence. However, even if there is a remote chance that damage may occur then ultrasound should not be used.

Dyson (1988) lists the following basic precautions to be taken to ensure that ultrasound is used effectively and safely:

1 Use ultrasound only if adequately trained to do so;
2 Use ultrasound to treat patients only with conditions known to respond favourably to this treatment (unless it is being used experimentally);
3 Use the lowest intensity that produces the required effect, because higher intensities may be damaging;
4 Move the applicator constantly throughout treatment, to avoid the damaging effects of standing waves;
5 If the patient feels any additional pain during treatment, either reduce the intensity to a pain-free level or abandon the treatment;
6 Use properly calibrated and maintained equipment;
7 If there is any doubt, do not irradiate.

Wound Assessment

It is vital that we have objective and sensitive techniques by which we can assess wound healing. Only when we have this can the rate and quality of repair of a patient's wound be optimized confidently.

Chronic wounds present additional problems with regards to wound assessment. Because these wounds heal so slowly it is often difficult to obtain an early indication whether they are healing, remaining static or deteriorating. Often, much time is wasted using ineffective therapeutic modalities.

There are numerous methods for evaluating wound repair, and these can be divided into two main groups: invasive, and non-invasive techniques.

Invasive

These techniques provide quantitative information regarding the wound and its stage in healing. These methods include:

1 Histological evaluation of excised tissue to identify and measure the number of cell types present during the healing process (Young, 1988);
2 Biochemical analysis of wound tissue biopsies and fluid to measure the various components involved in wound repair, e.g. collagen synthesis and deposition, mRNA synthesis, extracellular factors (Saperia, 1986);
3 Tensile strength may be analysed by tissue breaking point or 'wound rupture stress' (Charles et al., 1992);
4 Angiogenesis may be monitored by angiography (Young and Dyson, 1990c).

Although these methods are able to yield quantitative data regarding wound healing they are invasive, involving biopsy, which results in the destruction of the tissue under investigation, thereby delaying wound healing. In addition, many patients find this procedure, at best, uncomfortable.

Non-Invasive Methods

These techniques tend to be less quantitative than the invasive methods; however, they are more acceptable to patients. Non-invasive methods include:

1 Transparency Tracings: a double layer of sterile acetate or polythene film is placed over the wound, and the outline is traced using a permanent marker pen. By using a double-layer film, the side which has been in contact with the wound, can be discarded preventing contact infection. The surface area of the wound can then be measured by either placing the acetate tracing onto graph paper and counting the squares, or evaluated using a computer, which scans and digitizes the traced outline and calculates the surface area automatically. The disadvantages of using the tracing method is that it is very hard to define the edges of the wound and so the error can be high.
2 Photographic recording: wounds can be photographed instead of traced. The operator must place a ruler or some other object of known size next to the wound to provide a scale against which measurements can be made. The wound surface area can then be calculated from photographs using computerized image analysis. Although accuracy is increased using photographic rather than tracing methods, errors can still occur due, for example, to varying ambient light conditions leading to variations in exposure from film to film, or to distortions

of the vertical and horizontal axes which arise if the wound is on a curved surface.

3 Depth gauges: a device known as the Kundin gauge (Kundin, 1989), has been developed which is able to measure the length, width and depth of a wound; from these, area and volume are calculated. This method is more accurate when used to measure circular and elliptical wounds. When used for irregular wounds, in which there is tracking and underlying cavities, the method often underestimates area and volume; this is the main disadvantage of this method. However, the method is easy to use, disposable, objective and inexpensive.

4 Volume: the volume of wounds can be measured by making moulds of the wound. A variety of substances can be used, including hydrocolloid gel, silicone rubber, silastic foam, and alginates (Covington, 1989). The mould is then placed in water, and the volume displaced is the volume of the wound. The use of this method is restricted; it cannot be used over shallow wounds, or those which are circumferential around a limb, or for wounds with undermining and sinus formation. The orifice of the wound has to be sufficiently large to remove the material. Another method to measure volume, is the use of saline (Berg, 1990). The wound is covered by a film, and saline is injected into the wound. This is a simple and reproducible technique, but is not satisfactory for superficial sores.

5 Stereoscopic photography: this is used to overcome projection errors from the curved skin surface to a flat screen. This method uses two cameras, so that a photograph is produced from which depth measurements can be recorded (Bulstrode, 1986). The area and volume of the wound can be calculated by a computer. The method is accurate and reproducible, and measurements of irregular defects

in the wound, in three dimensions, can be made. However, the amount of specialized equipment and time involved restricts this method's application in clinical practice.

6 Thermal imaging: this method detects infrared radiation emitted from the skin. The emission of the wound, however will vary depending upon whether the wound has been exposed without a dressing, and if so for how long, and whether it is infected. It can be used to record temperature at the edges of a wound, to monitor blood perfusion, and it could also be useful for monitoring the effect of antibiotic therapy in an infected wound.

7 Video image analysis: video cameras can be used to record lesions from different angles to provide optimimum information, and to reduce the measurement problems caused by skin curvature (Smith, 1992). This method uses a video camera with a macrolens, linked to an image-processing computer which produce high-precision measurements of area, colour density and volume.

One major drawback exists with most of the non-invasive techniques discussed up to this point: they produce data which describes the outer surface of the wound and surrounding uninjured skin only – none of the techniques give any indication as to the quality of the underlying reparative tissue. However, there now exists a non-invasive method that allows the clinician to look deep into the wound bed, with a high degree of resolution, to assess the quality of the reparative tissue (Young et al., 1993; Whiston et al., 1993a, b; Karim et al., 1994). This technique involves the use of high-frequency ultrasound (Figure 15.7).

This is a simple procedure that is able to produce a high-resolution image of the dermis and wound bed (Figure 15.8). The scan can be carried out

Figure 15.7   Photograph showing a high frequency ultrasound scanner (K – keyboard, M – high-definition colour monitor, P – ultrasound probe). [Quality Medical Imaging Ltd.]

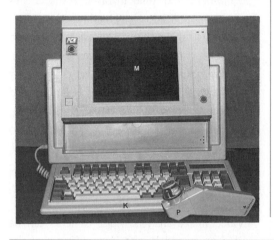

through certain wound dressings (e.g. Geliperm) when a coupling gel is applied, thereby avoiding risks of infection and also offering protection to the delicate wound surface during the scanning procedure. An axial resolution of 65 µm and a lateral resolution of approximately 200 µm can be obtained. The images produced can be analysed using software built into the scanner. Using image analysis it is possible to monitor even small changes in a wound, even before they become clinically evident, and to recognize whether the wound is deteriorating or improving. This early detection can lead to large savings in treatment times. Wound depth can also be calculated using

Figure 15.8   Ultrasound scan showing the structure of the skin, underlying tissue, and the extent of a surgical incised lesion. [Scale is in Millimetres].

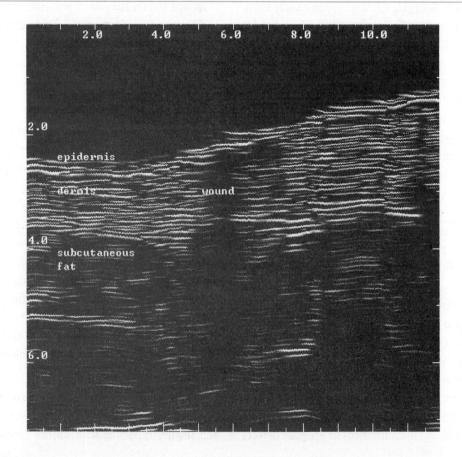

this technique, e.g. in burn injuries. This is a rapid, sensitive and repeatable method of quantifying wound healing.

Summary

In summary, it can be said that, if used correctly and at the right time after injury, ultrasound can be a very potent therapeutic force. 'Correctly' means using the lowest possible intensity to achieve the desired result (intensities above 1W/cm^2 should not be necessary), and the 'right time after injury' means during the inflammatory phase of repair. Bearing in mind clinical audit, clinicians should take advantage of the numerous wound assessment techniques which now exist to test the effectiveness of their therapies. Finally, ultrasound can be dangerous if used incorrectly, so users must understand fully the mechanisms by which it works.

Acknowledgements

I would like to thank the many physiotherapists I have met at lectures and meetings during the last few years. This interaction has provided me with a valuable insight as to how ultrasound is used clinically and also where the grey areas with respect to our knowledge of bioeffects exist.

I would like to thank all my colleagues in the Tissue Repair Research Unit at UMDS, who have given advice and support in the writing of this chapter.

Finally, I would like to thank Mary Dyson whose enthusiasm for research has eventually rubbed off on me.

References

Allman, RM (1989) Epidemiology of pressure sores in different populations. *Decubitus* 2: 30–33.

Bailey, AJ, Bazin, S, Sims, TJ, LeLeus, M, Nicholetis, C, Delaunay, A (1975) Characterisation of the collagen of human hypertrophic and normal scars. *Biochemistry and Biophysics Acta* 405: 412–421.

Berg, W, Traneroth, C, Gunnarsson, A, Lossing, C (1990). A method for measuring pressure sores. *Lancet* 335: 1445–1446.

Bulstrode, CJK, Goode, JW, Scott, PJ (1986). Stereophotogrammetry for measuring rates of cutaneous healing: a conventional technique. *Clinical Science* 71: 4–443.

Byl, NN, McKenzie, AL, West, JM, Whitney, JD, Hunt, TK, Scheuenstuhl HA (1992). Low-dose ultrasound effects on wound healing: a controlled study with Yucatan pigs. *Archives of Physical Medicine in Rehabilitation* 73: 656–664.

Byl, NN, McKenzie, AL, Wong, T, West, JM, Hunt, TK (1993). Incisional wound healing: a controlled study of low and high dose ultrasound. *Journal of Orthopaedic and Sports Physical Therapy* 18: 619–628.

Callam, MJ, Harper, DR, Dale, JJ, Ruckley, CV, Prescott, RJ (1987) A controlled trial of weekly ultrasound therapy in chronic leg ulceration. *Lancet* July 25: 204–206.

Chapman, IV, Macnally, NA, Tucker, S (1979) Ultrasound induced changes in the rates of influx and efflux of potassium ions in rat thymocytes in vitro. *British Journal Radiology* 47: 411–415.

Charles, D, Williams, K 3rd, Perry, LC, Fisher, J, Rees, RS (1992) An improved method of in vivo wound disruption and measurement. *Journal of Surgical Research* 52: 214–218.

Clark, RAF (1990) Cutaneous Wound Repair, in Goldsmith LE (Ed.) *Biochemistry and Physiology of the Skin.*, pp. 576–601. Oxford University Press, Oxford.

Collier, M (1990) A sore point. *Community Outlook*, October 29–30.

Covington, JS, Griffin, JW, Mendius, RK, Tooms, RE, Clifft, JK (1989) Measurement of pressure ulcer volume using dental impression materials. *Physical Therapy* 69: 68–72.

David, JA (1983) *An investigation of the current methods used in nursing for the care of patients with pressure sores.* Nursing Practice Research Unit. University of Surrey, Guildford.

Department of Health (1989) *Working for Patients. Medical Audit. Working Paper 6.* HMSO, London.

Dinno, MA, Dyson, M, Young, SR, Mortimer, AJ, Hart, J, Crum, LA (1989) The significance of membrane changes in the safe and effective use of therapeutic and diagnostic ultrasound. *Phys Med Biol* 34: 1543–1552.

Dyson, M (1981) The effect of ultrasound on the rate of wound healing and the quality of scar tissue, in (Mortimer, AJ and Lee, N, eds) *Proceedings of the International Symposium on Therapeutic Ultrasound (Manitoba, 1981)*, pp. 110–123. Canadian Physiotherapy Association, Winnipeg.

Dyson, M (1982) Nonthermal cellular effects of ultrasound. *British Journal of Cancer* 45(suppl. V): 165–171.

Dyson, M (1985) Therapeutic applications of ultrasound, in Nyborg WL, Ziskin MC (eds) *Biological Effects of Ultrasound (clinics in diagnostic ultrasound)*, pp 121–133. Churchill Livingstone, Edinburgh.

Dyson, M (1987) Mechanisms involved in therapeutic ultrasound. *Physiotherapy* 73: 116–120.

Dyson, M (1988) The use of ultrasound in sports physiotherapy, in Bromley I, Wattseries N (series eds) 25. *International Perspectives in*

Physical Therapy, and Grisogono, V (ed.) *Sports Injuries*, pp. 213–232. Churchill Livingstone, Edinburgh.

Dyson, M (1990) Role of Ultrasound in Wound Healing, in Kloth, LC, McCulloch, JM, Feedar, JA (eds) *Wound Healing: Alternatives in Management*, pp. 259–285. FA Davis, Philadelphia.

Dyson, M, Brookes, M (1983) Stimulation of bone repair by ultrasound, in Lerski, RA, Morley, P (eds) *Ultrasound 82, Proceedings 3rd Meeting World Federation of Ultrasound in Medicine and Biology*. Pergamon Press, Oxford.

Dyson, M, Franks, C, Suckling, J (1976) Stimulation of healing varicose ulcers by ultrasound. *Ultrasonics* 14: 232–236.

Dyson, M, Pond, JB, Joseph, J, Warwick, R (1968) Stimulation of tissue repair by pulsed wave ultrasound. *IEEE Transactions on Sonics and Ultrasonics* SU-17: 133–140.

Dyson, M, Pond, JB, Joseph, J, Warwick, R (1970) The stimulation of tissue regeneration by means of ultrasound. *Clinical Science* 35: 273–285.

Dyson, M, Pond, JB, Woodward, J, Broadbent, J (1974) The production of blood cell stasis and endothelial cell damage in the blood vessels of chick embryos treated with ultrasound in a stationary wave field. *Ultrasound and Medical Biology* 1: 133–148.

Dyson, M, Smalley, DS (1983) Effects of ultrasound on wound contraction, in Millner, R, Rosenfeld, E, Cobet, U (eds) *Ultrasound Interactions in Biology and Medicine*, pp.151. Plenum Publishing Corporation.

El Hag, M, Coghlan, K, Christmas, P, Harvey, W, Harris, M (1985) The anti-inflammatory effects of dexamethasone and therapeutic ultrasound in oral surgery. *British Journal of Oral Maxillofacial Surgery* 23: 17–23.

Enwemeka, CS, Rodriguez, O, Mendosa, S (1990) The biomechanical effects of low-intensity ultrasound on healing tendons. *Ultrasound Med Biol* 16: 801–807.

Fyfe, MC, Chahl, LA (1982) Mast cell degranulation: A possible mechanism of action of therapeutic ultrasound. *Ultrasound Med Biol* 8(suppl. 1): 62.

Fyfe, MC, Chahl, LA (1985) The effect of single or repeated applications of 'therapeutic' ultrasound on plasma extravasation during silver nitrate induced inflammation of the rat hidpaw ankle joint *in vivo* . *Ultrasound Med Biol* 11: 273–283.

Ginsberg, M (1981) Role of platelets in inflammation and rheumatic disease. *Adv Inflamm Res* 2: 53.

Goddard, DH, Revell, PA, Cason, J, Gallagher, S, Currey, HLF (1983) Ultrasound has no anti-inflammatory effect. *Ann. Rheum. Dis.* 42: 582–584.

Goode, FG *et al.* (1992) Vitamin C depletion and pressure sores in elderly patients with femoral neck fracture. *British Medical Journal* 305: 925–927.

ter Haar, G, Hopewell, JW (1982) Ultrasonic heating of mammalian tissue *in vivo*. *British Journal of Cancer* 45(suppl. V): 65–67.

ter Haar, G, Dyson, M, Oakley, EM (1985) The use of ultrasound by physiotherapists in Britain, 1985. *Ultrasound Med Biol* 13: 659–663.

Hart, J (1993) *The effect of therapeutic ultrasound on dermal repair with emphasis on fibroblast activity*. PhD Thesis, University of London.

Harvey, W, Dyson, M, Pond, JB, Grahame, R (1975) The stimulation of protein synthesis in human fibroblasts by therapeutic ultrasound. *Rheum. Rehabil.* 14: 237.

Hashish, I (1986) *The effects of ultrasound therapy on post operative inflammation*. PhD Thesis, University of London.

Heckman, JD, Ryaby, JP, McCabe, J, Frey, JJ, Kilcoyne, RF (1994) Acceleration of tibial fracture-healing by non-invasive, low-intensity pulsed ultrasound. *Journal of Bone and Joint Surgery (American Volume)* 76: 26–34.

Hibbs, P (1988) *Pressure area care for the City and Hackney health authority*. St Bartholomew's Hospital, London.

Hibbs, P (1989) The economics of pressure sores. *Care of the Critically Ill* 5: 6, 247–250.

HMSO (1994) *Annual Abstract of Statistics No. 194*, HMSO, London

Hogan, RDB, Burke, KM, Franklin, TD (1982) The effect of ultrasound on the microvascular hemodynamics in skeletal muscle: effects during ischemia. *Microvascular Research* 23: 370–379.

Hoogland, R (1986) *Ultrasound Therapy*. Enraf Nonius, Delft, Holland.

Hosseinpour, AR (1988) *The effects of ultrasound on angiogenesis and wound healing*. Bsc. Thesis, University of London.

Hustler, JE, Zarod, AP, Williams, AR (1978) Ultrasonic modification of experimental bruising in the guinea pig pinna. *Ultrasonics* Sept: 223–228.

Jackson, BA, Schwane, JA, Starcher, BC (1991) Effect of ultrasound therapy on the repair of achilles tendon injuries in rats. *Medicine, Science, Sports, Exercise.* 23: 171–176.

Karim, A, Young, SR, Lynch, JA, Dyson, M (1994) A novel method of assessing skin ultrasound scans. *Wounds* 6: 9–15.

Kaufman, GE, Miller, MW, Griffiths, TD, Ciaravino, V, Carstenson, EL (1977) Lysis and viability of cultured mammalian cells exposed to 1 MHz ultrasound. UMB 3: 21–25.

Kischer, CW, Schetlar, MR (1974) Collagen and mucopolysaccharides in the hypertrophic scar. *Connective Tissue Research* 2: 205–213.

Kitchen, S (1995) *Electrophysical Agents: Their Nature and Therapeutic Usage*, pp 2. PhD Thesis, University of London.

Knighton, DR, Hunt, TK, Scheuenstuhl, H, Halliday, BJ (1983) Oxygen tension regulates the expression of angiogenesis factor by macrophages. *Science* 221: 1283–1285.

Kundin, JI (1989). A new way to size up a wound. *American Journal of Nursing* 89: 206–207.

Lehmann, JF, Guy, AW (1972) Ultrasound Therapy, in Reid, J, Sikov, M (eds) *Interaction of Ultrasound and Biological Tissues*, pp. 141–152. DHEW Publication, (FDA) 73–8008, USA. Government Printng Office, Washington DC.

Lehmann, JF, DeLateur, BJ (1982) Therapeutic Heat, in Lehmann, JF (ed) *Therapeutic Healt and Cold* (3rd ed.), pp.404. Williams and Wilkins, Baltimore.

Leibovich, SJ, Ross, R (1975) The role of the macrophage in wound repair. *American Journal of Pathology* 78: 71–92.

Levenson, SM, Geever, EG, Crowley, LV, Oates, JF, Berard, CW, Rosen, H (1965) The healing of rat skin wounds. *Annals of Surgery* 161: 293–308.

Livesey, B, Simpson, G (1989) The hard cost of soft sores. *The Health Service Journal* 99: 5143, p. 231.

Loch, EG, Fisher, AB, Kuwert, E (1971) Effect of diagnostic and therapeutic intensities of ultrasonics on normal and malignant human cells *in vitro. American Journal of Obstetrics and Gynecology* 110: 457–460.

Lundeberg, T, Nordstrom, F, Brodda-Jansen, Eriksson, SV, Kjartansson, J. Samuelson, UE (1990) Pulsed ultrasound does not improve healing of venous ulcers. *Scandanavian Journal of Rehab. Med.* 22: 195–197.

McDiarmid, T, Burns, PN, Lewith, GT, Machin, D (1985) Ultrasound and the treatment of pressure sores. *Physiotherapy* 71: 66–70.

McDiarmid, T, Burns, PN (1987) Clinical applications of therapeutic ultrasound. *Physiotherapy* 73: 155.

Morison, MJ (1992) *A Colour Guide to the Nursing Management of Wounds.* Wolfe, London

Mortimer, AJ, Dyson, M (1988) The effect of therapeutic ultrasound on calcium uptake in fibroblasts. *Ultrasound Med Biol* 14: 499–506.

Mummery, CL (1978) *The effect of ultrasound on fibroblasts in vitro.* PhD Thesis, University of London.

NCRP Report No. 74. (1983). *Biological effects of ultrasound: Mechanisms and implications,* p. 82.

Nyborg, WL (1977) *Physical mechanisms for biological effects of ultrasound.* DHEW 78-8062. US Government Printing Office, Washington D.C.

Oakley, EM (1978) Applications of continuous beam ultrasound at therapeutic levels. *Physiotherapy* 64: 169–172.

Patrick, MK (1978) Applications of therapeutic pulsed ultrasound. *Physiotherapy* 64: 103–104.

Paul, BJ, Lafratta, CW, Dawson, AR, Baab, E, Bullock, F (1960) Use of ultrasound in the treatment of pressure sores in patients with spinal cord injuries. *Archives of Physical Medicine in Rehabilitation* 41: 438–440.

Peacock, EE (1984) Contraction, in Peacock, EE (ed) *Wound Repair,* 3rd ed., pp. 39–55. WB Saunders and Company.

Pilla, AA, Mont, MA, Nasser, PR, Khan, SA, Figueiredo, M, Kaufmann, JJ, Siffert, RS (1990) Non-invasive low-intensity pulsed ultrasound accelerates bone healing in the rabbit. *Journal of Orthopaedic Trauma* 4: 246–253.

Potter, MS (1994) Incidence of pressure sores in nursing home patients. *Journal of Wound Care* 3: 1, 37–42.

Reid, DC (1981) Possible contraindications and precautions associated with ultrasound therapy, in Mortimer, AJ, Lee, N (eds) *Proceedings of the international symposium on therapeutic ultrasound,* p. 274. Canadian Physiotherapy Association, Winnipeg.

Roche, C, West, J (1984) A controlled trial investigating the effect of ultrasound on venous ulcers referred from general practitioners. *Physiotherapy.* 70: 475–477.

Saperia, D, Glassberg, E, Lyons, RF (1986) Demonstration of elevated type I and II pro-collagen mRNA levels in cutaneous wounds treated with helium- neon laser. *Biochem. Biophys. Res. Commun.* 136: 1123–1128.

Scales, JT, Lowthian, PT, Poole, AG, Ludman WR (1982) 'Vaperm' patient support system : a new general purpose hospital mattress. *Lancet ii,* 1150–1152.

Smith, DJ, Bhat, S, Bulgrin, JP (1992) Video image analysis of wound repair. *Wounds* 4: 6–15.

Snow, CJ, Johnson, KJ (1988) Effect of therapeutic ultrasound on acute inflammation. *Physiotherapy Canada* 40: 162–167.

Sutherland, EW, Rall, EW (1968) Formation of cyclic adenine ribonucleotide by tissue particles. *Journal of Biol Chem* 232: 1065–1076.

Tsai, CL, Chang, WH, Liu, TK (1992a) Preliminary studies of duration and intensity of ultrasonic treatments on fracture repair. *Chinese Journal of Physiology* 35: 21–26.

Tsai, CL, Chang, WH, Liu, TK (1992b) Ultrasonic effect on fracture repair and prostaglandin E2 production. *Chinese Journal of Physiology* 35: 168.

Watson, R (1989) Pressure sores: a rational approach to treatment. *Nursing Standard* 39: 3, 23–24.

Webster, DF, Pond, JB, Dyson, M, Harvey, W (1978) The role of cavitation in the *in vitro* stimulation of protein synthesis in human fibroblasts by ultrasound. *Ultrasound Med Biol* 4: 343–351.

Webster, DF, Dyson, M, Harvey, W (1979) Ultrasonically induced stimulation of collagen synthesis *in vivo,* in Greguss P (ed.) Proceedings of the 4th Ultrasound in Biology and Medicine Symposium, vol I, pp. 135-140. Visegrad, Hungary.

Webster, DF (1980) *The effect of ultrasound on wound healing.* PhD Thesis, University of London.

Whiston, RJ, Melhuish, J, Harding, KG (1993). High Resolution Ultrasound Imaging in Wound Healing. 5: 116–121.

Whiston, RJ, Young, SR, Lynch, JA, Harding, KG, Dyson, M (1993) Application of high frequency ultrasound to the objective assessment of healing wounds, in *The 6th Annual Symposium on Advanced Wound Care,* pp. 26–29. Health Management Publications.

Williams, AR (1974) Release of serotonin from platelets by acoustic streaming. *Journal of the Acoustic Society of America* 56: 1640.

Williams, AR, Sykes, SM, O'Brien, WD (1976) Ultrasonic exposure modifies platelet morphology and function *in vitro. Ultrasound Med Biol* 2: 311–317

Williams, AR (1987) Production and transmission of ultrasound. *Physiotherapy* 73(3): 113–116.

Young, JB (1992) Aids to prevention of pressure sores. *British Medical Journal* 300: 1002–1004.

Young, SR (1988) The effect of therapeutic ultrasound on the biological mechanisms involved in dermal repair, pp. 169–174. PhD Thesis, University of London.

Young, SR, Dyson M (1990a) Macrophage responsiveness to therapeutic ultrasound. *Ultrasound Med Biol* 16: 809–816.

Young, SR, Dyson, M (1990b) The effect of therapeutic ultrasound on the healing of full-thickness excised skin lesions. *Ultrasonics* 28: 175–180.

Young, SR, Dyson, M (1990c). The effect of therapeutic ultrasound on angiogenesis. *Ultrasound Med Biol* 16: 261–269.

Young, SR, Lynch, JA, Leipins, PJ, Dyson, M (1993). Non-invasive method of wound assessment using high-frequency ultrasound imaging, in *The 6th Annual Symposium on Advanced Wound Care,* pp. 29–31. Health Management Publications.

Yurt, RW (1981). Role of the mast cell in trauma, in Dineen, P, Hildick-Smith, G (eds) *The Surgical Wound,* p-62. Lea and Febiger, Philadelphia.

F

Low-Frequency Currents

16

Low-Frequency Currents: An Introduction

TRACEY HOWE

Pulse Characteristics and Parameters Used During Neuromuscular Stimulation
•
Definitions of Terms
•
The Importance of Stimulation Parameters
•
Summary

Pulse Characteristics and Parameters Used During Neuromuscular Stimulation

Recent advances in miniaturized electronics have created increased interest in neuromuscular stimulation. However, many research papers do not state information regarding the parameters used. This makes it difficult to reproduce work or indeed to translate the results of published work into clinical practice. Singer *et al.* (1987) suggested that there is a need for standardization on the reporting of methodology. This chapter will outline the characteristics and parameters used during neuromuscular stimulation.

Neuromuscular stimulators produce electrical pulse trains that cause excitation of peripheral nerves and subsequently muscle tissue (Hultman *et al.*, 1983). These electrical pulses enter the body tissues via surface electrodes and hence all types of stimulators may correctly be called *transcutaneous neuromuscular stimulators*. The differences between them lies in their electrical output, which may be either constant-current or constant-voltage in nature. The electrical output, current or voltage, remains constant even with alterations in skin resistance or impedance caused by alterations in temperature or sweating etc. The characteristics and parameters of the pulse train produced by different neuromuscular stimulators varies. The parameters are fixed on some stimulators whereas others

271

allow them to be modified, within limits, by the operator.

Definitions of Terms

It is important at this point to define various terms commonly used, and misused, within the literature.

The *frequency* of a stimulus train is defined as the number of cycles per second and is usually expressed in hertz (Hz) or pulses per second (pps). This is the actual frequency of the stimulus train where pulses are produced at regular intervals. The mean frequency value is used for non-uniform stimulus trains where pulses are produced at irregular intervals, or for mixed frequency stimulation where more than one frequency is produced during a period of stimulation.

The *amplitude* of the waveform may be defined as the peak to peak amplitude of the cycle (Figure 16.1) and is expressed in milliamps (mA) or volts (V) depending on whether the stimulator produces a constant-current or a constant-voltage output. High voltage stimulators deliver peak outputs of around 150 V and low voltage stimulators 100 V or less.

The *pulse duration*, sometimes referred to as the pulse width, is defined as the duration of the

Figure 16.1   Peak to peak amplitude of a pulse.

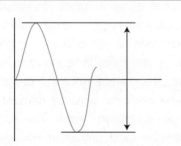

Figure 16.2   Pulse duration of a pulse.

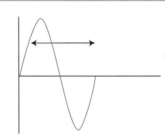

output pulse waveform at 50% of the maximum amplitude (BSI, 1988) (Figure 16.2) and is expressed in microseconds (μs).

The amount of energy applied to the stimulated tissue per pulse is termed the *charge density* and is the pulse duration multiplied by the current. Charge density is expressed in microcoulombs (μC).

There are two types of current: direct current (DC) and alternating current (AC), both of which have been described in greater detail in Chapter 1. *Waveform* refers to the shape of a pulse. Continuous unidirectional current is referred to as a galvanic current. If such a current is interrupted by periods when no current is flowing it is termed interrupted direct current (IDC). The series of pulses produced may vary in their shape (square or triangular), duration (short, < 1 ms or long, > 1 ms), and frequency of occurrence (1–200 Hz) (Figure 16.3). *Alternating current (AC)* is often delivered at high frequencies that lowers skin

Figure 16.3   Unidirectional pulses, a square and a triangular pulse.

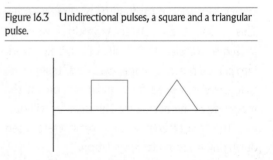

Figure 16.4   Interference-modulated current.

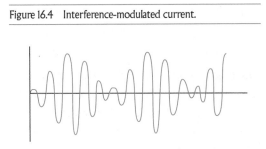

Figure 16.6   Symmetrical biphasic pulses, square and triangular.

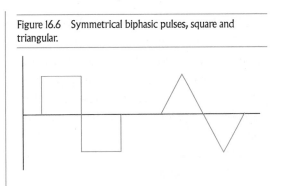

impedance and thus delivers more current to the motor nerves (Savage, 1984).

Figure 16.7   A sine wave, a symmetrical biphasic waveform.

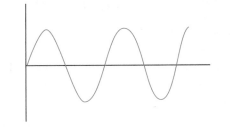

Interference-modulated current refers to the current produced by the interference pattern produced in the tissues by two slightly different high frequency (about 4000 Hz) sine waves; this is known as *interferential current* (Figure 16.4).

Burst-modulated alternating current is sometimes referred to as 'Russian stimulation' as it was first reported by Russian scientists. A high frequency (2500 Hz) carrier current is interspersed with 10 ms periods when no current is flowing, producing 50 bursts per second (Figure 16.5).

Biphasic waveforms may be discrete, a single pulse, or continuous, a series of pulses, in nature. When the shape and amplitude of the pulse is identical in both positive and negative directions it is termed a *symmetrical biphasic waveform* (Figure 16.6). A sine wave is a symmetrical continuous biphasic wave form, of which mains current (50 Hz) is an example of this (Figure 16.7). When the shape and amplitude of

the pulse is not identical in positive and negative directions it is termed an *asymmetrical* biphasic waveform (Figure 16.8). However, an asymmetrical pulse may be balanced, i.e. possesses a negative charge of zero, if the area under the curve is the same in both positive and negative direction.

The *duration of stimulation* may be defined as the time for which stimulation was applied, usually hours or minutes. The *duty cycle* of the stimulator is comprised of an 'on-time' reflecting the duration of pulse delivery, and an 'off-time' – the

Figure 16.5   Burst modulated current, 'Russian current'.

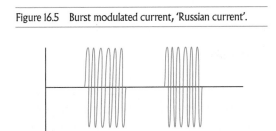

Figure 16.8   Asymmetrical biphasic pulses.

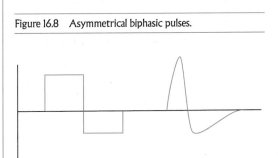

duration of quiescence. The total cycle time is the sum of the on and off-times.

Ramping may be used to gradually increase the charge applied to the tissue and hence increase the intensity of muscle contraction attained. This is achieved by a gradual increase in the amplitude (Figure 16.9) or the pulse width of the pulse train. This allows for accommodation of the nervous tissue-to-pulse delivery.

The Importance of Stimulation Parameters

Waveform — galvanic stimulation is only useful for stimulating denervated muscle whereas interrupted direct currents, including faradic stimulation is able to stimulate innervated muscle. However, both techniques create thermal and chemical reactions under the electrodes and are often painful and therefore should be used with caution.

Baker *et al.* (1988) investigated the effects on comfort of six different waveforms during neuromuscular stimulation. An asymmetric balanced biphasic square waveform (35 Hz) was reported to be comfortable and effective in stimulating the extensor and flexor muscles of the wrist. However, in the quadriceps muscles a symmetric biphasic square waveform (50 Hz) was preferred by subjects. Delitto and Rose (1986) reported that

Figure 16.9   Ramping by slowly increasing the intensity of the current.

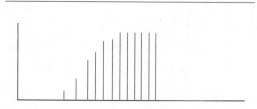

subjects' perception of discomfort alters with changes in waveform (at 50 Hz) and that individual preferences exist for different waveforms.

Amplitude — when stimulating a muscle at a constant frequency the only way to increase the force produced is to recruit more motor units by increasing the intensity (amplitude of the waveform) of stimulation.

Pulse duration — the most suitable pulse duration for motor stimulation of the triceps brachii was found to be between 20 and 200 μs, the most comfortable being 100 μs; pulse durations less than 100 μs were suitable for sensory stimulation (Alon *et al.*, 1983).

Electrodes — the size of electrodes may have an affect on the amount of muscle stimulated and hence the intensity of the contraction produced (Alon, 1989). Reversing the polarity of electrodes has little effect on force generated during stimulation with biphasic waveforms; however, changes greater than 20% were seen with monophasic waveforms (McNeal and Baker, 1988).

Percutaneous stimulation of healthy muscle selectively activates nerve endings and not the muscle fibres directly (Hultman *et al.*, 1983). It is postulated that slow rising pulses of long duration selectively stimulate denervated muscle, as opposed to fast rising pulses of short duration that stimulate innervated muscle. There is no scientific evidence to show that denervated muscle can be stimulated directly. However, neither is there any evidence to refute it (Belanger, 1991).

Summary

All stimulators which produce electrical pulses that enter the body tissues via surface electrodes may be classified as percutaneous neuromuscular stimulators. The type of output produced by such stimulators varies considerably. It is important to be aware of the differences in pulse characteristics and parameters and the relative effects that they may have. Accurate reporting of such information in the scientific literature will facilitate the transference of research work into clinical practice.

References

Alon, G (1989) Electro-orthopedics: A review of present electrophysiological responses and clinical efficacy of transcutaneous stimulation. *Advances in Sports Medicine and Fitness,* **2**: 295–324.

Alon, G, Allin, J, Inbar, GF (1983) Optimisation of pulse duration and pulse charge during transcutaneous electrical nerve stimulation. *The Australian Journal of Physiotherapy,* **29**(5): 195–201.

Baker, LL, Bowman, BR, McNeal, DR (1988) Effects of wareform on comfort during neuromuscular electrical stimulation. *Clinical Orthopaedics and Related Research,* **233**: 75–85.

Belanger, AY (1991) Neuromuscular electrostimulation in physiotherapy: a critical appraisal of controversial issues. *Physiotherapy Theory and Practice,* **7**, 83–89.

British Standards Institution (1988) *Medical electrical equipment: specification for nerve and muscle stimulators.* BS 5724: Section 2.10. British Standards Institution.

Delitto, A, Rose, SJ (1986) Comparative comfort of three waveforms used in electrically eliciting quadriceps femoris muscle contractions. *Physical Therapy,* **66**: 1704–1707.

Hultman, E, Sjoholm, H, Jaderholm, EKJ, Krynicki, J (1983) Evaluation of methods for electrical stimulation of human skeletal muscle in situ. *Pflugers Archives,* **398**: 139–141.

McNeal, DR, Baker, LL (1988) Effects of joint angle, electrodes and waveform on electrical stimulation of the quadriceps and hamstrings. *Annals of Biomedical Engineering,* **16**: 299–310.

Savage, B (1984) *Interferential therapy.* London: Faber & Faber Ltd.

Singer, KP, De Domenico, G, Strauss, G (1987) Electro-motor stimulation for research methodology and reporting: a need for standardisation. *The Australian Journal of Physiotherapy,* **33**(1): 43–47.

17

Neuromuscular and Muscular Electrical Stimulation

SHEILA KITCHEN

Introduction
•
Practical Application
•
Hazards
•
Contraindications

Introduction

Chapter 5 has described the normal contractile mechanisms of muscle and the role of nerve in producing that contraction, and Chapter 8 has examined the ways in which electrical stimulation may be used to replace normal function. The previous chapter, Chapter 16, has discussed the types of current which may be used to produce an electrical response in muscle and nerve and the parameters that may be varied to produce different responses.

This chapter will examine briefly the practical application of neuromuscular electrical stimulation (NMES) for innervated muscle, and electrical muscular stimulation (EMS) for denervated muscle.

Practical Application

Though both innervated and denervated muscle may be caused to contract through the use of current applied to the skin, most studies today focus on the use of electrical currents to stimulate innervated muscle. The method of application of treatment for both is, however, identical.

Skin Preparation

Prior to treatment the skin should either be washed with soap and water or cleaned with a proprietary, alcohol-based wipe. This is in order to remove skin debris (including dead epithelial cells and sebum), sweat and dirt. It is necessary to do this in order to facilitate good contact between the electrode and the skin and thus reduce the electrical resistance of the interface. ·

Electrode Types and Their Attachment

Electrodes are principally of two types:

1 Polymer-based electrodes: carbon—rubber electrodes have been introduced onto the market in recent years and are currently the most popular type due to their ease of use. They consist of carbon-impregnated silicone rubber (Figure 17.1). Such electrodes are re-usable, can be cut to size and can be moulded to the skin surface provided the surface is not too irregular. They are normally coupled to the skin through the use of an electrically-conductive gel and must be taped into place securely.

Figure 17.1   Carbon—rubber electrodes. (Photograph courtesy of Electro-Medical Supplies (Greenham) Ltd, Wantage.)

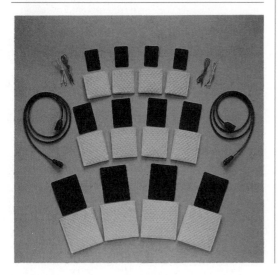

Other polymer-based electrodes are also available but are generally less efficient at transmitting electrical stimuli to the tissue (Nolan, 1991).

Recent advances in electrode design have further increased the ease with which they can be applied and improved their electrical contact with the skin. Such electrodes are considerably more malleable than those previously available and have an even layer of conductive material already in place; it is these particular qualities that allow them to make more effective contact with the skin. In addition, they are self-adhesive and reusable, factors which make them quick, easy and economical to use.

2 More traditional tin-plate or aluminium electrodes may also be used. These are coupled to the skin with saline water, which is normally retained within a cotton pad or sponge, and are securely located against the tissue. In addition, coupling may be achieved by placing both the part to be stimulated and the electrodes in a water bath. These electrodes may be cut to the required size and are re-usable; they are, however, less malleable than many of their commercial counterparts. A number of authors, including Nelson (1980) and Nolan (1991), have compared the efficiency with which various electrodes conduct stimuli to the tissues. Nelson (1980) demonstrated that metal electrodes are most efficient whilst Nolan (1991) showed that carbon—rubber electrodes are generally more efficient than many other polymer-based types. However, the final choice is determined by assessing all the factors mentioned above.

Both pad and hand-held electrodes are available. The first facilitates rapid movement of the electrode, which may be particularly useful when searching for the optimal stimulation point. The second is more useful for a prolonged period of stimulation.

Electrode Size

Fundamentally, choice of electrode size depends on:

- The size of the muscle to be stimulated;
- The intensity of the contraction to be elicited.

Small electrodes may be used to localize stimulation to small muscles or may be used to apply a stimulus over a nerve which supplies a muscle. Larger electrodes are needed to stimulate larger muscles, muscle groups and to act as dispersive terminals (see below).

Though the spread of the electrical current over the surface of electrodes may be irregular (for example, the intensity is often greater at the point where the current enters the electrode), it is generally true to say that the larger the electrode the lower the intensity of current per unit area. Thus, small electrodes tend to lead to stronger muscle contractions. However, it

should be remembered that the final stimulus received by the tissue is also dependent on other factors such as the point at which the current enters the electrode and the nature and efficiency of the contact medium.

Electrode Placement

Electrodes may be sited on muscles in a number of ways. First, a single electrode may be placed over the motor point of a muscle. This may be defined as the point on the surface of the skin that allows a contraction to occur using the least energy. In general, the motor point of a muscle is located over the belly of a muscle, often but not always at the junction between the upper and middle thirds of the belly. Figures 17.2–9 show the approximate positions of these points. It is important to remember, however, that these points act only as a guide; alternative placements may be both more effective and comfortable in certain subjects. When using this technique, a second dispersive, or indifferent, electrode must be placed elsewhere on the part, at a convenient location

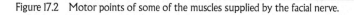

Figure 17.2   Motor points of some of the muscles supplied by the facial nerve.

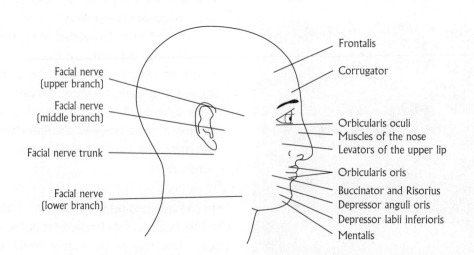

Figure 17.3   Approximate positions of some of the motor points on the anterior aspect of the hand.

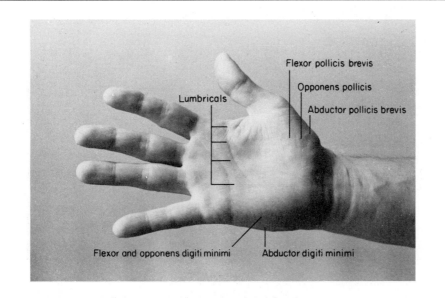

Figure 17.4   Approximate positions of some of the motor points on the anterior aspect of the right arm.

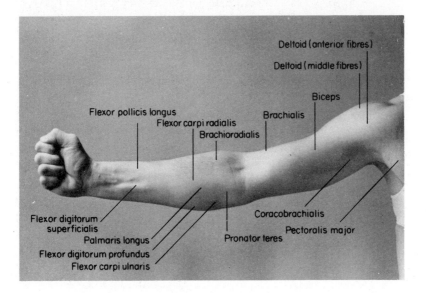

near to the muscle being treated. This electrode should be larger, resulting in the current density across it being lower and therefore making it unlikely to elicit either motor or sensory responses. This method is suitable for innervated muscle and is sometimes called a *unipolar technique*.

Second, electrodes may be placed at either end of a muscle belly. This method is suitable for both

Figure 17.5   Approximate positions of some of the motor points on the posterior aspect of the right arm.

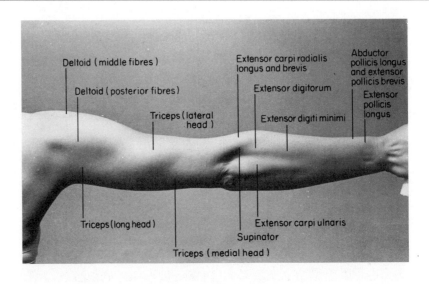

Figure 17.6   Approximate positions of some of the motor points on the posterior aspect of the hand.

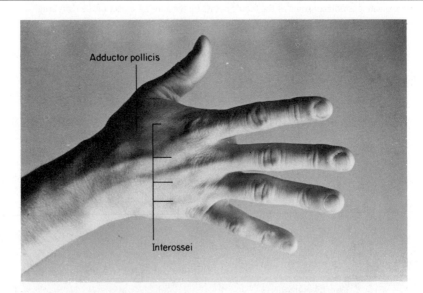

innervated and denervated muscle and may be termed *bipolar.* Two hand-held electrodes of similar sizes may be used or, if the treatment is to be for a longer period of time, two electrodes may be taped or adhered to the tissue.

Treatment Parameters

The treatment parameters affecting muscle and nerve response have been described in the last chapter. These include current wave form, pulse amplitude and duration, pulse frequency, duty

Figure 17.7 Approximate positions of some of the motor points on the anterior aspect of the right leg.

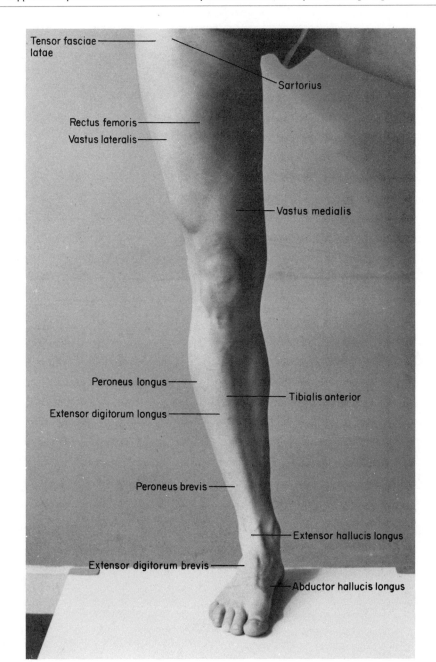

Figure 17.8   Approximate positions of some of the motor points on the posterior aspect of the left leg.

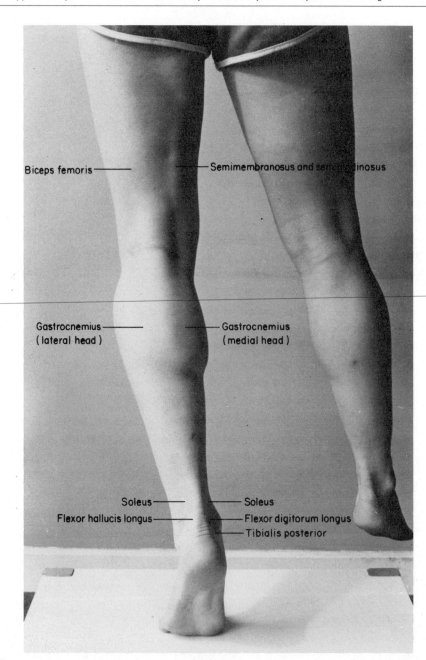

Figure 17.9   Approximate positions of some of the motor points of the back.

1 Trapezius (upper fibres)   6 Teres major and minor
2 Supraspinatus   7 Serratus anterior
3 Rhomboids   8 Trapezius (lower fibres)
4 Trapezius (middle fibres)   9 Latissimus dorsi
5 Infraspinatus

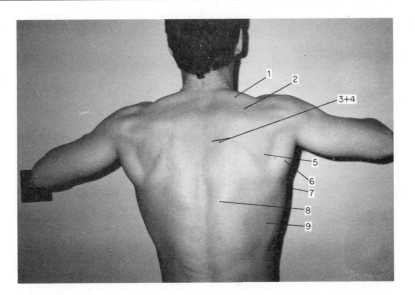

cycle, ramp modulation and duration of treatment.

Patient preference must also be borne in mind, though it is not clear from the literature which waveforms are most acceptable. Bowman and Barker (1985) suggest that symmetrical, biphasic waves are generally preferred, whilst Delitto and Rose (1986) reported there to be no significant differences between sinusoidal, rectangular and triangular waves. The therapist should therefore adjust the waveform in order to produce a satisfactory contraction in as comfortable a fashion as possible.

In order to produce a contraction of a designated intensity, it should be remembered that the shorter the pulse duration, the greater the pulse amplitude needed; this is demonstrated in the strength–duration curve shown in Figure 17.10a.

Figure 17.10b shows that the same relationship between pulse duration and amplitude exists for denervated muscle; however, the figure also shows that the whole curve is shifted to the right, such muscle requiring pulses of longer duration and greater amplitude than innervated tissue.

Force of contraction is determined by the amplitude, frequency, duration and shape of the stimulating waveform, and these factors are discussed in Chapter 16. A considerable number of researchers have examined the ways in which these parameters may be combined to produce optimal contractions, though to date no single combination of parameters has been shown to be most effective.

A number of authors have reviewed the studies which examine the efficacy of NMES (for

Figure 17.10 Strength–duration curves of (a) normally innervated and (b) completely denervated muscle.

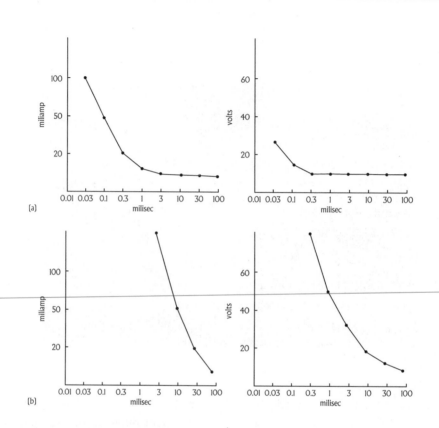

innervated muscle) and EMS (for denervated muscle). These include Delitto and Robinson (1989), Belanger (1991) and Delitto and Snyder-Mackler (1991).

NMES has become increasingly popular as a form of treatment for a variety of clinical problems since the beginning of the 1970s. Chapter 8 reviews the reasons for which it may be used in clinical practice. Delitto and Robinson (1989) suggest treatment parameters for use in muscle strengthening programmes and to increase the length of contracted tissues (see Table 17.1).

The frequency of sessions and number of contractions may be increased, and the intensity reduced when the aim is to increase joint range. Further work has been done to evaluate the effects of NMES on spasticity. Though a number of studies have suggested that it is an effective form of treatment, little is known about the underlying mechanisms leading to change. No clear guidelines are available to suggest appropriate treatment parameters and Delitto and Robinson (1989) conclude that the use of NMES for spasticity should be considered experimental at this time.

Despite the use of EMS to stimulate denervated muscle for more than a century, controversy over its use and efficacy still continues (Davies, 1983; Snyder-Mackler and Robinson, 1989). This is primarily due to the variety of treatment protocols which have been used to assess care. Though there is no current consensus about the duty cycle

Table 17.1

Parameters for use in NMES programmes for muscle strengthening

Type of current	Pulsatile or burst modulated AC
Amplitude of stimulation	Maximum tolerable
Phase duration	20–1000 μs
Waveform	Subject preference
Frequency of stimulation	30–50 pulses or bursts/s
Duty cycle	10–15 s on/50–120 s off
Type of contractions	Isometric
Number of contractions per session	10–20 at maximum tolerable intensity
Frequency of sessions	3–5 times/week minimum

which should be used, the frequency of stimulation or the number of contractions which should be employed, Snyder-Mackler and Robinson (1989) suggest that EMS can *delay* atrophy and its associated changes. However, they also note that there is no evidence to suggest that such a delay is significant in terms of final recovery.

Hazards

A number of hazards should be guarded against when using NMES. These include:

- Chemical damage due to inadequate skin protection when direct or interrupted direct current is used;
- Disruption of stimulating devices due to the proximity of diathermy equipment, which can result in altered output.

Contraindications

NMES should not be used, or used with caution, in patients with the following:

- Pacemakers;

- Peripheral vascular diseased, especially when there is the possibility of loosening thrombi;
- Hypertensive and hypotensive subjects; NMES may affect the autonomic responses of these patients;
- Areas of excess adipose tissue in obese subjects; these subjects may require high levels of stimuli which may lead to autonomic changes;
- Neoplastic tissue;
- Areas of active tissue infection;
- Devitalized skin; for example, after treatment with deep x-ray therapy;
- Patients who are unable to understand the nature of the intervention or provide feedback about the treatment.

In addition, treatment should not be applied over the following areas:

- Carotid sinus;
- Thoracic region; it has been suggested that NMES may interfere with the function of the heart;
- Phrenic nerve;
- Trunk of a pregnant subject.

Electrical stimulation of innervated muscle continues to be a popular form of treatment, though stimulation of denervated muscle is less popular. However, as with many other electrophysical agents, there are still major gaps in our knowledge about the effects it has, the most effective parameters to use and its long-term efficacy.

References

Bowman, BR, Barker, LL (1985) Effects of waveform parameters on comfort during transcutaneous neuromuscular electrical stimulation. *Annals of Biomedical Engineering*, 13: 59–74.

Davies, HL (1983) Is electrostimulation beneficial to denervated nerve? A review of results from basic research. *Physiotherapy (Canada)*, 35: 306–310.

Delitto, A, Rose SJ (1986) Comparative comfort of three wave forms used in electrically elicited quadriceps femoris contractions. *Physical Therapy*, 66: 1704–1707.

Delitto, A, Robinson, AJ (1989) Electrical stimulation of muscle: techniques and applications. In Snyder-Mackler, L, Robinson, AJ (eds) *Clinical electrophysiology: electrotherapy and electrophysiological testing*. Baltimore: Williams and Wilkins.

Delitto, A, Snyder-Mackler, L (1991) Two theories of muscle strength augmentation using percutaneous electrical stimulation. *Physical Therapy*, 70: 158–164.

Nelson, H, Smith, M, Bowman, B *et al.* (1980) Electrode effectiveness during transcutaneous motor stimulation. *Archives of Physical Medicine and Rehabilitation*, 61: 73–77.

Nolan, MF (1991) Conductive differences in electrodes used with transcutaneous electrical nerve stimulation devices. *Physical Therapy*, 71: 746–751.

18

Transcutaneous Electrical Nerve Stimulation (TENS)

VICTORIA FRAMPTON

Introduction
•
TENS Parameters
•
Mechanisms by which TENS may Inhibit Pain
•
Hazards
•
Application and Operation of TENS
•
Discussion

Introduction

The development of transcutaneous electrical nerve stimulation (TENS) is based directly on Melzack and Wall's (1965) innovative work on the spinal gate control theory and pain modulation (see Chapter 5, page 85). Research examining pathological changes occurring in nerves following injury led to the scientific justification for applying electrical impulses to damaged nerves in order to modify their abnormal responses. These findings and the gate control theory form the basis of much of our understanding of pain mechanisms and clarify the therapeutic value of electrical nerve stimulation. For centuries, electrical stimulation has been reputedly used for pain relief, e.g. electric eels were used by the Ancient Egyptians to treat gout and headaches.

Transcutaneous electrical nerve stimulation is a low-frequency current when compared to the full spectrum of electrical current frequencies available for therapeutic uses.

TENS Parameters

Energy Source

All portable TENS machines are powered by an alkaline 1.5 volt battery.

Amplitude

This is adjustable from 0 to 50 mA (milliamperes) into an electrode impedance of 1kΩ (kiloohms).

Wave Form

The most commonly produced wave form is a biphasic, asymmetrical, balanced square wave with a zero net DC component (Figure 18.1). The area under the positive wave is equal to the area under the negative wave. No net polar effects are produced, preventing the build-up of long-term positive–negative ion concentrations beneath each electrode, or within the tissues (Mannheimer and Lampe, 1984). Consequently, there are no adverse skin reactions due to polar concentrations.

Adequate Stimulus

In order for a stimulus to be effective it must reach a certain intensity, be of a certain duration, and reach its maximum intensity at a certain minimum speed. It is the relationship of the amplitude and pulse width that will determine an adequate sti-

mulus. Short pulse widths require high amplitudes to produce adequate stimuli, while wider pulse widths require lower amplitudes to produce adequate stimuli. If the pulse width is increased, the energy within the pulse is raised by an increase in the surface area along the horizontal axis (Figure 18.2). Aβ afferent nerve fibres can be recruited by impulses of low-amplitude, high-frequency and short duration. Aδ afferent nerve fibres can be recruited by impulses of higher amplitude, lower frequencies and longer pulse widths.

In a biphasic waveform, the positive portion of the wave is omitted at one electrode of a two electrode system (single channel) and a negative portion omitted at the other. Although a zero net-DC current is produced, one electrode may be more active. If the amplitude is increased, the potential of the wave form is increased in both waveforms, but in different ways; the *vertical* axis of the negative wave portion is increased, but the *horizontal* axis of the positive wave portion is increased (Figure 18.3). This tends to make the electrode on the negative wave portion more active, although not significantly so in most commercially available machines.

Figure 18.1 Biphasic asymmetrical square wave with zero net DC component.

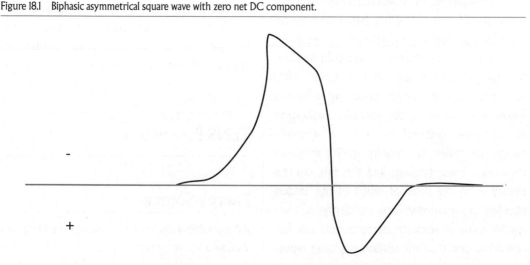

Figure 18.2   Increase in pulse width — results in an increase in energy / increase in wave surge area along horizontal axis.

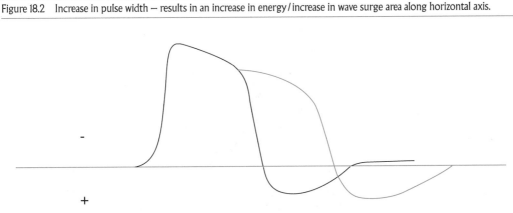

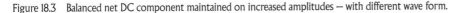

Figure 18.3   Balanced net DC component maintained on increased amplitudes — with different wave form.

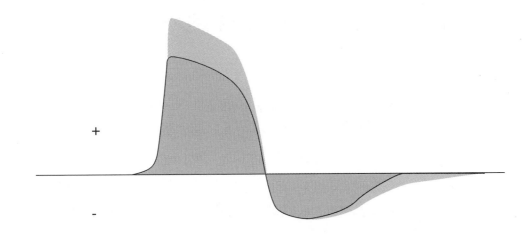

Sensory Action Potentials (SAP)

The peripheral nerve membrane has a resting potential that is negative inside and positive out- side. When an adequate stimulus is applied, a change in membrane potential takes place — a reversal of its resting potential. This change is brought about by the sodium pump mechanism: on the application of an adequate stimulus, sodium ions flood into the area, thus altering the potential inside the membrane; this change in potential is then conducted along a nerve fibre through its own metabolic inertia (Figure 18.4).

Pulse Frequency or Rate

This is variable in all machines, and the range of variation of the parameters vary, on average from 1–150 pulses per second or hertz (Hz). A slow rate at around 10 pulses per second is described by the patient as a slow ticking sensation, whereas a fast or high rate is expressed as a continuous buzzing sensation (Figure 18.5).

Figure 18.4 Sodium-pump mechanism — evoking change in SAPs.

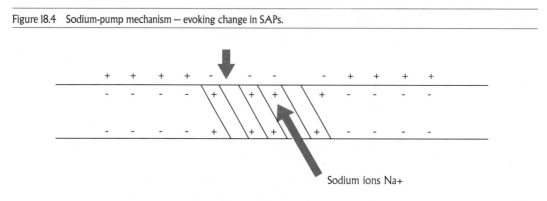

Sodium ions Na+

Figure 18.5 Pulse types (figures are not drawn to scale but illustrate the differences between pulse patterns). (a) Continuous pulse — slow rate, e.g. 10 pulses/second. (b) Continuous pulse — fast rate, e.g. 150 pulses/second. (c) Burst-type pulse — in this example, 2.3 bursts/second. The impulse has been interrupted. (d) Frequency-modulated pulse — constant stimulus with a variable frequency.

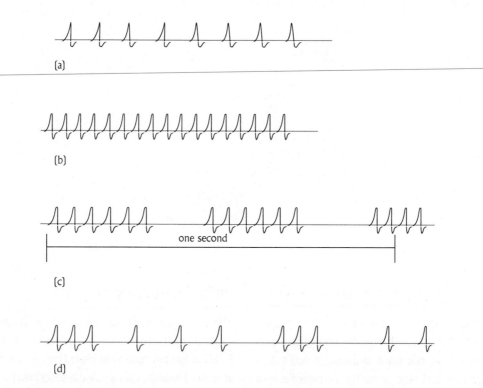

Continuous-burst Variable-frequency Stimulation

A large number of researchers (Anderson *et al.*, 1976; Linzer and Long, 1976; Mannheimer and Carlsson, 1979; Woolfe *et al.*, 1981; Sjolund, 1985; Omura, 1987; Johnson *et al.*, 1991a–c; Tulgar *et al.*, 1991a) have tried to investigate the effects of different parameters. Certainly there is an indication that the benfits of TENS tend to fall with time (Loeser *et al.*, 1975; Eriksson *et al.*, 1979 ; Long *et al.*, 1979; Taylor *et al.*, 1981; Bates and Nathan,

1980). It is possible that this is due to the adaptation of the nervous system to regular repetitive stimuli (Thompson, 1987; Pomeranz et al., 1987). However, prescriptive parameters cannot be given as the results of the different trials are not consistent (Tulgar et al., 1991a,b; Johnson et al., 1991a; Sjolund, 1985; Eriksson et al., 1979; Sjolund and Eriksson, 1979).

The different types of frequency-modulated current available on some machines can be seen in Figure 18.5 (a–d). A double-blind, controlled, long-term clinical trial by Tulgar et al. (1991b) indicated that patients preferred burst-mode stimulation and frequency-modulated stimulation (Figures 18.5c,d). In the four different modes of stimulation that were tried, their conclusions showed that most patients in their study preferred high-rate, frequency-modulated and burst-type stimulation. The analgesic affects of different pulse patterns of TENS on cold-induced pain in normal subjects was investigated by Johnson et al. (1991a). Five frequencies of pulse delivery and four patterns of pulse delivery together with two sizes of electrodes were examined. From the outcome of this trial, the authors concluded that frequencies of 20–80 Hz produced the greatest analgesia, and the greatest statistical reliability was observed at 80 Hz. A continuous-pulse pattern was shown to be optimal. Eriksson et al. (1979) showed that bursts at high intensity and low frequency (so called 'acupuncture-like TENS') were more effective in pain relief than continuous-pulse TENS. One theory suggests that burst-mode TENS mimics acupuncture in producing analgesia by stimulating the release of endogenous opioid peptides (Sjolund and Eriksson, 1979), whereas high-frequency continuous-mode TENS is thought to relieve pain by activating gating mechanisms (Melzack and Wall 1965; Wall and Sweet, 1967).

In summary, Johnson et al. (1991b) concluded, following an in-depth study of long-term users of TENS with a variety of chronic pain problems, that there was remarkably little correlation between patient, the site or cause of pain with the stimulator and outcome variables. This finding was consistent with those reported by other researchers (Bates and Nathan, 1980; Woolfe, 1981; Frampton, 1994). A subsequent study by Johnson et al. (1991c) suggested that individual patients used a specific pulse frequency but consistently there was a significant variation in the pulse frequency used by different patients; the majority, however, preferred a continuous-pulse pattern. It would appear in this study that patients used pulse frequencies and pulse patterns which were unique to the individual to control their pain. It appears the patients turn to such frequencies and patterns for reasons of comfort which may be unconnected with specific pain control mechanisms (Frampton, 1994). Patients should try a variety of different frequencies and modes of stimulation to find the parameters that are most appropriate for the relief of their pain. If TENS is successful initially but then ceases to have any effect, burst mode should be tried to overcome adaption and accommodation.

Lead Wires

Electrical potential or electric current generated by TENS is transmitted via the lead wires from the TENS machine to the electrode which is applied to the patient's skin. It is important that these wires or cables are robust enough to withstand daily-living activities. Most cables plug into a single output socket. A single cable then bifurcates to insert into the two electrodes.

Electrodes

The most common form of electrodes supplied as standard with most machines are black, carbon impregnated, silicone rubber electrodes. They are available in several sizes, which include standard 4 cm $\times$ 4 cm electrodes, and large 4 cm $\times$ 8 cm pads. The carbon electrodes require electroconductive gel to be spread over the surface area of the pad and then applied to the skin and fixed with tape. A variety of different self-adhesive and hypoallergenic pads are also available. These pads do not require gel or tape, but they do tend to be more expensive and are not indefinitely reusable. Small button electrodes are useful for treatment of small difficult areas, and sterile electrodes are available for postoperative pain control. Allergic response to electrodes, tape or gel provides the greatest problem in TENS application and it is essential that the recommended electroconductive gel is used with the carbon-silicone electrodes. Other mediums such as ultrasound jelly are unsuitable as they do not possess the same cohesive properties of the TENS gel. The recommended electroconductive gel will remain spread over the electrode pad for long-term stimulation, whereas other mediums will dry up and contract to the centre of the carbon pad. Electroconductive TENS gel has high conduction, non-allergenic, cohesive properties, and is designed specifically for use with the TENS equipment.

Single- and Dual-channel TENS Units

A single-channel unit is one with a single amplitude parameter and one pair of electrodes. A dual-channel unit has two output channels providing for two variable amplitude parameters and two pairs of electrodes. The choice of single- or dual-channel unit is dependent upon the site and extent of painful area. In most cases, where one site of pain is identified, a single-channel unit is adequate. Rationale of treatment and application of TENS relies upon the ease of application, operation and cost effectiveness. Dual channel application is indicated when the pain is widespread, e.g. back pain with bilateral leg pain. TENS machines range from the basic, single-channel continuous-mode stimulator to dual-channel, burst, and variable-frequency machines.

Some models provide autoscanning for pulse frequency and pulse width. These models have a reset facility which automatically returns the pulse frequency to 80 Hz and a pulse width of 210 microseconds. Multifrequency (random) output modes also help to overcome accommodation and adaptation (one example of this type of TENS is the Xenos produced by Neen Pain Management Systems). The frequency spectrum spans from the minimum of 8 Hz to a maximum preset by the frequency setting when on the continuous mode. Clearly, the more sophisticated the machine the more expensive it becomes and initial application should be restricted to the basic model. If unsuccessful, progression can be made to the more sophisticated models.

Mechanisms by which TENS may Inhibit Pain

The extensive use of TENS over the past 25 years has established this inexpensive, non-invasive technique as an accepted modality for pain relief. Clinical trials, however, are often poorly controlled and lack long-term follow-up. The difficulty in establishing conclusive placebo trials still exists. The complexity of the chronic pain sufferer and the lack of adequate numbers of trials prevents the identification of ideal prescriptions for any particular pain problem. Recent work by Johnson *et al.* (1991b) and Tulgar *et al.* (1991a) have made significant contributions to identify optimum parameters for electrical stimulation. In many cases, application of TENS is very similar. The exact mechanism of how pain is inhibited relies on a full understanding of the pathology of the injury and the subsequent changes which may take place in the nerve pathway and the central nervous system.

Modulation of normal physiological pathways can lead to pain relief. TENS may be working in one of several ways to inhibit or relieve pain:

Gate Control Theory – Presynaptic Inhibition

Large, myelinated Aβ fibres provide the pathway for TENS. These fast-conducting fibres are highly sensitive to electrical stimulation and quickly conduct the electrical impulse to the spinal cord. Small, slower-conducting non-myelinated C fibres carrying noxious (painful) stimuli are unable to pass on their message. The mechanism by which nociceptive fibres (pain-carrying fibres) are prevented from passing on their message to the spinal cord is described as presynaptic inhibition (Wagman and Price, 1969; Handwerker *et al.*, 1975; Woolfe and Wall, 1982; Chung *et al.*, 1984). The 'opening' or 'closing' of the gate to noxious or painful stimuli will dictate an individual's awareness to a painful stimulus. Stimulation of the afferent fibres by TENS may provide one mechanism to keep the gate closed to painful stimuli. This inhibitory process possibly modulates the sensory input entering the spinal cord. The use of TENS may distort the function of the nervous system by jamming one of its inputs (Woolfe, 1989). The closer to the damaged area TENS can

be applied, the greater the chance that noxious stimuli will be inhibited appropriately. The inhibitory circuits mediated by Aβ fibres are segmentally arranged, so low-intensity segmental stimulation is required. Other polysegmental inhibitory circuits, which are mediated by Aδ and C afferents, require higher-intensity stimuli (myofascial or trigger-point acupuncture) (Frampton, 1994; Bowsher, 1994; Alltnee, 1994) for activation.

Direct Inhibition on an Excited Abnormally Firing Nerve

A small but significant proportion of people experience pain following nerve injury. When a peripheral nerve is damaged, the proximal end forms the seat of spontaneous electrical discharges. The spontaneous firing may spread from the cut end where the sprouting nerve has formed a knot of nerve fibres (neuroma site) proximally along the whole length of the nerve. Nerve sprouts are very sensitive to slight mechanical stimuli. They are spontaneously active, and tapping over the neural sprouts in a regenerating nerve reproduces referred sensation into the part of the skin that used to be supplied by the nerve (Tinel 1915; Moldaver 1979). The nerve sprouts are also sensitive to noradrenaline released by sympathetic nerve endings in the tissues (Loh and Nathan, 1978). The sympathetic system is itself normal, but it may be that an abnormal response of C fibre sprouts produce a reflex increase in sympathetic activity and may lead to the symptoms of sympathetic disturbance (Wallin *et al.*, 1976). This may give the basis for the symptoms seen in reflex sympathetic distrophy. Pain experienced following nerve injury presents as an abnormally painful response to light touch

(Wynn Parry, 1981; Withrington and Wynn Parry, 1984).

Experimental work on animals (Wall and Gutnik, 1974) demonstrated that proximal application of vibration or electrical stimulation damps down or stops abnormally firing electrical discharges occurring at damaged ends of nerve or neuromata. It may be that TENS relieves pain by directly inhibiting the electrical firing occurring at damaged nerves, e.g. in a nerve crush injury, nerve root compression following prolapsed disc, or in carpal-tunnel compression. Long-term irritation or pressure from a disc prolapse on a nerve root may lead to chronic firing at the site of irritation and along the length of the nerve distal to the dorsal horn (Wall and Devor, 1981).

In conjunction with the peripheral pathophysiological changes that take place following nerve damage, simultaneous central changes in the spinal cord may contribute to the painful state. Central effects from nerve damage may include increased firing of cells in the dorsal horn of the spinal cord (Wall and Devor, 1981) morphological changes and sprouting of neurons. These central changes, together with the peripheral responses to nerve injury, may ultimately lead to abnormal central patterns being set up, leading to the autonomous painful cycle being established (Figure 18.6).

Restoration of an Artificial Afferent Input in Diafferentation and Central Pain

Loeser and Ward (1967) demonstrated spontaneous firing in the dorsal horn cells following severance of the trigeminal nerve of the cat. The frequency of these spontaneous, abnormal firings increased over a three-week period until cells fired continuously. It may be that the barrage of firing could result from normal afferent input being lost from the severed nerve. Input to the spinal cord results often in central inhibition, and loss of normal input may lead to the unsuppressed firing of cells in the dorsal horn. Patients with deafferentation lesions, e.g. avulsion injuries of the brachial plexus, phantom limb pain following amputation or spinal cord injuries, experience severe pain of a characteristic nature (Wynn Parry, 1980; Frampton, 1990 and 1994). The pain

Figure 18.6 Pathophysiological changes in damaged peripheral nerves. The resultant central changes and abnormal central patterns may in turn exacerbate the changes occurring peripherally, and so establish the 'pain cycle'.

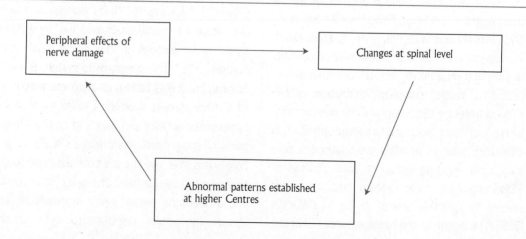

is not immediate following injury but onset may be up to 2–3 weeks after injury (Wynn Parry, 1981). The clinical observation is consistent with experimental findings (Loeser and Ward, 1967). It may be that TENS relieves pain by artificially restoring an afferent input to the spinal cord, albeit at a different level to the damaged level. Clearly there would be no input via the pathway that had been destroyed.

The Role Played by Endogenous Opioid Peptides

Eriksson *et al.* (1979) and Salar *et al.* (1981) demonstrated an increase in opioid peptides in lumbar CSF with transcutaneous nerve stimulation.

An understanding of chronic pain includes those changes that occur in the central nervous system and the peripheral nervous system. It may be that abnormal central changes which take place may result from those peripheral changes, and that the two become autonomous to support the chronic pain cycle. It is vital that the role played by central and peripheral nervous systems is understood if chronic pain is to be managed successfully (Devor, 1989).

Applying an Understanding of Pain Mechanisms in the Clinical Situation

An understanding of the ways in which TENS may work to relieve pain will prevent it being applied randomly, and greater knowledge of the pain mechanisms and a comprehensive examination and assessment of the patient will direct the physiotherapist where best to focus treatment (Frampton, 1994). It is important to note that TENS can form only part of a treatment programme for patients with chronic pain (Framp-

ton, 1994), and central changes of nerve injury promoting abnormal movement and behaviour must be reversed or modified (Withrington and Wynn Parry, 1984). Failure with TENS may often be due to failure in considering pain management as part of a full, comprehensive rehabilitation programme. Short-term TENS prescribed for analgesia may be adequate for acute pain, but, at the same time, inadequate to modify complex changes that have established themselves as a result of the chronic pain state.

Hazards

TENS is an extremely safe modality; contraindications are based generally on common sense, and are quoted by manufacturers to avoid possible litigation. Those most commonly quoted include:

Do not use TENS on people who have:

- Pacemakers;
- Heart disease or dysrhymmias (unless recommended by a medical practitioner after their evaluation of the patient).
- Undiagnosed pain (unless advised by Medical Practitioner after full evaluation).
- Epilepsy, without due care and advice for its use from a Medical Practitioner.
- In the first three months of pregnancy.

Do not use TENS on the following areas of the body:

- The mouth;
- The cartoid sinus;
- Broken skin;
- Anaesthetic skin;
- The abdomen during pregnancy.
- Near the eyes.

(There is little research data to support the statement by some manufacturers that TENS has unproven safety in pregnancy. Indeed, many obstetric physiotherapists recommend TENS as preferable to strong analgesic drugs during pregnancy and lactation (Polden, 1994). In conclusion, pending further research, TENS may be used on areas other than the abdomen, such as the neck (Manaheimer and Lampe, 1984), during pregnancy.)

Basic safety principles quoted include:

- Keep TENS appliances out of the reach of children;
- Do not use TENS while operating vehicles or potentially hazardous equipment;
- Switch the appliance off before applying and removing electrodes;
- After prolonged application, local skin irritation or allergic rash can occur beneath or around the electrodes and skin area after stimulation. Care of the skin can be assured if the application site and electrodes are washed after stimulation to prevent skin rash and the rubber electrode from perishing.

The allergic response and skin irritation are the most common problem experienced in TENS. There are really very few reasons why anyone may not use TENS, and it forms one of the most non-invasive pain relieving techniques available.

Application and Operation of TENS

Electrode Placement

As a general guide, the following principles in electrode placement are:

- Pads are placed over the nerve where it is most superficial and proximal to the site of pain;
- Pads are placed over the painful dermatome or the adjacent dermatome;
- Pads are placed over the nerve trunk;
- Pads are placed above and below or either side of the painful area;
- Pads are never placed on anaesthetic areas;
- Pads are placed so that normal use of the limb is still permitted and not limited by the pad or lead wire;
- Pads may be placed over trigger points (Melzack et al., 1977).

Accurate placement of pads is often time consuming. It is important to understand fully the cause of pain so that electrode placement can be based on a sound knowledge of the pain mechanisms involved. For example, the patient suffering from deafferentation pain will have a better response if large pads are used. Similarly, pads should be placed on skin with equivalent sensibility. For example, a pad placed on normal skin and one pad placed on skin with loss to light touch will result in no perception of electrical stimulus under the pad with the area of skin that has diminished sensation. It would be better to place both pads on the skin with diminished sensation to create an effect of pain relief. There has been a minimal amount of work to confirm conclusively ideal electrode placements for specific conditions (Johnson et al., 1991a). However, systematic placement of electrodes over repetitive sessions increase the success of the outcome (Woolfe et al., 1981; Frampton, 1982 and 1994).

Operation

TENS can commence once the electrodes have been secured to the skin adequately. First, prior to switching on the machine, the patient must be told how the machine works, and what the stimulus will feel like, emphasizing that it is mild and can not harm them; many patients are alarmed by the term 'electric current'. It should be pointed out that the only way in which the patient will perceive an unpleasant experience is if they accidentally knock the dials to give a suddenly increased output. However, this is unlikely to happen on modern machines which have press buttons or protective shutters.

With all settings on zero, the machine is switched on and the output increased until the patient perceives a mild buzzing or pulsating sensation. The pulse frequency should then be scanned from minimum to maximum to demonstrate the range to the patient. The patient can then be asked to vary the rate until the level which is most comfortable and most effective in relieving the pain is found. Quite often the patient ceases to feel the stimulus after a few minutes and it is necessary to turn the output up again until the buzzing is felt. The principle that the stimulus does not have to be strong to have an affect must be reinforced with the patient – it should not be too strong or painful. As has already been described, the widening of the pulse width can increase the intensity of the stimulus. However, this may recruit some of the motor fibres, an effect which is not required.

In patients with denervated muscles and very poor sensory input (e.g. in avulsion lesions of the brachial plexus) it may be that an increased pulse width together with an increased output may be necessary in order that the patient perceives the stimulus (Frampton, 1990).

Treatment Time

Inadequate periods of stimulation have led to failure with TENS, and this is the most common reason for poor or unsustained pain relief with TENS. Experimental work has shown that TENS can have an accumulative effect (Sjolund and Eriksson, 1979; Woolfe *et al.*, 1981; Wynn Parry, 1980). The major pathophysiological effects fol-

lowing nerve damage and the complexities of the pain mechanisms involved in chronic pain would support the suggestion that prolonged periods of stimulation are necessary; to allow normal functional stimuli to be fed back to the spinal cord, a prolonged period of pain relief is essential for more normal patterns of movement to replace the abnormal central patterns that have been built up over a long period of time. Initially, stimulation should be for a minimum of 8 hours. However, the following principles form a guideline for treatment time:

- A minimum of 8 hours continuous stimulation per day;
- In severely painful conditions, continuous stimulation should be applied for 3 weeks, after which a reduction in treatment time can commence;
- If TENS stimulation has been reduced to 3 hours a day and the pain returns, it is essential to return to the increased period of stimulation, e.g. 4 hours a day for a further week before once again commencing reduction;
- Treatment time should be reduced slowly until no further stimulation is required;
- Ideally, TENS machines should be retained by the patient for a further month after treatment before returning it, in case the pain returns;
- Twenty-four hour stimulation maybe indicated in some severe pain cases;
- In some cases of chronic pain, TENS may be required on a long-term basis;
- TENS may be used at night only, e.g. in phantom limb pain the pain is often more severe at night when the patient is trying to get to sleep; it may also be necessary for the patient to wear a prosthesis during the day not only to allow walking but also to restore some afferent stimulation to the stump.

Discussion

Of recent trials, one by Johnson *et al.* (1991b) reviewed 179 patients who were long-term users of TENS. The results were as follows:

- 47% of patients reported their pain reduced by half or more;
- 13.7% reported no relief from pain;
- 15.% reported total relief of pain;
- Two thirds of the patients who reported complete failure had none the less continued to use TENS on a daily basis;
- 25% of patients used daily stimulation (TENS was used between 39.7 and 19.8 hours per week, i.e. 6.1 days per week for between 6.3 and 2.5 hours each day);
- Onset of pain relief occurred within 0.5 hours in 75% of patients and within 1 hour in over 95%;
- 30% of patients received 1 hour of analgesia post TENS;
- 51% of patients had less than 30 minutes analgesia post TENS.

No significant difference was reported of the time for onset of pain relief or for the time of post-TENS pain relief between burst or continuous modes of stimulation. The authors of this study suggested that patients with rapid pain relief, but rapid cessation of pain relief following TENS, may have been demonstrating the gate control mechanism, whereas those whose pain relief was more prolonged may be demonstrating the endorphin release mechanism. Patients appear to choose parameters for reasons of comfort (Johnson, 1991c); it is essential therefore that the patients try different parameters and different electrode placements systematically over successive treatment periods. Manufacturers providing a free loan service enables the patient to try the TENS at no expense before deciding to purchase their own equipment.

Troubleshooting – Reasons for Poor Results

Poor results may be attributed to a number of different factors which, though seemingly trivial individually, in combination are the most common reason for abandoning TENS as apparently unsuccessful.

Specific factors that can lead individually or in combination to poor results are summarized in

Table 18.1
Sources of poor results with TENS.

Factor relates to	Common Factors
1. Patient	• Inappropriate patient selection, e.g. hysterical or unreliable
2. Therapist's technique	• Electrodes wrongly positioned
	• Too little/much electroconductive gel used
	• Treatment time insufficient
	• Therapist did not adapt technique to maximize therapeutic effectiveness in the individual patient – e.g. systematically alter electrode placement stimulation parameters or size of electrodes
3. TENS equipment	• Batteries were flat or poorly connected to the machine
	• Worn electrode pads were not replaced
	• Flimsy cables were used
	• Variations in current were not tried
4. Interpretation	• Results were inadequately monitored/documented for comparison and follow-up

Table 18.1. It is worth noting that a failure to consider TENS as being part of what must be a comprehensive rehabilitation programme may lead to it giving poorer results than expected.

Machine Selection

The following factors are important to consider when selecting a machine. It should ideally:

- Be compact, small and light in weight;
- Be robust and durable;
- Have low-profile casing;
- Have easy-to-operate dials with protective shielding to prevent accidental knocking;
- Have a variety of electrode sizes and types, and resilient leads that don't break easily;

Figure 18.7   (a) Pain behaviour chart.

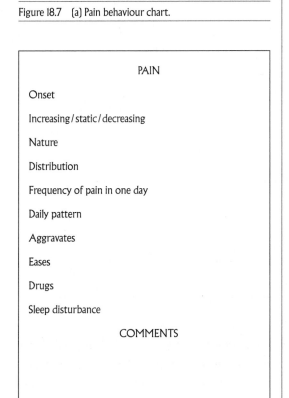

- Have a good service and maintenance back-up service from the manufacturer;
- Offer burst, continuous or frequency modulated units.

Other specialist machines available are the obstetric TENS which have been modified to meet needs of acute spasmodic pain and incorporate a patient hand-held facility which can alter the pulse.

Monitoring

Following full assessment of the patient, it is essential to focus on the pain profile and pain behaviour (Figure 18.7a). A change in a pain pattern may be the treatment goal identified, and the success of TENS may be evaluated by comparing the changes that occur with successive treatments. For example, in a patient suffering from severe burning pain which is constant and a sharp shooting pain which is spasmodic, TENS treatment may result in a reduction of the spasmodic pain to once an hour as opposed to once every five minutes. It may not be possible to alter the whole behaviour of the pain, but only facets of its characteristics. A quantitative analysis of pain using a 10 cm visual analogue scale is a good way of measuring objective pain relief (Figure 18.7b). In contrast, a verbal score of 0–10 may not be as accurate, but is still a useful baseline from which to analyse treatment. A score before and after treatment is helpful, though this may not always be possible if the patient takes the TENS machine away with them. A week's trial is essential for the reasons described previously, and a record of placement of electrodes is essential so that one may record successive placements (Figure 18.8a). Also, a data chart is needed to record time of treatment, the electrode placement, the parameters used and the response (Figure 18.8b). The record charts should also include a comments

Figure 18.7 (b) Visual analog scale chart. On a full-sized VAS chart the scale measures 10 cm in length. This enables the physiotherapist to obtain accurate data of the patient's pain after each treatment session.

Name: . . . . Medical record number: . . . . Date: . . . .

Date: . . . .

Before stimulation
No pain _____ Maximum pain

After stimulation
No pain _____ Maximum pain

Date: . . . .

Before stimulation
No pain _____ Maximum pain

After stimulation
No pain _____ Maximum pain

Date: . . . .

Before stimulation
No pain _____ Maximum pain

After stimulation
No pain _____ Maximum pain

Date: . . . .

Before stimulation
No pain _____ Maximum pain

After stimulation
No pain _____ Maximum pain

Date: . . . .

Before stimulation
No pain _____ Maximum pain

After stimulation
No pain _____ Maximum pain

Date: . . . .

Before stimulation
No pain _____ Maximum pain

After stimulation
No pain _____ Maximum pain

Date: . . . .

Before stimulation
No pain _____ Maximum pain

After stimulation
No pain _____ Maximum pain

column to allow recording of drug intake, since it may be that success with TENS is indicated by the reduction of analgesic medication. It is essential to review outpatients the day following the initial application of TENS. It is helpful to request that the patient reapply the TENS at home so that a more accurate assessment of his/her technique and placement of the electrodes can be made. If

Figure 18.8 (a) Body chart for TENS Electrode Placement.

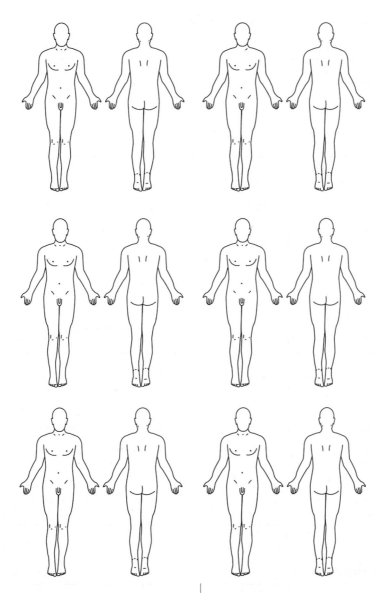

unsuccessful initially, it may be more helpful for the patient to attend on a daily basis in an attempt to find the most successful electrode position. For that reason, a Friday appointment should be avoided if review at the weekend is not possible.

Philosophy of Treatment

Many patients who have been suffering from chronic pain for a long period of time have over-optimistic expectations of pain relief. It is therefore essential that clear and obtainable objectives are set prior to treatment, and it must be emphasized that the pain may be relieved but not

Figure 18.8   (b) TENS data chart.

Date	Tens Make & Number	Time on	Time off	Total h Stimulation	Electrode Position/ Size	Most Effective Position			Comments
						Ouput	Frequency	Pulse Width	

Table 18.2

Common chronic painful conditions

- Brachial plexus avulsion injuries, peripheral nerve injuries, e.g. painful neuroma, reflex sympathetic dystrophy and nerve compression injuries, such as Carpal tunnel syndrome
- Stump and/or phantom limb pain
- Post herpetic neuralgia
- Back and neck pain with associated leg or arm pain respectively
- Trigeminal neuralgia
- Post-operative pain
- Pain in the terminally ill
- Obstetric pain

Figure 18.9 Electrode placement: 1. Carpal tunnel compression low median nerve irritation. 2. Low back pain. 3. Brachial plexus injury with anaesthesia below elbow (C5-T1), 4. Low back pain with L5 root pain in left leg. 5. Below-knee amputation right leg position (i). 6. Below-knee amputation right leg position (ii). 7. Post-operative TENS for low abdominal wound. 8. Back pain with bilateral leg pain (left leg S1 root; right leg L5 root) 9. Post-hepatic neuralgia includingT4, 5 roots. 10. Obstetric TENS for pain control in labour. 11. Hypersensitive scar right knee following knee surgery. 12. Neck pain.

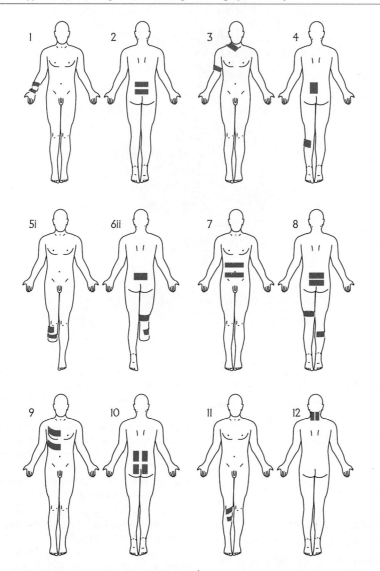

completely eliminated. Different goals may be set for different conditions, e.g. a patient with an 11-year history of low back pain is unlikely to have the same outcome as a patient with only a 1-month history of pain. The patients' expectations must be rationalized without dampening their hope and morale, which may already be at a low level; gaining patients' confidence is vital since motivation and encouragement are an essential ingredient of treatment for chronic pain patients.

Some chronic painful conditions for which TENS might be used are listed in Table 18.2.

Figure 18.10 *Lifetime* obstetric TENS showing electrode positioning for the relief of obstetric pain. (Photograph courtesy of NEEN Healthcare, Norfolk.)

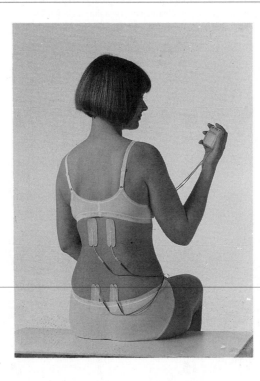

Some examples of electrode placement can be seen in Figure 18.9 and also Figure 18.10, which shows TENS used for the relief of obstetric pain. Detailed case histories are beyond the scope of this book. [Frampton, 1994].

Conclusion

TENS provides a cheap, non-invasive modality for pain relief. It is essential that it is properly monitored and evaluated and is considered in the context of a complete rehabilitation programme for the management of chronic pain [Frampton, 1994]. Inadequate information and instruction to patients, without proper follow-up and monitoring, will deny the chronic pain sufferer the opportunity to appreciate fully the scope of this small machine.

References

Altree, J (1994) Acupuncture, in Wells, PE, Frampton, VM, Bowsher, D (eds) *Pain Management by Physiotherapy*, p 104.. Butterworth Heinemann, London.

Anderson, SA, Hansson, G, Holmgren, E, Renberg, O (1976) Evaluation of the pain suppressing effect of different frequencies of peripheral electrical stimulation in chronic pain conditions. *Acta Orthopaedica Scandinavia* **47**: 149–57.

Bates, JAV, Nathan, PW (1980) Transcutaneous electrical nerve stimulation for chronic pain. *Anaesthesia* **35**: 817–22.

Bowsher, D (1994) Modulation of nociceptive input, in Wells, PE, Frampton, VM, Bowsher, D (eds) *Pain Management by Physiotherapy*, p 56. Butterworth Heinemann, London.

Chung, JM, Lee, KH, Haar, Y, Endo, K, Willis, WD (1984) Factors influencing peripheral nerve stimulation produced inhibition of primate spinothalamic tract cells. *Pain* **19**: 277–293.

Devor, M (1989) The pathophysiology of damaged peripheral nerves, in Wall, PD, Melzack, R (eds) *Textbook of Pain*, pp. 63–81. Churchill Livingstone, Edinburgh.

Eriksson, MBE, Sjolund, BH, Neilzen, S (1979) Long term results of peripheral conditioning stimulation as an analgesic measure in chronic pain. *Pain* **6**: 335–47.

Frampton, VM (1982) Pain control with the aid of transcutaneous nerve stimulation. *Physiotherapy* **68**(3): 77–81.

Frampton, VM (1990) Therapist's management of brachial plexus injuries, in Hunter, Schneider, Mackin and Callahan (eds) *Rehabilitation of the Hand: Surgery and Therapy*, pp. 630–639. CV.Mosby, St.Louis.

Frampton, VM (1994) Transcutaneous electrical nerve stimulation and Chronic Pain, in Wells, PE, Frampton, VM, Bowsher, D (eds) *Pain Management by Physiotherapy.* Butterworth Heinemann, London.

Handwerker, HO, Iggo, A, Zimmermann, M (1975) Segmental and supraspinal actions on dorsal horn neurons responding to noxious and non-noxious skin stimuli. *Pain* 1: 147–65.

Johnson, MI, Ashton, CH, Bousfield, DR, Thompson, JW (1991a) Analgesic effects of different pulse patterns of transcutaneous electrical nerve stimulation on cold-induced pain in normal subjects. *Journal of Psychosomatic Research* 35(2/3): 313–321.

Johnson, MI, Ashton, CH, Thompson, JW (1991b) An indepth study of long term users of transcutaneous electrical nerve stimulation (TENS). Implications for clinical use of TENS *Pain* 44: 221–229.

Johnson, MI, Ashton, CH, Thompson, JW (1991c) The consistency of pulse frequencies and pulse patterns of transcutaneous electrical nerve stimulation (TENS) used by chronic pain patients. *Pain* 44: 231–234.

Linzer, M, Long, DM (1976) Transcutaneous neural stimulation for relief of pain. *IEEE Transactions on Biomedical Engineering* 23: 341–345.

Loeser, JD, Ward, AA (1967) Some effects of deafferentation on neurons of the cat spinal cord. *Archives of Neurology* 17: 629–36.

Loeser, JD, Black, RG, Chirstman, A (1975) Relief of pain by transcutaneous stimulation. *Journal of Neurosurgery* 42: 308–314.

Loh, L, Nathan, PW (1978) Painful peripheral states and sympathetic blocks. *Journal of Neurology, Neurosurgery and Psychiatry* 441: 664–671.

Long, DM, Campbell, JN, Gurer, G (1979) Transcutaneous electrical stimulation for relief of chronic pain, in Bonica, JJ, Liebeskind, JC, Albe-Fessard, DG (eds) *Advances in Pain Research and Therapy* (3rd ed.), pp. 593–599. Raven Press, New York.

Mannheimer, C, Carlsson, C (1979) The analgesic effects of transcutaneous electrical nerve stimulation (TNS) in patients with rheumatoid arthritis. A comparative study of different pulse patterns. *Pain* 6: 329–334.

Mannheimer, JS, Lampe, GN (1984) *Clinical Transcutaneous Electrical Nerve Stimulation.* FA Davis, Philadelphia.

Melzack, R, Wall, PD (1965) Pain mechanism: a new theory. *Science* 150: 971–978.

Melzack, R, Stillwell, DM, Fox, EJ (1977) Triggerpoints and acupuncture points for pain. Correlations and implications. *Pain* 3: 3–23.

Moldaver, J (1979) Tinel's sign its characteristics and significance. *Journal of Bone Joint Surgery* 60A: 412.

Omura, Y (1987) Basic electrical parameters for safe and effective electro-therapeutics (electro-acupuncture TES TENMS (or TEMS) TENS and electro-magnetic field stimulation with or without drug field) for pain neuro-muscular skeletal problems and circulatory disturbances. *Acupuncture and Electrotherapy* 12: 201–225.

Polden, M (1994) Pain relief in obstetrics and gynaecology, in Wells, PE, Frampton, VM, Bowsher, D (eds) *Pain Management by Physiotherapy.* Butterworth Heinemann, London.

Pomeranz, B, Niznick, G (1987) Codetron, a new electrotherapy device overcomes the habituation problems of conventional TENS devices. *AMJ Electromed.* First quarter 22–26.

Salar, G, Job, I, Mingrino, S *et al.* (1981) Effects of transcutaneous electrotherapy on CSF b-endorphin content in patients without pain problems. *Pain* 10: 169–172.

Sjolund, B, Eriksson, MBE (1979) The influence of naloxone on analgesia produced by peripheral conditioning stimulation. *Brain Research* 173: 295–301.

Sjolund, BH (1985) Peripheral nerve stimulation suppression of C fibre-evoked flexion reflex in rats. *Journal of Neurosurgery* 63: 612–616.

Taylor, P, Hallett, M, Flaherty, L (1981) Treatment of osteoarthritis of the knee with transcutaneous electrical nerve stimulation. *Pain* 11: 233–246.

Thompson, JW (1987) The role of transcutaneous electrical nerve stimulation (TENS) for the control of pain, in Doyle, D (Ed.) *International Symposium on Pain Control*, pp. 27–47. Royal Society of Medical Services, London.

Tinel, J (1915) he signe de "fourmillement" dans les lesions des nerfs peripherique. Press Med. 47: 388.

Tulgar, M, McGlone, F, Bowsher, D, Miles, JB (1991a) Comparative effectiveness of different stimulation modes in relieving pain. Part I A Pilot Study. *Pain* 47: 151–155.

Tulgar, M, McGlone, F, Bowsher, D, Miles, JB (1991b) Comparative effectiveness of different stimulation modes in relieving pain. Part II A double blind controlled long-term clinical trial. *Pain* 47: 157–162.

Wagman, IH, Price, DD (1969) Responses of dorsal horn cells of M. Mulatta to cutaneous and sural nerve A and C fibre stimulation. *Journal of Neurophysiology* 32: 803–817.

Wall, PD, Sweet, W (1967) Temporary abolition of pain in man. *Science* 155: 108–109.

Wall, PD, Gutnik, M (1974) Properties of afferent nerve impulses originating in a neuroma. *Nature* 248: 740.

Wall, PD, Gutnik, M (1974) Ongoing activity in peripheral nerves. The physiology and pharmacology of impulses originating from a neuroma. *Experimental Neurology* 43: 580–593.

Wall, PD, Devor, S (1981) The effect of peripheral nerve injury on dorsal root potentials and on transmission of afferent signals into the spinal cord. *Brain Research* 209: 95–111.

Wallin, G, Torebjork, E, Hallin, RG (1976) Preliminary observation on the pathophysiology of hyperalgesia in the causalgic pain syndrome, in Zotterman, Y (ed) *Sensory functions of the skin in primates*, pp. 489–502. Pergamon Press, Oxford.

Withrington, RH, Wynn Parry, CB (1984) The management of painful peripheral nerve disorders. *Journal of Hand Surgery* 9B(1): 24–28.

Woolfe, SL, Gersh, HR, Rao, VR (1981) Examination of electrode placements and stimulating parameters in treating chronic pain with conventional transcutaneous electrical nerve stimulation (TENS). *Pain* 11: 37–47.

Woolfe, CJ, Wall, PD (1982) Chronic peripheral nerve section diminishes the primary afferent A-fibre mediated inhibition of rat dorsal horn neurones. *Brain Research* 242: 77–85.

Woolfe, CJ (1989) Segmental afferent fibre-induced analgesia. Transcutaneous electrical nerve stimulation (TENS) and vibration, in Wall, PD, Melzack, R (eds) *Textbook of Pain*, pp. 884–896. Churchill Livingstone, Edinburgh.

Wynn Parry, CB (1980) Pain in avulsion lesions of the brachial plexus. *Pain* 9: 41–53.

Wynn Parry, CB (1981) *Rehabilitation of the Hand.* Butterworths, London.

19

Interferential Therapy

DENIS MARTIN

Introduction
•
Interferential Therapy
•
Indications for Use
•
Treatment Guidelines
•
Conclusion

Introduction

Interferential therapy is an aspect of electrotherapy which is widely used but poorly understood. Although it has many similarities with other electrotherapy devices (and these will be acknowledged throughout the text), this chapter seeks specifically to address interferential therapy as a distinct treatment modality in its own right and discusses its value in physiotherapy from this basis. Figure 19.1 shows a modern interferential stimulator.

Definition of Interferential Therapy

While the actual definition of interferential therapy is not standardized in the literature, it may be described as the transcutaneous application of alternating medium-frequency electrical currents, amplitude modulated at low frequency for therapeutic purposes. From this definition it should be seen that interferential therapy is a form of transcutaneous electrical nerve stimulation. It is, however, rarely included in discussions concerning the ubiquitous TENS machines. Where such similarities arise the reader is referred to more detailed discussion in Chapter 18. Interferential therapy is also seen as a means of

Figure 19.1   A modern interferential stimulator. (Photograph courtesy of Central Medical Equipment Ltd, Nottingham).

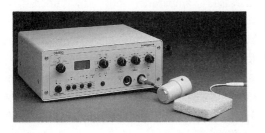

applying low-frequency current within the so-called therapeutic range. Again, the reader is referred to Chapter 18 to avoid repetition.

Interferential Therapy

In the 1950s Hans Nemec sought to overcome the problems of discomfort caused by low-frequency currents whilst maintaining their claimed therapeutic effects [Nelson and Currier, 1991]. The skin's resistance to the low-frequency currents in use at the time was too high to permit penetration of the current into deeper tissue without causing undue levels of patient discomfort.

Skin impedance to electricity is inversely proportional to the frequency of the electrical current.

The following equation describes the relationship between the two:

$$Z = 1/2fC,$$

where Z = skin resistance, f = current frequency, and C = skin capacitance.

Medium-frequency currents, associated with a relatively lower skin resistance, are believed generally to be more comfortable than low-frequency currents; thus, using a medium frequency, a more tolerable penetration of current through the skin is possible. Nemec, utilizing the principles of amplitude modulation, argued that medium-frequency currents could be used to produce low-frequency current. It was claimed that, in this way, the effects of low-frequency stimulation could be obtained while improving the comfort factor. These claims, however, are not accepted by all [Alon, 1989].

Amplitude Modulation

Amplitude modulation is a term used to describe the transmission of an information-containing signal by varying the amplitude of a carrier wave. The process is used in telecommunications where an electrical signal of audio frequency is transmitted along a carrier wave of a much larger

Figure 19.2   (a) Amplitude modulation of the radiofrequency wave   (b) to transmit audiofrequency wave.

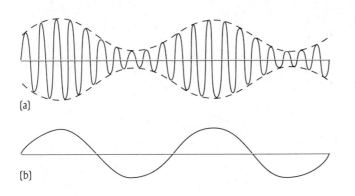

(a)

(b)

Figure 19.3 Algebraic summation of two waves in phase: wave (a) plus wave (b) produces a wave of increased amplitude, (c).

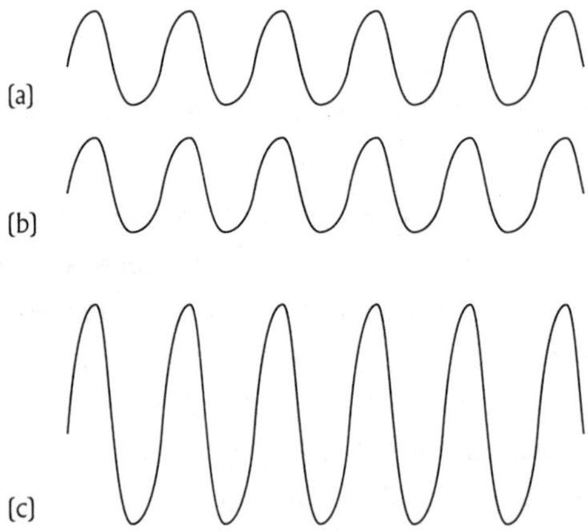

(a)

(b)

(c)

radio frequency. By varying the amplitude of the higher frequency wave at regular intervals, the smaller frequency is created (Figure 19.2).

In interferential therapy, the process of amplitude modulation is achieved by mixing two out-of-phase medium-frequency currents. The individual currents interfere with each other where they meet, and set up a new waveform. Due to wave interference, the current amplitudes sum algebraically.

Two waveforms of equal frequency and in phase with each other have both peaks and troughs that coincide. A new waveform is created with an increased amplitude but an unchanged fre>quency (Figure 19.3). If, however, the two currents are of slightly different frequencies they are not in phase and the peaks and troughs of the current do not coincide. The resultant current is shown in Figure 19.4. This current has a frequency equal to the mean of the two original frequencies.

Because the peaks and troughs of the two currents do not coincide, the amplitude of the resultant current increases and decreases in a regular cycle. The frequency of this cycle is equal to the difference between the two original frequencies and is termed the *beat frequency* or *amplitude modulation frequency* (AMF).

At the most simple level, therefore, interferential current can be considered to consist of a medium frequency current which is amplitude modulated at a low frequency.

Current Distribution

The traditional method of applying interferential therapy uses four electrodes to supply two cir-

Figure 19.4 Amplitude-modulated wave (c) produced by interference between two out-of-phase waves, (a) and (b).

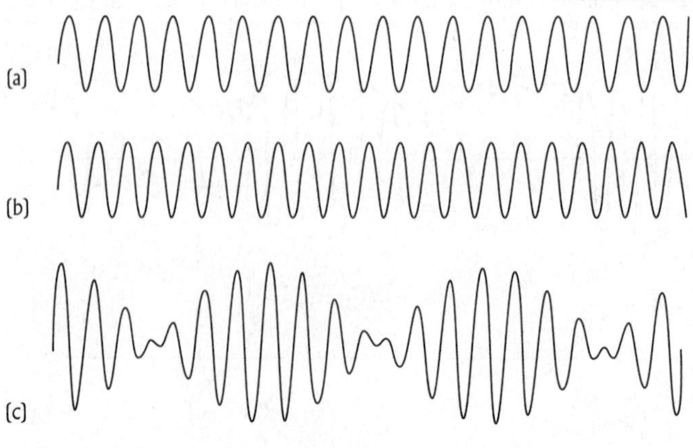

(a)

(b)

(c)

Figure 19.5   Two circuits arranged perpendicularly to each other to intersect at the target area.

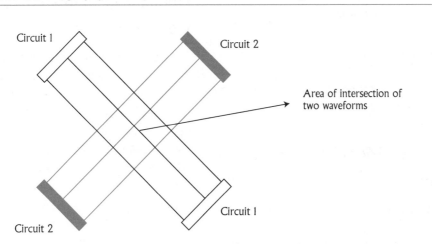

cuits. The circuits are arranged perpendicularly to each other so that they intersect at the intended area of stimulation (Figure 19.5). DeDomenico (1981) summarized a theoretical description of the nature of the amplitude-modulated current in a homogeneous medium. He described how the amplitude-modulated current is contained chiefly in a flower-shaped pattern between the sets of electrodes (Figure 19.6). A more detailed description of the field pattern by Treffene (1983) suggests that the original flower-shaped pattern is an oversimplification. Treffene concluded that an interferential field was set up at all areas of the medium – including at the electrodes – rather than exclusively within the described area originally. All present theories, concern a homogeneous medium. How accurately such ideas transfer to the strongly heterogeneous medium of body tissue is unclear, although work carried out by Meyer-Waarden, Hansjurgens and Friedmann (1980) suggests that they have some validity. Demmink (1995), however, presented findings

Figure 19.6   Amplitude-modulated current within a flower-shaped area between the two circuits.

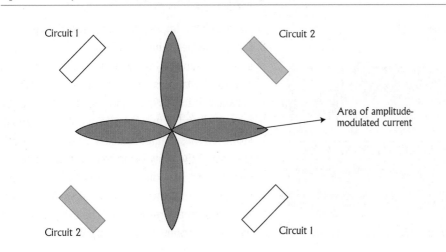

which suggest strongly that the degree of modulation is highly irregular.

Machine Settings

Figure 19.7 shows the settings that are present on most interferential machines.

Amplitude Modulation Frequency (AMF)

Interferential stimulators use two medium-frequency currents, one at a fixed frequency of 4000 Hz and another adjustable between 4000 and 4250 Hz. (These figures can vary between different machine models.) The inclusion of the adjustable frequency permits the selection of a range of amplitude-modulated low frequencies – the medium-frequency current will change accordingly. For example, selection of an amplitude modulation frequency of 100 Hz will produce a resultant medium frequency of 4050 Hz.

Frequency Modulation / Sweep Frequency

The amplitude modulation frequency can itself be modulated by frequency. The AMF can be made to alternate over a set range by manipulation of the sweep-frequency control – the original AMF becomes the base frequency, e.g. 100 Hz. Applying a sweep frequency of 10 Hz will result in an AMF varying between 100 Hz and 110 Hz. The medium frequency will vary correspondingly between 4050 Hz and 4055 Hz. Many machines also allow the sweep rate to be adjusted.

Machines vary in the sweep frequency available to the practitioner, but range between 0 and 250 Hz.

Intensity

The intensity of the current can be adjusted on the machine and, on some units, by remote control as well. As the intensity increases, the patient will feel a tingling sensation. With more intensity, a muscle contraction will occur. If the current is applied at a high-enough intensity, the patient may feel discomfort or pain. This progression of sensation / effect is concomitant with selective stimulation of nerve types (den Adel and Luykx, 1991).

Although it is impossible to be prescriptive about the intensities which will produce therapeutic effects in subjects, work on normal subjects has suggested that sensory effects are likely to arise at between 4 and 10 mA and motor responses at between 8 and 15 mA (Martin and Palmer, 1995a). However, these values are likely to vary with both the area of the body being treated and the individual subject. In addition, it is impossible to identify 'optimum' treatment values as these can vary according to the response of the the patient and to the philosophy of the therapist.

Figure 19.7   A commonly used interferential unit showing selection of machine settings.

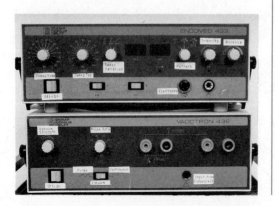

Figure 19.8   Vector-sweep facility to allow the area of amplitude-modulated current to cover a larger area.

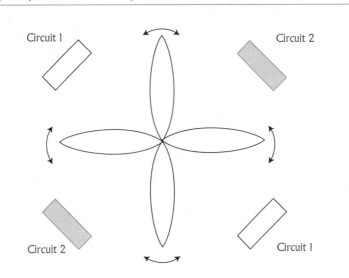

Figure 19.8   Vector-sweep facility to allow the area of amplitude-modulated current to cover a larger area.

Rotating Vector

A rotating vector design is incorporated into some machines to vary the strengths of the currents relative to each other. By doing so, the interference pattern will rotate to ensure that a wide area can be covered by the interferential current (Figure 19.8). Thus, treatment is not restricted in its distribution to the areas previously described and shown in Figure 19.6.

Electrodes

Current can be applied through flexible electrodes taped or bound to the skin or by vacuum electrodes which use suction to maintain contact (Figure 19.9). Vacuum electrodes provide a useful means of applying interferential current to areas relatively inaccessable to flexible electrodes. Some users state that vacuum electrodes offer a therapeutically beneficial massage effect in addition to any effects of the current itself. Such claims have not been tested and would appear to lack authenticity.

Interferential therapy is usually applied using four electrodes; however, it is also possible to use two electrodes. Here, amplitude modulation occurs inside the machine before application to the tissues. The reader is referred to Chapter 18 for discussion of electrode placement.

Indications for use

The general indications for interferential therapy are relief of pain, the promotion of healing in

Figure 19.9   Suction electrodes (a)   or flexible electrodes (b) can be used. In both cases, water-soaked sponges are required.

(a)   (b)

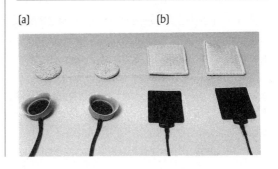

tissue, and the production of muscle contraction (e.g. Savage, 1981; Niklova 1987; Low and Reed, 1990; Goats, 1990).

Pain

The claims of pain relief share their origins with the use of TENS. Some authors state that the low-frequency components of the interferential current, i.e. the beat frequencies, cause nerve stimulation. In practice, it is clear that when there is no beat frequency, i.e. when the current is purely unmodulated 4000 Hz, there is still a similar level of stimulation. What the beat frequency may do is influence the rate of firing of the nerve. The reader is referred to Chapter 18 for discussion of the possible importance of this.

To recap, interferential current consists primarily of a medium-frequency current of approximately 4000 Hz. At 4000 Hz, the pulse duration will be 0.125 ms. On the strength–duration principle (Howson, 1978), such a low pulse duration renders the current useful as a stimulator of Aβ nerve fibres with stimulation of the motor nerves occurring with sufficient intensity of current. With sufficient pulse charge, small diameter afferents may be stimulated although, from a theoretical viewpoint, interferential current would appear to be an inefficient method of stimulation of Aδ/C nerve fibres. On this argument, the beat frequency, therefore, is of little or no importance in determining the type of structure stimulated.

DeDomenico (1982) voiced claims that interferential current could relieve pain by producing a peripheral blockade of activity in nerve fibres carrying noxious inpulses. On the basis that A and C fibres have impulse transmission rates of 40 Hz and 15 Hz respectively, he argued that they would become overloaded if stimulated at frequencies above this rate. He advocated that this

would be achieved with interferential therapy using AMFs of approximately 100 Hz. Some researchers have suggested the possibility of peripheral blocking with electrostimulation (e.g. Inglezi and Nyquist, 1976). This claimed mechanism has yet to be confirmed for interferential current by appropriate evidence. Any neurally mediated effect on pain perception would appear to be argued more logically from the basis of large diameter stimulation as opposed to blocking of small diameter afferents. By stimulation of large diameter Aβ sensory fibres, interferential therapy can act similarly to TENS to relieve pain.

Despite the popularity of interferential therapy in clinical practice and the clinical claims of efficacy, the published evidence of the pain-relieving effect of interferential therapy is scant. Taylor et al. (1987) could not show any difference between interferential therapy and placebo on the intensity of jaw pain in a group of 40 patients. Using a submaximum-effort tourniquet test to produce sensations of pain in normal subjects, Scott and Purves (1991) reported no difference in pain perception among control, placebo or treatment subjects. It would be unwise to be judgemental on two studies, however. Given that interferential current is capable of the stimulation of Aβ fibres, the reader is again referred to the more substantial work in the related area of TENS.

Tissue Healing

Because of its low-frequency component (due to amplitude modulation), interferential current is claimed to offer similar therapeutic benefits to the healing process as low-frequency electrical stimulation. For a detailed discussion of these effects the reader is referred to the appropriate chapter. Niklova (1987) claimed to have produced evidence that interferential currents could effect healing activity due to cellular effects. While much of her work is difficult to assess, her available reports suggest that her claims arose from poorly conducted, often uncontrolled trials open to bias. Replication of the findings are required before such claims can be accepted.

Muscle Stimulation

Interferential current has also been used as a muscle stimulator (DeDomenico, 1986). While it is often quoted as being more comfortable than other waveforms for muscle stimulation, a study by Baker *et al.* (1988) suggested that a symmetrical, biphasic square wave was more comfortable than either interferential current or a monophasic, paired, spike waveform. The authors did state, however, that there appeared to be a subgroup who found interferential current to be most comfortable. They recommended that interferential current should be used for patients who could not tolerate other current types. One area of muscle stimulation where interferential current is used is in the treatment of incontinence; variable results have been reported, e.g. Van-Poppel *et al.* 1985; Wilson *et al.*, 1987; Laycock and Green, 1988; Olah *et al.*, 1990.

Treatment Guidelines

A problem in interferential therapy, common to all forms of electrotherapy, is the determination of appropriate control settings on the machines. The literature is often unhelpful about this issue, but guidelines dictating specific settings for specific conditions are frequently quoted in texts (e.g. Savage, 1981). While, on the surface, such prescriptions appear to be useful, it is possible that such an approach has led to confusion and

has inhibited proper scientific development of electrotherapy. No evidence is offered to substantiate these guidelines and their choice appears to be arbitrary. The following account, therefore, does not offer prescriptive guidelines. Theoretical principles are used to attempt to enable the reader to make reasoned choices of machine settings. As research evidence becomes available more rigid guidelines may then be possible.

Pain Relief

Perhaps the most commonly asked question is which beat frequency should be selected. The question may be best answered by considering which is the therapeutically effective component of interferential therapy for nerve stimulation — the medium-frequency current or the beat frequency? As stated above, the beat frequency has been considered traditionally to be the effective parameter, mimicking the effects of low-frequency electrical current. There is little valid support for this in the literature. Claims of the importance of beat frequency in nerve stimulation are difficult to support. From a physiological perspective, it is arguably more justifiable to cite the medium frequency (approximately 4000 Hz) as being of most importance (Alon, 1989). However, beat frequency has been suggested as influencing patient comfort (den Adel and Luykx, 1991). The best use of the therapy may be achieved by selecting the most comfortable beat frequency for the patient. The higher beat frequencies (>50 Hz) are reported as being most comfortable (den Adel and Luykx, 1991), but the patient is best placed to decide which is the most comfortable setting.

The necessity of the sweep frequency is questionable. The parameter has been suggested to be useful in that it allows a scanning of the tissues with a number of the therapeutic beat frequencies. However, these claims must remain unsubstantiated until the beat frequencies have been shown to have therapeutic importance. With regard to nerve stimulation, it is claimed that adding a sweep frequency prevents the adaptation of nerves to the stimulus. Such claims are not necessarily accurate (Martin and Palmer, 1995b). The changes in the medium-frequency current due to amplitude modulation are relatively minimal. At an AMF of 10 Hz, the medium frequency is 4005 Hz. At an AMF of 100 Hz the medium frequency is 4050 Hz — a difference of 45 Hz. In the range of 4000 Hz, such a difference is minimal and the medium frequency may be considered to remain constant in practical terms. Increasing the intensity at regular intervals is probably the most effective means of preventing adaptation to the stimulus. Again, on this line of argument, the rate of beat-frequency change — the sweep rate — is no longer of importance.

The choice of four electrodes or two electrodes is also a matter of debate. In practical terms, it is probably easier to use two electrodes although this is a matter of personal preference.

The issue of intensity of current is, perhaps, best dealt with by drawing from research into TENS.

Healing

Healing effects are claimed for interferential currents. Activation of Aβ fibres can be used to modulate activity of the autonomic nerve system with the possibility of influence on the healing process. Here, the recommendations regarding nerve stimulation for the relief of pain apply.

Interferential current is also claimed to have a direct effect on cells. In this case, the beat frequency may be of value in producing effects specific to low frequencies. Such claims require that the AMF can be demodulated in tissue to produce effects. As stated by Deller (in Savage, 1984) this requires cells to have non-linear properties to demodulate the AMF from the signal. While Patterson (in Stillwell, 1983) strongly doubted this possibility, Charman (1990), summarizing work in the field of bioelectromagnetics, quoted evidence to suggest that demodulation is possible. Cellular demodulating mechanisms have been described for the other electrotherapy devices mentioned above, although the position is very unclear in these more widely researched fields.

It is difficult to provide useful guidelines on the selection of intensity and AMF for direct cellular effects due to the lack of a research basis. Proposed settings may be gleaned tentatively from research into other modalities. For example, supporters of the use of microcurrent therapy may argue that low-intensity, even subliminal, levels of current offer the best chance of success. It may be better practice clinically, however, to use other more established modalities until such possibilities of interferential currents have been properly tested.

Muscle Stimulation

For muscle re-education, it would appear to be appropriate to use the most comfortable settings for the individual. As stated previously, while this may differ between people, the higher AMFs may be of most use.

Contraindictions and Safety of Use

There do not appear to be any singular contraindications to the use of interferential therapy, and the reader is again referred to the Chapter 18 for contraindications and safety of use.

Conclusion

Based on the available evidence, interferential therapy can be argued as being a useful means of stimulation of Aβ fibres for pain relief and a means of stimulating muscle at relatively comfortable levels. The equipment is expensive and bulky, however, and has not been shown to be any better than cheaper, less complex modalities, such as TENS or portable muscle stimulators. As such, it may be viewed as being superfluous at present. With regard to its efficacy in promoting healing, research is well behind that of other modalities, e.g. ultrasound. If future research does provide supporting evidence, then interferential therapy could provide an extremely versatile tool, being capable of nerve stimulation and cellular effects to relatively deep tissue levels.

References

Alon, G (1989) Electro-orthopaedics: a review of present electrophysiological responses and clinical efficacy of transcutaneous stimulation. *Advances in Sports Medicine and Fitness* 2: 295–324.

Baker, LB, Bowman, BR, McNeal, DR (1988) Effects of waveform on comfort during neuromuscular electrical stimulation. *Clinical Orthopaedics and Related Research* 233: 75–85.

Charman, RA (1990) Bioelectricity and electrotherapy – towards a new paradigm. Part 2: Cellular reception and emission of electromagnetic signals. *Physiotherapy* 76(9): 509–516.

DeDomenico, G (1982) Pain relief with interferential current. *Australian Journal of Physiotherapy* 28: 14–18.

DeDomenico, G, Strauss, GR (1986) Maximum torque production in the quadriceps femoris muscle group using a variety of electrical stimulators. *Australian Journal of Physiotherapy* 32: 51–56.

Demmink den Adel, RV, Luykx, RHJ (1991) *Low and Medium Frequency Electrotherapy*. Enraf Nonius, Delft.

Goats, GC (1990) Interferential current therapy. *British Journal of Sports Medicine* 24(2): 87–91.

Howson, DC (1978). Peripheral neural excitability. Implications for transcutaneous electrical nerve stimulation. *Physical Therapy* 58(12): 1467–1473.

Ignelzi, RJ, Nyquist, JK (1976) Direct effect of electrical stimulation on peripheral nerve evoked activity: implications in pain relief. *Journal of Neurosurgery* 45: 159–165.

Low, J, Reed, A (1990) *Electrotherapy Explained*. Butterworth-Heinemann, Oxford.

Low, J, Reed, A (1994) *Physical Principles Explained*. Butterworth-Heinemann, Oxford.

Meyer-Waarden, K, Hansjurgens, A, Friedmann, B (1980) Representation of electric fields in homogeneous biological media. *Biomedizinische Technik* 25: 295–297.

Nelson, RM, Currier, DP (eds) (1991) *Clinical Electrotherapy*, 2nd ed. Appleton & Lange, California.

Nikolova, LT (1987) *Treatment With Interferential Current*. Churchill Livingstone, Edinburgh.

Olah, KS, Bridges, N, Denning, J, Farrar, DJ (1990) The conservative management of patients with symptoms of stress incontinence: a randomized, prospective study comparing weighted vaginal cones and interferential therapy. *American Journal of Obstetrics Gynecology* 162(1): 87–92.

Savage, B (1984) *Interferential Therapy*. Faber & Faber, London.

Scott, SM, Purves, CE (1991) The effect of interferential therapy in the relief of experimentally induced pain: a pilot study, in *Proceedings of the World Confederation for Physical Therapy 11th International Congress Book II*.

Stillwell, GK (ed.) (1983) *Therapeutic Electricity and Ultra-Violet Radiation*, 3rd ed. Williams and Wilkins, Baltimore, London.

Taylor, K, Newton, RA, Personius, RA, Bush, FM (1987) Effects of interferential current stimulation for treatment of subjects with recurrent jaw pain. *Physical Therapy* 67(3): 346–350.

Treffene, RJ (1983) Interferential currents in a fluid medium. *Australian Journal of Physiotherapy* 29(6): 209–216.

Van-Poppel, H, Ketelaer, P, Van-DeWeerd, A (1985) Interferential therapy for detrusor hyperreflexia in multiple sclerosis. *Urology* 25(6): 607–12.

Wilson, PD, Al-Samarrai, T, Deakin, M, Kolbe, E, Brown, AD (1987) An objective assessment of physiotherapy for female genuine stress incontinence. *British Journal of Obstetrics and Gynaecology* 94(6): 575–582.

20

Diagnostic Applications

OONA SCOTT

Introduction
•
Electromyography (EMG) Studies
•
Sensory and Motor Nerve Conduction Studies
•
Human Muscle Function Studies
•
Summary

Introduction

This chapter provides an overview of a number of electrophysiological tests used in the clinical setting to assist both in the diagnosis and in the evaluation of response to therapeutic intervention in peripheral nerve and muscle disorders. The past thirty years have seen major advances both in our understanding of the basic and applied physiological properties of peripheral nerves and skeletal muscles and in the development of tools used to investigate these properties. The bibliography at the end provides a list of key texts used as source material.

Electromyography (EMG) Studies

Electromyography refers to methods of studying the electrical activity of muscles. Recordings are made of muscle unit action potentials (MUAPs) as they pass from the neuromuscular junctions along muscle to activate the individual muscle fibres within motor units. The output is recorded on an electromyogram (EMG). The introduction of the concentric needle electrode in 1929 (see section *Recruitment of Motor Units in Voluntary Contractions* in Chapter 4) meant that it was possible to record the electrical activity that accompanied the activation of particular parts of a muscle.

Clinically, it was useful to be able to demonstrate

when a particular muscle was contracting. The normal pattern of electrical activity could be recognized, and it also became possible to recognize departures from normal, and to associate these with nerve–muscle disorders. Needle electrodes record activity from a much smaller area than surface electrodes and have made it possible to study the activity of single motor units. Because all of the muscle fibres for a given motor unit discharge almost simultaneously, one aggregate spike is picked up, usually the output of the greater density of fibres from the same motor unit nearest to the tip of the electrode wire. The waveform may be complex as additional spikes will have different amplitudes and sizes depending on the distance of the active fibres from the electrode.

Surface electrodes (discs, usually silver–silver chloride) are attached to the skin overlying the muscle or nerve from which the activity is to be recorded. More recently, malleable, self-adhesive electrodes have been developed commercially. These have the advantage of being both very light and easy to apply. The potential difference between the two electrodes is recorded through a differential amplifier, a third electrode being used to connect the patient to earth. The recorded signal represents the sum of the individual potentials produced by all of the nerve or muscle fibres that are activated.

The muscle unit action potentials (MUAPs) or potential differences are very small, usually only a few microvolts. These signals are fed into an amplifier which is connected to a cathode-ray oscilloscope or a computer screen, to a loudspeaker system, and to some form of recorder so that they can be monitored both visually and acoustically, as well as being stored for further analysis at a later date.

More recently, different researchers have developed a number of quantitative techniques for analysing the raw signal and it is now often processed for comparison with other biomechanical signals. A commonly used term is that of a 'rectified integrated signal'. Rectification means that the EMG signal is converted into a signal that only contains positive voltages and is then filtered with a low-pass filter (Winter, 1990). This provides a linear envelope or 'moving average' because it follows the trend of the EMG. However, great care has to be taken in interpreting the relationship between tension generated by the muscle and this signal.

The Tendon Jerk

The tendon jerk, or monosynaptic stretch reflex, is a spinal reflex and is used clinically to observe the response of a muscle to percussion (a tap) on its tendon and to determine neuronal status at a spinal level. Conventionally, two types of neurones were thought to be involved. A tap to the tendon initiates a burst of impulses passing along the Group Ia afferent nerve fibres from the primary sensory endings in the muscle spindle (see section *Afferent Input to the Central Nervous System* in Chapter 4). These are the fastest-conducting afferent neurones. Among the spinal connections of the afferent nerves are excitatory synapses on motoneurones supplying the same muscle. These motoneurones are the second type of neurone involved in the reflex; they complete the reflex arc by forming the efferent pathway via the α motoneurones, neuromuscular junctions and resulting contraction of the skeletal muscle fibres.

The afferent axons project directly onto the motoneurones without necessarily involving interneurones. The motoneurones so activated innervate the extrafusal or skeletal fibres of the muscle that was originally stretched and the action potentials relayed down the motor nerves cause the muscle to contract.

The afferent neurones branch within the dorsal horn of the spinal cord. A side branch (collateral) projects to an inhibitory interneurone in the spinal chord. This inhibits motoneurones innervating the antagonist muscles. The time delay between the afferent input recorded in the dorsal root and the excitatory postsynaptic potential in the excited motoneurone is about 1 ms. A further 1 ms elapses before the inhibitory postsynaptic potential is recorded in the motoneurones supplying fibres in the antagonist muscle.

The H Reflex

The H reflex is a monosynaptic reflex response to electrical stimulation of spindle afferent (1a) fibres and was first described by Hoffman in 1926. Hoffman stimulated the tibial nerve with a low-intensity stimulus which mediated a monosynaptic

response in the soleus muscle. This low-intensity stimulus selectively activates the 1a afferent fibres. Figure 20.1 shows the typical M and H waves elicited in human soleus muscle by stimulating the tibial nerve.

It was originally thought that the H reflex was analogous to the stretch reflex. Essentially, the H reflex stimulates the 1a afferent fibres, bypassing the muscle spindles which are directly stimulated by the tendon tap. It is thought that the H reflex provides an indication of the excitability of the α motoneurone pool.

The stimulus used to evoke the H reflex should be of lower intensity than is required to elicit a maximal M response (see the next section), otherwise the H reflex will be blocked. Blocking occurs because antidromic (opposite direction) impulses evoked in motoneurones by direct stimulation collide with orthodromic (same direction) impulses evoked reflexly in these axons in response to stimulation of the spindle afferent

Figure 20.1   The typical M and H waves elicited in human soleus muscle by stimulating the tibial nerve.

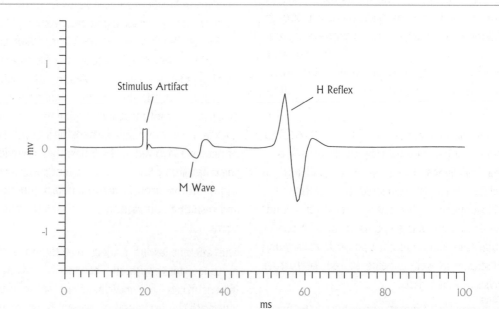

fibres. Latency depends on the site of stimulation and is approximately 30 ms for the soleus and 16 ms for the flexor carpi radialis.

A means of standardizing the intensity of stimulation is to present the results in terms of an H/M ratio. Use of the direct motor response (M wave) is well documented in studies investigating human H reflexes. If the position and intensity of the stimulating electrode is not altered, the size of the M wave has been found to be consistent.

The M Wave

If the motor fibres of a peripheral nerve are stimulated electrically, a response is evoked in the muscles that they supply. This potential is called the M wave. The interval (latency) from the time of application of the signal to muscle contraction represents the conduction time, i.e. the time the impulse takes to travel along the nerve fibres, across the neuromuscular junction and to travel along the muscle fibres to the recording electrodes.

The latency of a submaximal response may be longer than a maximal response. The stimulus must evoke a maximal motor response because, with an inadequate signal, an H reflex may be elicited and mistaken for an M response of prolonged latency. A maximal M response is accomplished by increasing the intensity gradually until the response is maximal, and then increasing the intensity by an additional 30 per cent.

The F Wave

This is evoked in muscle by electrical stimulation of the peripheral nerve by which it is supplied. It occurs as a result of a motoneurone discharge elicited by antidromic (opposite direction) activation rather than by any reflex phenomenon. It has a latency similar to that of the H reflex (see above), but it requires a more intense stimulus and is not blocked if the stimulus evokes a maximal M response in the muscle. It is smaller than the M response and may not be elicited by every stimulus that is applied, even if they are of the same intensity. It can be elicited in deafferented muscles and its latency decreases as the electrode is moved proximally.

Sensory and Motor Nerve Conduction Studies

Both sensory and motor nerve conduction velocities can be recorded and this measurement is routinely performed in patients where peripheral nerve problems are suspected. The passage of an action potential along a nerve fibre generates a change in potential in the surrounding extracellular field. This potential is smaller than the action potential recorded across the membrane of the nerve and is initially negative because sodium ions are leaving the extracellular fluid to enter the axoplasm.

Sensory Nerve Conduction

To account for the neural events involved in the perception of touch, we can start by recording signals from a neurone that terminates in the skin. Brief electrical pulses of 0.1 V amplitude, lasting for 0.001 second (1 millisecond) move up the nerve at a speed up to 80 m/s. Although the impulses in a cell responsive to touch are virtually identical with those in other nerve cells, the significance and meaning are specific for that cell, e.g. they convey to the brain that a particular part of the skin has been pressed.

Adrian (1946) showed that the frequency of

impulse firing in a nerve cell is a measure of the intensity of the stimulus. The stronger the pressure applied to the skin, the higher the frequency and the better maintained the firing of the cell. Information is provided about the modality of the stimulus (by the particular type of sensory neurone it influences), its location (by the position and the connections of the sensory cell), and its intensity (by the frequency of firing).

Techniques have been developed for stimulating the sensory digital nerves using ring electrodes while recording the impulses either as they pass under a pair of electrodes placed more proximally from the nerve trunk or with reference to a single electrode placed over the nerve and another placed at a distance from the nerve. The position of the nerve trunk is located using a stimulating electrode and then finding the point at which the muscle potential is minimal.

The detection of the nerve action potential is facilitated by using an electronic averaging technique. The wave form is typically triphasic with a small positive onset which coincides with the arrival of the impulse at the more distal of the two electrodes. However, latency is often more satisfactorily measured to the peak of the negative deflection, which is best used directly as a measure of latency rather than being converted into conduction velocity (Buchtal and Rosenfalck, 1966). Peak-to-peak amplitude of the potential should also be measured. The amplitude relates to the number of sensory nerve fibres activated, the distribution of their conduction velocities and the distance of the nerve from the recording electrodes.

Motor Nerve Conduction Studies

These involve the use of electrical stimulation and either surface or needle electrodes. Nerves are stimulated where they are relatively superficial with surface electrodes. Deeply situated nerves such as the sciatic nerve at the gluteal fold need to be stimulated with needle electrodes. If bipolar stimulation is used, two small stimulating electrodes, the anode (positive) and cathode (negative), are placed 2–3 cm apart over the nerve with the cathode distal to the anode. For monopolar stimulation, the cathode is positioned over the nerve and a large anode is placed more distally and at a significant distance from it.

Pulse duration can be varied from 0.05–2 ms; the frequency of stimulation is also variable, but 1 Hz or 2 Hz is often used. The two recording electrodes are placed on the muscle innervated by the nerve that is being stimulated, with one being as close to the motorpoint of the muscle as possible (see section *Basis for the Therapeutic Use of Electrical Stimulation* in Chapter 8). The motor point, the position on the skin where maximum contraction can be achieved, is often found at the junction of the proximal third with the distal two thirds of the muscle belly.

The response is typically biphasic, with a negative onset. Conventionally, the negative phase is recorded as an upward deflection. The amplitude of the negative component is usually slightly reduced when the nerve is stimulated proximally rather than distally. This is attributable to variation in time of the action potentials, because of their differing conduction velocities. The amplitude is recorded as a *compound action potential* since it is compounded of contributions from the many action potentials of individual nerve fibres.

The velocity at which the impulse is propagated along the fastest-conducting motor fibres can be determined by stimulating the nerve at two separate points and recording the evoked responses of the muscle it supplies. The stimulus is given at two points and the distance between the two points is measured. To determine the conduction velocity, the distance between the two points is measured and divided by the time difference.

Magnetic Stimulation

Magnetic stimulation is one of the most recent developments in the field of electrodiagnosis. Originally designed (Merton *et al.*, 1982) for the stimulation of peripheral nerves, magnetic stimulation has been applied widely for painless stimulation of the brain, spinal chord and nerve roots. Magnetic stimulators use a magnetic field that varies over time and which passes unchanged through skin and bone, to induce currents in excitable tissue. When such activation applied to the brain, neurones in the cortex can be activated and a motor response elicited in the targeted muscle. Magnetic stimulation has been used to examine central motor pathway conductivity and to assess excitatory and inhibitory influences of descending nerve pathways.

Strength–Duration curves

By applying rectangular pulses of differing pulse widths to a peripheral nerve and recording the current required to produce a muscle twitch, the relationship between the intensity of the current required to produce a muscle contraction and the time for which it is applied, the strength–duration relationship can be determined. This test has clinical applications and can be used to determine the state of innervation and to monitor reinnervation of skeletal muscle following trauma to peripheral nerves (see section *Motoneurone to Muscle Activation* in Chapter 4).

Human Muscle Function Studies

Early studies of human muscle function were limited to evaluating maximum strength or maximum voluntary force (MVC) and estimating energy metabolism during work; the latter involves measurement of oxygen consumption, carbon dioxide production and calculation of

Figure 20.2 A typical trace of force measurements of the human tibialis muscle showing maximum voluntary contraction and the response to stimulation at 1, 10, 20 and 40 Hz, before and after fatigue testing, and the response to fatigue testing by stimulation at 40 Hz for 250 ms, every second for 5 minutes.

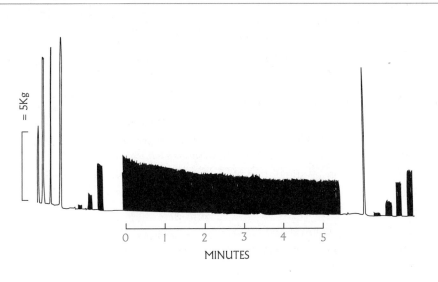

whole body respiratory quotient (see Astrand, 1977).

The 1970s brought major advances in histochemical techniques (Dubowitz and Brooke, 1973) together with more acceptable methods of taking biopsy samples from human subjects. In the past 20 years, methods have been developed to monitor individual or group muscle performance in either isometric or isokinetic contractions; whole muscle cross-sectional area can be measured with ultrasonography and computerized axial tomography; and other methods allow the measurement of the contractile properties of living human muscle using electrically elicited contractions. Figure 20.2 shows the response of the tibialis anterior muscle to electrical fatigue testing. At the same time, rapid developments in molecular biochemistry and immunocytochemical techniques have made it possible not only to identify the histochemistry of different types of fibre but also to relate changes in muscle mass and contractile characteristics of skeletal muscle to overall function and metabolism.

Techniques developed to measure the isometric tensions developed in both voluntary and electrically elicited contractions were first described by Merton (1954) and Desmedt et al. (1968), and more recently by Edwards et al. (1977b). Other studies Scott et al (1990) have shown that it is possible to measure:

1 Maximum voluntary contraction (MVC) with and without superimposed twitches;
2 Response to short trains of stimulation at 1, 10, 20 and 40 Hz;
3 Response to fatigue testing by stimulation at 40 Hz for 250 ms, every second for 5 minutes;
4 The time course of muscle contraction;
5 Loss of force and changes in integrated EMG activity during a 60 s voluntary fatigue test.

Summary

Using a selection of these testing procedures it is now possible for comprehensive studies to be undertaken of the effects of electrical stimulation on human skeletal muscle.

References

Adrian, ED (1946) The physical background of perception. Clarendon Press, Oxford.

Aminoff, MJ (1987) Electromyography in Clinical Practice, 2nd edition Churchill Livingston, New York.

Astrand, PO, Rodahl, K (1970) Textbook of Work Physiology. McGraw-Hill, New York.

Basmajian, JV, Luca, CJ (1985) Muscles alive. Their functions revealed by Electromyography, 5th edition. Williams & Wilkins, Baltimore.

Buchtal, F, Rosenfalck, A (1966) Spontaneous electrical activity of human muscle. Electroencephalography and Clinical Neurophysiology 20: 321.

Desmedt, JE (1967) The isometric twitch of human muscle in the normal and dystrophic states in Exploratory Concepts in Muscular Dystrophy and related disorders (Ed). Milherat AT, Excepta Medica Foundation, Amsterdam 224–231.

Dubowitz, V (1985) Muscle Biopsy. A Practical Approach, 2nd ed. Baillière Tindall, London.

Dubowitz, V, Brooke, MH (1973) Muscle Biopsy. A modern approach. WB Saunders Co., Philadelphia.

Edwards, RHT, Young, A, Hoskings, GP, Jones, DA (1977) Human Skeletal muscle function: Description of tests and normal values. Sci Mol Med 52: 283–290.

Merton, PA (1954) Voluntary strength and fatigue. Journal of Physiology WB Saunders Co., Philadelphia.

Merton, PA, Morton, HB, Hill, DK, Marsden, CD (1982) Scope of a technique for electrical stimulation of human brain, spinal chord and muscle The Lancet Sept II: 597–600.

Rothwell, J (1994) Control of Human Voluntary Movement, 2nd ed. Chapman & Hall, London.

Scott, OM, Hyde, SA, Vrbova, G, Dubowitz, V (1990) Therapeutic possibilities of chronic low frequency electrical stimulation in children with Duchenne muscular dystrophy. Journal of Neurological Sciences 95: 171–182.

Winter, DA (1990) Biomechanics and Motor Control of Human Movement 2nd ed. John Wiley & Sons Inc.

21

Electrical Stimulation for Wound Healing

TIM WATSON

Introduction
•
Historical Review
•
Electrical Activity in the Skin Related to Wounds and Healing
•
Becker's Global DC theory
•
Cellular and Animal Studies
•
Main Approaches
•
Conclusions and Clinical Implications

Introduction

Problems Associated with Chronic Wounds

A relatively small proportion of wounds present with healing problems and most will heal spontaneously without major therapeutic intervention, including electrotherapy. Some wound types are notoriously slow to heal, e.g. chronic venous ulcers and pressure sores. These tend to be lesions of long duration and are often resistant to many forms of treatment. They can result in significant problems medically, socially and eco-nomically for the patient, their relatives and the medical professionals involved.

The factors responsible for poor wound healing are legion and clearly beyond the scope of this chapter, but they must remain central to the philosophy of the use of electrical stimulation as a healing-enhancement tool. Interference with one or more levels of the cascade of events associated with any healing process can lead to inadequate healing / repair responses. Frank and Szeto (1983) summarized the possible general factors thus:

- Inability to form a blood clot or mount an adequate inflammatory reaction;
- Inability to produce new cells or scar components in adequate quantity or quality;

- Inability to organize the scar into an appropriate functional or cosmetic unit.

These factors can be considered on both a local and systemic level. The local factors include infection, inadequate blood flow and nutrition, resulting in low oxygen levels and poor inflammatory response. Repeated wound stresses can also make a significant contribution. The systemic effects which may be detrimental include age-related changes, concurrent disease states, and hormonal problems. Clearly, one could continue to add to these lists with ever more detailed categories, but in principle there are a large number of factors which might be responsible for the interruption of one component of the healing process, and in doing so achieve a major healing dysfunction due to the cascaded nature of the normal events and the complex interactions between components of the processes.

Risk Groups

The main groups of patients with superficial (i.e. skin) wounds likely to suffer from this delayed or prolonged healing can be divided into three major categories (after Vodovnik, 1992):

1 Spinal cord injury (with problems related to decreased movement, decreased sensation and disturbances in peripheral blood flow);
2 Peripheral vascular disease (with ischaemia, tissue congestion and altered tissue viability);
3 The elderly (with decreased movement, altered blood flow, and possibly additional multipathology).

Other groups have been identified using alternative criteria (e.g. Biedebach, 1989), but the high-risk patients are recognized as those presenting with concurrent problems which in some way inhibit or reduce the efficiency of the normal healing responses.

Variety of Approaches

One of the main problems in reviewing the literature in this field is the wide variety of approaches adopted by the various research groups involved in both laboratory and clinical research. For the purposes of this review, the use of electrical stimulation to enhance or stimulate wound healing has been divided into three main approaches. As with any categorization, this does not achieve a universal acceptability, but does provide a useful framework from which the interested reader can investigate further. Each approach described has reported beneficial clinical effects, and it does not appear possible to identify the preferred approach at this stage of the development of the therapeutic modality.

This chapter sets out to consider the effects of electrical stimulation on chronic skin wounds, particularly chronic venous ulcers, pressure sores and allied lesions. There is also a tremendous amount of work concerning electrical stimulation for promoting bone healing, which is equally important. Brief reference is made to this work throughout the chapter, but it is not discussed in any detail. The interested reader is referred to several recent reviews which will provide an excellent platform for further investigation (Black, 1987; Rubinacci *et al.*, 1988, Albert and Wong, 1991).

Historical Review

The use of electrical stimulation as a means of enhancing wound healing is not a new or revolutionary approach. Reports dating back to the 1600s record the use of gold-leaf applications to cutaneous lesions associated with smallpox.

DuBois Reymond (1860) presented an early

description of injury currents leaving human skin wounds, in which the injured bleeding finger was found to be electrically positive compared with an uninjured finger (reviewed in Borgens, 1982).

Burr *et al.* (1938) demonstrated changing wound potentials alongside healing in laboratory animals and then in 1940 measured surface electropotentials over the healing incision sites in patients after abdominal surgery. It was found that the electrical potentials over the wounds were initially positive, but became negative after the fourth day and remained negative until healing was complete. The negative wound potential was associated with the proliferative phase of healing (see Weiss, 1990 for review).

Barnes (1945) measured the wound potentials in humans in an attempt to study the rate of healing. Differences in potential between homologous uninjured finger tips (left and right) were measured, following which fingertip lesions were produced with sandpaper (sufficient to cause bleeding) on the 4 fingers of the left hand. Potential measurements were made immediately following injury and daily thereafter until healing had occurred. The preinjury potentials from 70 subjects (all male) averaged less than 1 mV. The potentials immediately following injury ranged from 15–50 mV (injured fingers more positive). It was also demonstrated that this positive potential disappears once the wound closes over.

More recently, Illingworth and Barker (1980) measured injury currents in children (10) who had accidentally amputated the tip of their finger. The currents reached their peak density some days after the initial injury, gradually returning to zero over a period of up to 45 days.

Electrical interference with externally applied currents in a variety of forms can reasonably be expected to have some interaction with these naturally occurring electrical events that appear to be associated with skin healing. A more detailed consideration of the internal (endogenous) electrical activity of the skin under normal and injured conditions follows as an introduction to the principle of electrotherapeutic intervention with that same process. For a recent review, see Vanable, 1989.

Electrical Activity in the Skin Related to Wounds and Healing

Skin Batteries

There is good reason to believe that the human epidermis contains a skin battery capable of driving substantial currents into wounds. If wound healing is mediated at least in part by electrical signals, then the artificial exposure of wounds to electrical stimulation could be expected to alter the healing process (Weiss, 1990).

Living tissues possess direct current electropotentials that appear to regulate, at least in part, the healing process. Following tissue damage, a current of injury is generated that is thought to trigger biological repair. Exogenous electrical stimuli have been shown to enhance the healing of wounds in both human subjects and in animal models (e.g. Weiss, 1990; Carley and Wainapel, 1985; Griffin *et al.*, 1991).

The mammalian skin battery is quite powerful (at least in humans and guinea pigs) and it can maintain transcutaneous potential voltages of up to 80 mV (internally positive), and has a current-driving capacity of the order of 1 μA/mm of wound length (Jaffe and Vanable, 1984).

The work on skin batteries in mammals achieved a

major forward step after the publication of the paper by Barker *et al.* (1982) describing the skin battery of the guinea pig. They demonstrated a transcutaneous skin potential of 40–80 mV, with the external surface being electrically negative compared with the subdermal tissues. The behaviour of the skin potential was then investigated following skin incision and it was established that the greater part of the skin resistance occurs across the stratum corneum, but that the potential is generated across the living epidermal layers (the stratum granulosum and basement membranes).

The potential across the skin at a wound that cuts right through the epidermis is zero, whilst a few millimetres away, there is a normal transcutaneous voltage of 40–80mV. There is a lateral voltage gradient therefore between the wound and the adjacent epidermis. This voltage gradient is steep, with an average value of 140±20 mV / mm. Close to the wound, the outer surface of the living layer is electrically positive with respect to the outer surface of the living layer further from the wound (Jaffe and Vanable, 1984).

This work was extended by Foulds and Barker (1983) when they measured the transcutaneous potentials in 17 non-injured human volunteers. The surface potential was measured at 121 pre-determined points in each subject, referred to a common reference point which was subepidermal. The average potential for all sites on all subjects was 23±9 mV, with the surface always being negative with respect to the reference point. A consistent anatomical variation was demonstrated with the greatest potentials measured at the hands and the feet. No significant correlations were found between skin potential, age and sex.

The skin potentials measured by Foulds and Barker were similar in magnitude and orientation to those measured in the guinea pig and some amphibian species. This skin potential appears to be capable of driving substantial currents into wounds and it is expected that lateral voltage gradients demonstrated in the guinea pig would also exist in human skin. It is suggested (Foulds and Barker, 1983; Jaffe and Vanable, 1984) that the lateral voltage gradients may be responsible for the epidermal cell migration across a healing wound.

Mammalian wounds heal more slowly when they are dry compared with when they are kept moist (Eaglstein and Mertz, 1978). Jaffe and Vanable (1984) note that when wounds were allowed to become dry, the current is 'switched off' and the lateral voltage gradient is eliminated. Drying of the wound causes the resistance at the wound to increase and eliminated the potential drop at the wound margin (Barker *et al.*, 1982).

It is against this background that the electrical enhancement of wound healing is framed. The essential tenet is that normally healing wounds demonstrate electrical characteristics which can be superimposed on wounds which are not healing at the normal rate in a variety of ways in an attempt to trigger the healing / repair process.

It has been suggested (Gentzkow and Miller, 1991) that the cascade of events which occurs during and after inflammatory / proliferative healing process may have been arrested in cases of chronic wounds. It is further suggested that the external electrical stimulation of these wounds produces effects that can 'restart' or 'jump start' the healing phase.

The lateral voltage gradients associated with skin injury are within the limits of field strengths found to influence a variety of cells in several *in vitro* experiments. In addition to skin batteries, piezoelectric potentials (stress-generated potentials), pyroelectric potentials (thermal-related potentials) and streaming potentials (interaction of

Figure 21.1 Current path with full-thickness wound in mammalian skin (after Jaffe and Vanable, 1984); current represents the movement of positive ions.

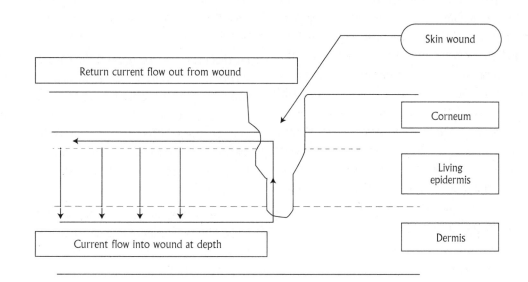

charged fluids) can also be considered to exert an influence on the healing tissue (Dayton, 1989; Charman, 1990).

Skin Battery Changes on Injury/Healing

Bioelectric changes following injury have been demonstrated in several tissue types (predominantly bone, skin and nerve). The recorded potentials are different from those normally present in these tissues, though there does not appear to be any widely accepted explanation for the generation of such potentials (Watson, 1995). Their existence is generally accepted as being significant rather than just an epiphenomenon (Borgens, 1984) and additionally it is considered by most authors that these potentials and subsequent current flow have a major role to play in initiating, controlling, and terminating the repair process (Becker *et al.*, 1962a, b, 1967, 1974a, b; Borgens, 1982; Foulds and Barker, 1983; Hinkle

et al., 1981; Illingworth and Barker, 1980; Patel and Poo, 1982).

The bioelectric disturbances that occur on injury persist for various lengths of time depending on the tissue involved and the extent of the injury. Friedenberg and Brighton (1966), Wilber (1978), Illingworth and Barker (1980), Chang and Snellen (1982) and Chakkalakal *et al.* (1988a, b) are amongst those who have monitored the electrical activity of damaged tissues as it progresses through its proliferative and healing processes. Each of these groups have reported progressive changes associated with the healing process and have obtained results from mammalian tissue.

The surface of a recent skin wound is electrically positive in relation to surrounding skin (Barnes, 1945; Illingworth and Barker, 1980) and, generally, it has been shown that this potential magnitude diminishes as healing progresses.

Additionally, many workers have considered the bioelectric correlates of injury/repair/

regeneration in amphibians and other lower vertebrates. Borgens (1982, 1984) has established clear patterns of behaviour in amphibians following limb amputation and subsequent regeneration. Becker (1961) has demonstrated a difference in electrical behaviour in regenerating and non-regenerating species. In regenerating systems, i.e. where the lost tissue is actually replaced with similar tissue, the initial injured positive polarity reverses to a high negative polarity and progressively returns to normal when the regeneration process is complete. In non-regenerating systems, the initial positive polarity slowly returns to normal with no phase of negative polarity (Becker, 1967) (Figure 21.2).

Whether this electrical activity is a consequence of local metabolic and physiological processes, or whether it acts as an initiator / control mechanism for the reparative process has yet to receive unequivocal confirmation. Barker *et al.* (1982), Weiss *et al.* (1990), Becker (1974a, b), Borgens and McCaig (1989), and Vanable (1989) are amongst a growing body of researchers who present evidence for the latter view.

Further evidence to support the initiator / control theory is derived from studies (in animal models) where the natural electrical activity associated with tissue repair is inhibited or subjected to polarity reversal. The effect of this type of manipulation is to either significantly slow down, or more usually to completely inhibit the normal repair process (Borgens, 1981).

The use of exogenous electrical potentials, fields and currents in order to facilitate tissue healing (in bone, nerve and skin) is becoming a clinically accepted technique. More than 40 papers have been identified which report research in this area. The results vary with tissue type, subjects and

Figure 21.2   Difference between injury from regenerating and non-regenerating species (after Becker, 1974).

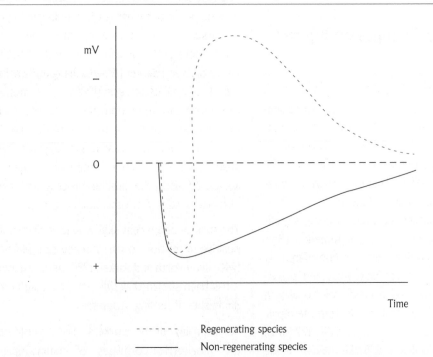

type of applied stimulus, but a high proportion claim significant enhancement of tissue healing.

One is led to the conclusions that tissues are electrically active, that following injury the behaviour of this electrical activity is modified, and that as the repair process proceeds, there is a progressive return to a normal pattern of bioelectric behaviour. Without necessarily considering the wider implications of the initiator/control concept, the physiological evidence is strong and gaining widespread acceptance.

Becker's Global DC Theory

In addition to the evidence for local bioelectric phenomena (such as the skin battery described above) a more global bioelectric view is taken by some researchers in the field. Becker has produced a large volume of literature expounding this aspect of bioelectric activity, highlighting the body-wide electric fields and current flow. Becker suggests that there are a series of equipotential lines that can be mapped from the body surface which reflect the organization of a complex field with a spatial configuration which has a close relationship to the gross distribution of the central and peripheral nervous systems. In several species, including man, the cranial, brachial and lumbar neuraxes were found to be electropositive, with an increasingly negative potential along the peripheral outflow (Becker, 1962a). A complex pattern of axodendritic polarization is proposed, with the steady DC potentials being transmitted by the Schwann cells in the periphery and the glial cells in the central nervous system. The nerves are thought to be capable of carrying both action potentials (equated to digital signals) and slow DC potentials (equated to analogue signals). Local injury, trauma or disease is thought to lead to a disturbance of this body-wide potential pattern, acting as a stimulus for the healing, regenerative or reparative process appropriate to the tissue concerned (Figures 21.3 and 21.4).

Becker and Spadaro (1972) proposed a theoretical framework to model these events. An injury to living systems initiates a series of complex electrical currents at the site of injury which are directly responsible for changes in both cell types and numbers. Secondly, the local electrical effect

Figure 21.3   Axio-dendritic polarization of nerves (after Becker).

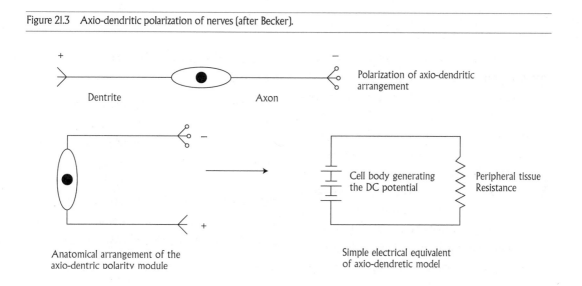

Polarization of axio-dendritic arrangement

Cell body generating the DC potential

Peripheral tissue Resistance

Anatomical arrangement of the axio-dentric polarity module

Simple electrical equivalent of axio-dendretic model

Figure 21.4   Physiologic and electrical model of a neurone pair forming an elementary circuit (after Becker, 1962).

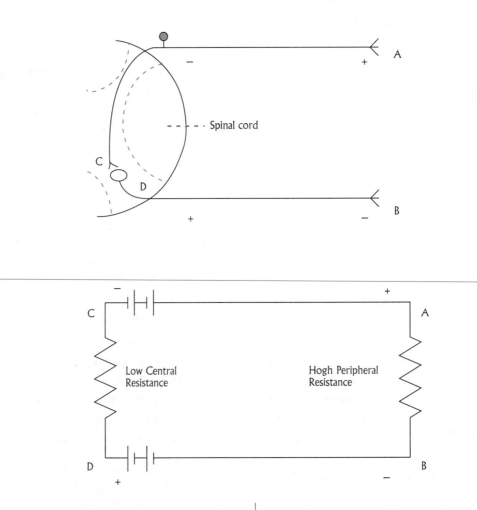

(the current of injury), is the primary response that is responsible for the appearance of new cells. The combination of these first two effects constitutes Phase I of the model. Phase II involves the transmission of data to these new cells facilitating their ability to achieve the required repair and organization into a self-regulating system. This theory does not deny the role of hormones and the numerous mediators involved in healing; instead, it suggests that there is a central, monitoring and controlling role, which is electrical in nature, responsible for the initiation and manage-

ment of the process (see Frank and Szeto, 1983 for a review).

The concept can be considered as a demand control model, with the injured tissue giving rise to an 'abnormal' potential which initiates the tissue response. As healing/repair occurs, the stimulus (the injury potential) diminishes, thus reducing the intensity of the stimulus for repair. This principle is illustrated below as a simple control diagram (after Black, 1987) (Figure 21.5).

Becker's research remains controversial, but to

Figure 21.5   Control diagram for tissue repair stimulus / response (after Becker; Black, 1987).

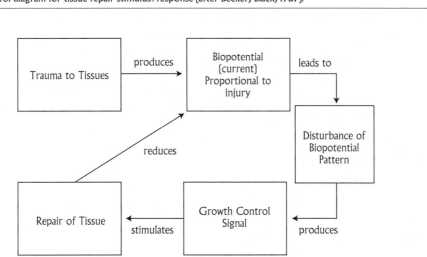

many involved with electrical stimulation as a method of promoting tissue repair, it is an attractive concept. The idea that the normal electrical activity of the tissues forms part of a global electrical network, which on disturbance provides a stimulus for repair, and by means of simple feedback control, the reparative processes can be controlled, is attractive. Disturbance of this normal situation could be involved in delayed wound healing, thereby offering the opportunity to facilitate or enhance the process by external electrical intervention. Many studies have used this tenet as a convenient starting point. Several studies have provided indirect evidence to support this theory including Chakkalakal, 1988a, b; Chang and Snellen, 1982; Weiss et al., 1990.

Cellular and Animal Studies

There is a substantial volume of published work concerning the effects of electrical stimulation on cell cultures and in vivo animal experiments. Numerous studies have demonstrated cellular responses to direct current, often at magnitudes comparable with those found physiologically.

Fibroblasts have been investigated by several groups, though not all studies have used human fibroblast cultures. Dunn et al. (1988) used DC stimulation when investigating fibroblast invasion of a collagen matrix placed in a skin wound in the guinea pig. They found that the fibroblast ingrowth and collagen fibre alignment were increased with DC stimulation when compared with controls. The currents used were between 20 and 100 µA. Maximal fibroblast response was observed near the cathode.

Erickson and Nuccitelli (1984) also used fibroblasts (from quail embryo) and demonstrated cell migration towards the cathode when the cells were exposed to a DC field. The threshold field strength was found to be between 1 and 10 mV / mm. In addition to cell migration, they demonstrated cell orientation changes, the fibroblasts realigning with their long axis perpendicular to the field direction. Field strengths of up to 10 times greater than those necessary to induce fibroblast responses have been measured in vivo.

Ross et al. (1989) used human (adult) fibroblasts which were exposed to an electric field. Cellular alignment was noted with field strengths of 0.1 to

1.5 V/mm (100–1500 mV/mm), though they were unable to demonstrate mobility changes.

Gentzkow and Miller (1991) have reviewed several further studies involving fibroblasts. These include the work of Bassett et al. (1968) who showed that increases in DNA synthesis of 20% and of collagen synthesis (of up to 100%) occurred when fibroblasts were exposed to DC electric fields.

It has recently been suggested (Vodovnik et al., 1992) that cellular proliferation is modified by DC stimulation. If the proliferative rate is too low, it can be increased and, conversely, if the rate is too high, then downregulation occurs with a reduced proliferative rate.

Cooper and Schliwa (1985) used epidermal cells (from fish) exposed to DC electric fields. The epidermal cells were observed to orientate in relation to the field and then to migrate towards the cathode. Chemotactic gradients were eliminated as a causal mechanism. The threshold for these effects was in the region of 0.5 V/cm (50 mV/mm), which represents some 1–4 mV per cell diameter. The demonstration by Winter (1964) that epithelial cells migrating from the periphery of an ulcer move in response to the voltage gradient is also pertinent to the discussion on the effects of electrical stimulation for wound healing.

In addition to fibroblasts and epidermal cells, several other cell types have been shown to respond to electrical stimuli. Cultured cartilage cells have shown an increase in cellular metabolism in response to a 1 μA DC stimulation (Okihana et al., 1985) and mast cell numbers in healing wounds have been shown to be modified with DC stimulation (Reich et al., 1991). It was noted that a decrease in mast cell numbers followed pulsed electrical stimulation. No evidence

was presented to show that the electrical stimulation had induced mast cell degranulation. The galvanotactic effect on neutrophils has been investigated by several groups (see Gentzkow and Miller, 1991). One interesting finding was that when tissues were inflamed, neutrophils are attracted to the cathode suggesting a link between chemically mediated events and electrical responsiveness.

Experimental results (predominantly from in vitro work) with neurones have demonstrated strong effects with DC electrical fields. Although not necessarily directly concerned with wound healing per se, it is important in the context of tissue repair, rather than simply skin lesion repair. Borgens (1988a, b) discusses at some length, the relationship between nerve injury potentials, degenerative events, and regenerative events. Long-term persistent injury potentials are thought to play a role in neuronal development and regeneration and, in addition, may have a modulating effect on the response of neurones to injury.

Patel (1986) demonstrated that neurites are attracted towards the cathode (-ve) pole in a DC field, and are repelled from the anode (+ve pole). Patel discusses and develops a theoretical model which considers these effects in relation to the endogenous currents that could be present in damaged tissue. Pomeranz (1986) suggests that DC fields may enhance nerve growth in adult mammals. The significant results were achieved with cathodal (-ve) stimulation. Control and anodal stimulation experiments showed no effect. The effect was stronger for sensory than for motor nerves.

Other recent neuronal studies of interest include a well cited paper by Hinkle et al. (1981) describing neurite growth patterns in response to DC stimulation. Neurites were found to grow preferentially towards the cathode with field strengths of 7–190 mV/mm. The lower value appeared to be a threshold for their experiments (using frog neurites *in vitro*). In addition to the galvanotactic response, it was shown that greater numbers of neurons sprouted in the DC stimulation experiments and that fibroblasts were also stimulated, resulting in increased differentiation. Myoblasts were found to be responsive to greater field strengths (36–170 mV/mm) resulting in elongation and the development of a growth axis perpendicular to the field direction.

Finally, Patel and Poo (1982) demonstrated similar effects with cathodal galvanotaxis and preferential growth with neurons. The effects were reversible and did not appear to be related to electrode contaminants. This adds weight to the evidence for the effects of DC stimulation of neuronal cells.

Some results are conflicting, and not all publications report the exact stimulation parameters. Common features include cellular orientation in relation to the field and cellular movement (galvanotaxis), usually towards the cathode.

Animal Studies

Before considering the effects of electrical stimulation for wound healing in the clinical environment, it is pertinent to review some of the evidence generated from numerous animal experiments. It is difficult to extrapolate directly from this animal work as the wound healing process is not identical, and although there are similarities between species, there are no directly equivalent animal healing models. The experimentation does provide useful background material for the principles supporting clinical intervention.

A substantial number of studies have considered the electrical correlates of healing and regeneration in amphibian species. It is beyond the scope of this chapter to consider them in any depth, but the interested reader can read excellent recent reviews by Sisken (1983), Borgens *et al.* (1977), and Borgens (1981, 1982).

Chang and Snellen (1982) investigated the regenerative capacity in rabbit ears, noting that the naturally occurring potentials presented a similar pattern to the amphibian species in which true regenerative limb capacity had been retained. This pattern consists essentially of an initial wound-positive phase which lasts for approximately 1 week in the rabbit, which is followed by a wound-negative phase during the proliferative repair. The magnitude of the negative wound potential varied, and this variation appears to correlate with the regeneration, in that those animals who exhibited the largest negative wound potentials demonstrated the most complete regeneration. The animals with negative potentials of smaller magnitude had less complete regeneration. Chang and Snellen (1982) summarize their report with the observation that negative bioelectric activity accompanies growth and that whilst growth continues, the negative bioelectric potentials persists.

In an earlier series of experiments with rabbits (Wu *et al.*, 1967) the effects of electrical stimulation through a metallic suture in abdominal muscle lesions was investigated. Two suture materials were compared for effects: stainless steel and platinum. DC stimulation at 40–400 µA was used, and it was found that the rabbits with steel sutures gained greater wound strength than those with platinum sutures. The increases in wound strength did not appear to be related to stimulation polarity or intensity, and it was suggested therefore that the benefits of stimulation might be due to electrode products (Fe^{2+}) rather than the stimulation itself.

Skin incision work in rabbits is reported by

Konikoff (1976) who used bilateral, full-thickness paravertebral incisions, with one side receiving DC stimulation whilst a sham treatment was delivered to the contralateral wound. A DC current of 20 µA was used and the wounds were tested at 1 week for tensile strength. The treated lesions required an average 53% increase in loading compared with the sham-treated wounds before separation. The electrical stimulation polarity was for the wound electrode to be made negative relative to the subcutanenous positive distal electrode.

Experiments with rats also feature in the animal-model research. Politis et al. (1989) developed a full-thickness skin excision and replacement model. A necrotic area of skin resulted under control conditions following this procedure. After one week, the size of the necrotic area was compared in a control group and two treatment groups who had received DC stimulation with opposite polarity currents. The group with the anode to the skin surface and the cathode implanted deep to the wound showed least necrosis (50%), whilst the reverse polarity stimulation group and the sham treatment group both having 80–90% necrosis after the same time period. The electrical stimulation was at 4.5 µA for 4 days following the operation.

Bach et al. (1991) also used a rat-skin wound model, comparing the effects of DC, AC and sham treatments on wound strength. The DC stimulation group used 1 V, 20 µA stimulation for 1 hour a day on days 4–8. The AC stimulation group used a sinusoidal current at 1 V peak, 100 µA, 300 Hz for 15 minutes/day on days 2–4. Neither type of electrical stimulation had a significant effect on wound strength when compared with controls, but both electrical stimulation groups showed significant collagen content increases in and around the wound compared with the sham

group. Some doubt has been raised as to the validity of measuring wound healing in terms of tensile strength alone (Forrest, 1983), although it has been used in numerous studies as a useful indicator.

Wound healing in pig skin has been extensively studied as it provides an animal model which more closely resembles human skin. Amongst the more recent studies, Im et al. (1990) raised bilateral bipedicle skin flaps in pigs, the central portion of which is known to become ischaemic without intervention. This central zone was treated with electrical stimulation (pulsed DC) at 35 mA, 128 Hz, for 30 minutes twice a day over 9 days. The treatment protocol involved negative stimulation on days 1–3, positive stimulation on days 4–6 and negative again for days 7–9. The necrotic area in the treated animals was significantly less (13.2%) compared with that for the control group (28%).

The experimental work of Alvarez et al. (1983) also used a pig model, and compared the effects of DC stimulation, sham stimulation and no treatment on skin wounds which were evaluated for re-epithelialization and collagen synthesis. The collagen content increased in the DC stimulation group and the epithelial covering was more rapid in the treatment group compared with the sham and no-treatment groups. In these experiments, the wound electrode was positive, with a dispersive (negative) electrode plate some distance from the lesion.

Stromberg (1988) reported the results of different electrical stimulation protocols on 13 skin wounds in pigs. They measured wound contraction and the open wound area. The stimulation groups either received DC stimulation with 35 mA unipolar square-wave stimulation for 30 minutes twice a day with the negative electrode at the wound, or an identical electrical stimulation but with the wound electrode polarity reversed every

3 days. The group with the consistently negative wound electrode appeared to have gained no benefit from the treatment, with a trend towards a retarded healing process. The stimulated wound receiving alternating wound electrode polarity demonstrated wound size decreases to 18% of the original size in 2 weeks, and down to 5% of the original size by the end of 3 weeks treatment.

One animal study, which is not concerned directly with tissue healing, is of interest in that it demonstrates a fundamental physiological change associates with electrical stimulation. Reed (1988) investigated the effects of electrical stimulation on the microvascular permeability changes in the hamster. The cheek pouch of the hamster offers a suitable model for microvascular changes which are observed relatively easily. Animals were given a dose of histamine in order to produce a vasodilation and increased vascular permeability. The animals were divided into two groups, and one group were given electrical stimulation in addition to the histamine. The stimulation consisted of a twin-pulse direct current given at 120 double pulses per second at peak voltages of 10, 30 and 50 volts (giving currents of 10, 20 and 50 mA with average current densities of 0.02, 0.04 and 0.11 mA/mm^2) The pulses were of short

duration and are shown in Figure 21.6 below. The effect of the electrical stimulation was to reduce the leakiness from the vessels when compared with the histamine-only animals. It is suggested that electrical stimulation of this type may be capable of retarding oedema formation.

There are many more animal studies reporting a wide variety of effects of electrical stimulation, and a more complete review is beyond the scope of this chapter. Further references are included in the bibliography.

Main Approaches

One of the problems with reviewing the literature concerning electrical stimulation (ES) for wound healing is that there are multiple approaches, several variations with each area, and a lack of controlled trials with large sample sizes. The mechanisms by which ES achieves its results are still poorly understood, and although there are clearly links that can be established between the hypothetical effects of the treatment and the outcome of the intervention, the theoretical basis for the treatment remains tenuous in places. Nevertheless, the general trend of the

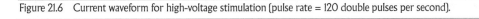

Figure 21.6   Current waveform for high-voltage stimulation (pulse rate = 120 double pulses per second).

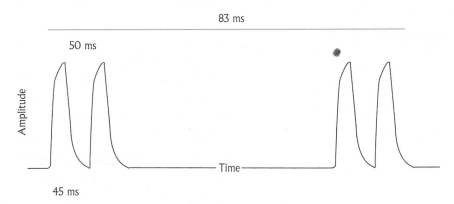

clinical research reports is for the beneficial effects to dominate, with a minority of trials reporting zero or negative effects.

In clinical studies, there are three main approaches to ES, though the differences within each group make direct comparison of the studies all but impossible. The main approaches are:

- The use of low-intensity direct current (LIDC);
- The use of pulsed low-intensity direct current;
- The use of high-voltage pulsed galvanic stimulation (HVPGS) (also known as high-voltage pulsed current – HVPC).

Carey and Lepley (1962) have demonstrated that positive polarity stimulation attracts inflammatory cells to a wound site with an increase in the inflammatory reaction. Alvarez et al. (1983) have shown beneficial effects of ES on wound epithelialization and collagen synthesis, encouraging cellular migration and stimulating collagen synthesis.

Decreased bacterial counts in wounds with negative-pole stimulation has been demonstrated by several groups working with patients in the clinical setting, often followed by stimulation of the healing response itself with the use of positive-pole stimulation (Wolcott et al., 1969; Gault and Gatens, 1976; Carley and Wainapel, 1985; Dayton, 1989). This approach has become popular, with several groups using combinations of negative-pole stimulation initially to reduce or eliminate bacterial infection, followed by positive pole stimulation in order to enhance the proliferative process. This is sometimes further modified with alternating positive- and negative-pole stimulation when a healing plateau is reached.

Low Intensity Direct Current (LIDC)

The measurement of small DC potentials associated with injury and the repair processes following musculoskeletal lesions (Barnes, 1945; Illingworth and Barker, 1980; Jaffe and Vanables, 1984) has resulted in a number of research groups using low-intensity direct currents (LIDC) as a therapeutic tool in the management of non-healing or delayed-healing wounds.

DC stimulation was one of the first forms of ES to be used clinically, with reports from the 1600s concerning the application of charged gold leaf to smallpox lesions (see Dayton, 1989). Many of the animal studies outlined above have used DC stimulation with encouraging results. The philosophy for the use of DC exogenous stimulation is that it can supplement or enhance the naturally occurring DC potentials associated with repair, and thereby stimulate the healing process, particularly in cases where the process is slow or appears to have stopped, as in the case with chronic wounds such as venous ulcers and chronic pressure sores.

One of the first of the more recent research reports that involved the use of LIDC was by Assimacopoulos (1968) who treated chronic leg ulcers (which had been resistant to all previous forms of therapy) with DC stimulation. The ulcers were treated with negative polarity stimulation at currents up to 0.1 mA intensity. Complete healing was reported in 6 weeks. The main problem with this study was the very small sample (N=3) and lack of any control group, thus limiting the strength of the results.

Soon after this, Wolcott et al. (1969) published the results of a more extensive study, in which 83 ischaemic ulcers were investigated. The DC stimulation involved 3 sessions a day, each of which was for 2 hours using current intensities of between 0.2 and 0.8 mA. One electrode (copper mesh) was placed in the wound, and the other on the skin surface proximally. The intensity of the stimulation was determined empirically as it was found that stimulation with too great an intensity resulted in a bloody exudate from the ulcer and stimulation with too low an intensity resulted in a serous exudate. The intensity was used which fell between these two limits, being determined for each patient individually.

The wound electrode was made negative initially, and maintained so for at least 3 days. If the ulcer was not infected at this stage, the electrode polarity was reversed such that the wound electrode was made positive. Infected ulcers were stimulated with a negative wound electrode until the infection had cleared, and then for threee further days; only then was the wound electrode made positive. All patients had the polarity of the wound electrode reversed each time a plateau was reached in the healing process.

The results from the 75 patients with a single ulcer were encouraging. 34 (45%) achieved 100% healing over 9.6 weeks with an average healing rate of 18.4% per week. Of the remaining 41 ulcers, the mean healing rate was 9.3% per week and these patients achieved an average 64.7% healing over 7.2 weeks. Additional data was derived from a group of patients who presented with bilateral ulcers of comparable size and aetiology. These patients only received ES to one of the ulcers, the other acting as a control lesion. The results from these patients showed that 6 of the 8 treated ulcers healed completely and the remaining two achieved 70% healing. The control ulcers from the same patients healed less well with 3 of the 8 showing no healing, a further 3 healing less than 50% and the remaining two healing by 75%. The average healing rate for the treated ulcers was 27% per week and for the control ulcers was 5% per week.

Although the trial results are more convincing due to the increased sample and to the fact that there was a control group for part of the work, there are a number of pertinent issues which need to be highlighted. The control ulcers did show signs of healing and this may be due to the natural healing process at work, or may be due to the effects of the ES to one ulcer causing the release of a systemic mediator substance which in turn stimulated the contralateral ulcer. It is not possible with the experimental design to differentiate between the possibilities. A placebo effect can not be discounted.

In addition to the encouraging healing effects, the authors noted that there appeared to be a strong antimicrobial effect associated with the initial wound-negative current application. Follow-up work on the bacteriostatic effects of LIDC (Rowley et al., 1974) demonstrated that the application of low-level direct electrical current to infected soft tissues retards the growth of bacteria which, coupled with normal defence mechanisms, enhances the destruction of an infecting microorganism. Further studies (Rowley, 1985) showed that LIDC enhances the destruction of infecting bacteria by retarding the growth of the bacteria and opening the capillary beds, therefore allowing the normal biological defences to act. In both of these reports, negative polarity stimulation was responsible for the bacteriostatic effects.

The work of Wolcott et al. is one of the most frequently cited in the field of ES for wound healing, and although there have been criticisms of the design and protocol (e.g. Vodovnik, 1992) it remains an important paper. It is of interest that although in principle the treatment was based on supplementing or enhancing the naturally occurring currents associated with healing, the polarity reversal on reaching a growth plateau does not appear to be based on a recognized physiological phenomenon. The published works, which have measured rather than manipulated the potentials occurring with repair, do not report multiple polarity reversals during the healing process, and although in this study the effects were beneficial, the rationale for the approach is questioned.

A similar trial to that of Wolcott et al. was conducted by Gault and Gatens (1976) involving 76 patients with a total of 106 ischaemic ulcers of differing aetiology and site. Six patients presented with bilateral ulcers, providing a small control group, as with the previous work. The treatment protocol was the same in that the wound electrode was negative initially and was changed to positive stimulation either after three days in the case of non-infected wounds or three days after the infection had been cleared in the case of infected wounds. The difference in this protocol was that once the positive stimulation had begun, there was no reversal to the negative stimulation if a healing plateau was reached. For the patients with a single ulcer, the mean healing rate was 28.4% per week (an improvement on the unilateral ulcer result from Wolcotts study). For the patients with bilateral ulcers, where one was treated with ES and one acted as a control, the mean healing rate of the control ulcers was 14.7% per week, and the treated ulcers was 30% per week. Wound asepsis was achieved typically in 3–7 days.

The third significant trial involving LIDC was a more rigorously controlled study by Carley and Wainapel (1985), using a similar but not identical protocol as Wolcott et al. (1969) and Gault and Gatens (1976). Thirty hospital inpatients were involved in the study, divided equally into a treatment and a control group by random selection. In addition to the equal size of groups, the patients were matched (paired) on the basis of age, diagnosis, and wound aetiology, location and size.

The patients in the control group received conventional conservative therapy. The LIDC group received (in addition to conventional therapy), 2 hours of ES twice a day, 5 days a week. The two stimulation sessions were separated by a 2–4-hour rest period when the machine gave no output but remained in situ. One electrode was placed at the wound site, and an indifferent or dispersive electrode was placed on the skin 15–25 cm proximally. The wound electrode had negative polarity for the first three days of the trial after which time the polarities were reversed, with the wound electrode made positive. The wound-positive arrangement was maintained until the wound healed or until there was a healing plateau, in which case, the wound electrode was made negative again for a further three days, then reverted to wound-positive stimulation. The current intensity was between 300 and 700 µA, determined empirically in the same manner as Wolcott et al. Wounds were measured and photographed on a weekly basis, and the programme continued for five weeks or until the ulcer had healed.

The results of the study showed that the patients in the LIDC group showed healing rates that were 1.5–2.5-times faster than those of their paired controls. The overall healing rate was two-times greater. There was no significant difference between the wounds in the two groups at the commencement of the study and, in fact, the differences did not become apparent until week 3 of the study, after which the difference became progressively more significant.

In addition to the increased rate of healing, the scar tissue from the treatment group appeared to be stronger and there were fewer problems with wound infection. Control group healed tissue appeared thin and fragile and reopened in some patients. No patients in the treatment group required wound debridement during the trial period, whilst the control group patients typically required repeated debridement. Patients in the LIDC group also reported decreased pain and discomfort compared to the control group patients.

The rationale for the alternating wound electrode polarity appears to be derived from the report by Rowley *et al.* (1974) concerning the effects of opposite polarities on rabbit wound healing. It is suggested that a negative polarity wound electrode appears to encourage the resolution of infection, but does not stimulate healing. The wound positive electrode stimulates both infection and healing. The suggestion, therefore, that the wound electrode should be made negative until the infection has cleared, then positive to promote the repair has a rational basis. The alternating wound electrode polarity on reaching a healing plateau can not be traced to the published literature.

Pulsed LIDC

Two recent publications have reported the use of pulsed LIDC for the treatment of chronic wounds. Mulder (1991) and Feedar *et al.* (1991) both report the results from a randomized, double-blind, multicentre study with results presented from 47 patients with a total of 50 wounds. These wounds were of several different pathologies, covering nine different sites and at stages II–IV. Of the 50 wounds, 24 were allocated (randomly) to the control group and 26 to the treatment group.

Patients in both groups were treated twice daily (with real or sham stimulation) using a small battery-powered device. Each session was for 30 minutes with a rest period of 4–8 hours between sessions. Treatment was thus applied seven days a week for the first 4 weeks of the trial. The stimulation protocol was variable according to wound state (infected or non-infected) and wound stage (II–IV). The two pulse frequencies applied to the lesions are shown in Figure 21.7 below.

Infected wounds were treated at 128 pulses per second (pps) at a nominal current of 35 mA (measured at 29.2 mA through a 1 kΩ load) with the wound electrode having negative polarity. This stimulation was continued until the wound was infection free, and then continued for a further three days. Following this initial phase, the polarity of the wound electrode was alternated every 3 days until the wound reached Stage II. After this time, the pulse repetition rate was reduced to 64 pps and the wound electrode polarity was reversed daily.

The initial part of the trial was conducted on a double-blind basis with neither the patient nor the investigator knowing whether real or sham treatment had been applied. After completion of this element, patients from the sham treatment (control) group were allowed to join the full-treatment programme along with any patient from the treatment group who had not achieved full healing.

The results are presented for the initial four-week period and, additionally, for the follow-up study, with wound size being reported as a percentage of the original size. Following the four-week blind element, the treatment group wounds were 44% of their original size on average, whilst the control wounds averaged 67% of their initial size. The mean healing rate of the treated lesions was 14% per week compared with the control healing rate of 8.25% per week. No wounds in the treatment group increased in size, compared with 5 wounds in the control group.

Figure 21.7   Pulse characteristics of monophasic pulsed currents used by Feedar *et al.*, 1991.

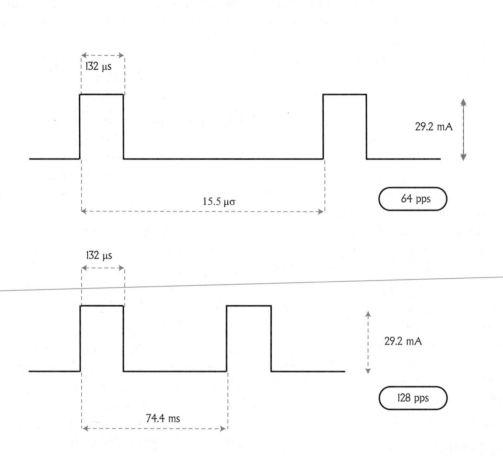

In the second phase, 14 wounds were crossed over to the stimulation protocol. The mean reduction in wound size during the sham treatment had been 11.3% at an average rate of 2.9% per week. After four weeks of active ES these wounds had reduced to 49% of their size at cross over and had demonstrated a mean healing rate of 12.8% per week. With the exception of the ES parameters, all wounds in both groups were treated identically. The authors concluded that the results support

the use of pulsed LIDC in the management of chronic dermal wounds at stages II, III and IV. The strength of the results is enhanced by the cross-over group improvements.

Weiss *et al.* (1989) compared scar thickness and hypertrophic scar formation at skin graft donor site in a small study of four patients. Each patient had bilateral split skin grafts taken from the anterior thigh. One site was given ES whilst the other acted as a control. The ES started on the day of surgery, and consisted of two sessions daily, each of 30 minutes' duration, which was continued for seven days. The stimulation was delivered by a small unit as a pulsed DC stimulation at 128 pulses per second, the pulses being 150 µs duration, at a peak current of 35 mA. The wound electrode was maintained at positive polarity throughout the study. A combination of evaluation by independent (3) physicians and donor site punch biopsies at 2–3 months post-surgery provided data for the analysis.

The subjective findings strongly suggested that the scar at the donor sites which had been subjected to ES were softer, flatter and more cosmetically acceptable than the untreated scars. These differences were apparent by 1 month post-surgery and were persistent, but less marked at 6 months.

The biopsy data supports the subjective (blinded) findings, with the treated scars being an average 46% of the thickness of the untreated scars. Biopsies also showed fewer mast cells in the stimulated scars. The effect of ES under these conditions suggests that it can decrease fibrosis, possibly by means of mast cell number reduction.

HVPGS

A more recent development in the use of ES for wound healing utilizes a pulsed DC current applied at a high voltage – known as high-voltage pulsed galvanic stimulation (HVPGS) or high-voltage pulsed current (HVPC). The pulses are commonly 'twin pulses' of short duration and high intensity (100–500 V).

A study by Akers and Gabrielson (1984) reports the results of a comparative trial involving three treatment protocols with pressure ulcers in 14 patients. It is unfortunate that much of the critical information needed to replicate this study is omitted from the published report. The three treatment groups were whirlpool therapy once daily, whirlpool therapy and ES twice daily, and ES alone twice daily. There was no control group and the initial condition of the patients in the three groups were not comparable in that the patients in the group receiving ES alone had sensory loss whilst those in the other groups had some sensation. The treatment parameters are not reported, i.e. electrode placement or polarity, stimulation intensity, characteristics, duration or patient numbers in each group. The results did not achieve statistical significance, but the underlying trend appears to be that the group receiving ES alone achieved the best results, followed by the combined ES and whirlpool therapy group and least effective of the three treatments appears to have been the whirlpool therapy alone. The lack of significance was attributed to the wide variability of the results (and one assumes to the relatively small sample size).

A far more rigorous trial concerning the effects of HVPGS is reported by Kloth and Feedar (1988). A group of 16 patients with stage IV decubitus ulcers were recruited for the trial. All had lesions that had been unresponsive to previous treatment. Patients were allocated randomly to a treatment group (N=9) or control (sham treatment) group (N=7). The ES consisted of monophasic twin pulse at 105 pulses per second delivered at a voltage just below that required to achieve visible muscle contraction (100–175 V). These stimulation parameters are reported as being arbitrarily set. ES was given for one 45-minute session a day for 5 days a week. Control group patients had electrodes placed in the same way, but the machine output was set to zero.

Electrode polarity was set initially for the wound electrode to be positive, with the negative electrode placed on the skin surface proximally. If a healing plateau was reached during the trial, the wound electrode was made negative and the treatment continued. If a second plateau was reached, the electrode polarity was reversed daily thereafter. Whichever electrode was placed at the wound site, the relative arrangement was maintained in that the positive electrode was always placed cephalad in relation to the negative electrode.

All patients in the treatment group achieved complete healing of their ulcers (in an average 7.3 weeks at a mean healing rate of 44.8% per week). The control group patients did less well, with a mean wound size increase of almost 29% between the first and last treatments. A subgroup of patients who were in the control group went on to complete a course of ES following the main trial. The three patients achieved full healing of their ulcers over 8.3 weeks with an average healing rate of 38% per week.

Griffin et al. (1991) assessed the effects of HVPC on pressure ulcer healing in a group of patients with spinal cord injury. Seventeen patients were assigned randomly to either a treatment or a control (sham treatment) group. ES treatments were carried out for one hour a day for 20 consecutive days with repeated wound assessments during this period. HVPC was delivered by means of a negative wound electrode with the stimulator delivering 100 pulses per second at an intensity of 200 volts using similar twin pulses to the previous studies. The percentage change (decrease) in ulcer size for the treatment group was significantly greater at days 5, 15 and 20. The average change for all ulcers in the treatment group was an 80% size reduction compared with a 52% decrease for the control group.

Interestingly, Kincaid (1989) published a series of results highlighting the effects of HVPC on cultured bacterial species in a series of in vitro experiments. Three commonly isolated bacterial strains were exposed to positive and negative HVPC. All three strains were affected equally by 2 hours HVPC above 250 volts. Cathodal (-ve) exposure resulted in bacterial death, whilst at the anode (+ve), toxic electrochemical end products appeared to be responsible for the bacterial demise. The authors suggest that HVPC could have significant antibacterial effects in the clinical environment. Figure 21.8 shows one type of HVPC stimulator available in the UK.

Comparative Studies

Stefanovska et al. (1993) conducted a comparative study involving three patient groups (DC stimulation, AC stimulation and a control group). Of 250 patients, 170 were spine-injured patients

Figure 21.8   The JACE Tri Stim produces a twin-peak monophasic waveform, adjustable from 0–330 V in 5 V increments. The polarity can be controlled, as can the stimulation pattern of the two channels, the stimulation rate, on time, off time, and the ramp times, both up and down.

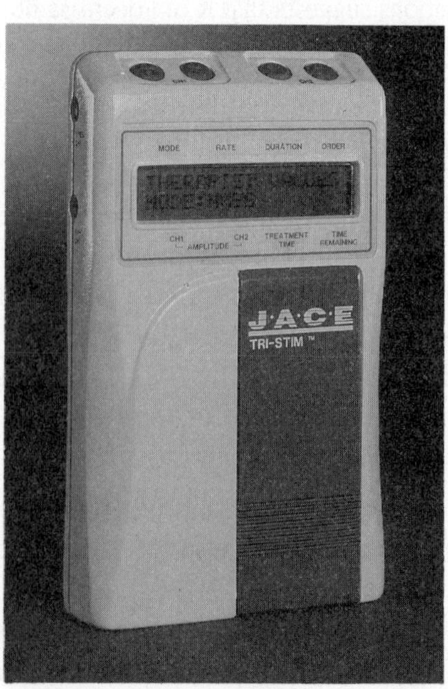

with 'pressure wounds'. As this constituted a common aetiology, this subset of the results were considered in more detail. Careful analysis of the non-equivalent initial factors (age, sex, wound size, duration) is included in the published report. The ES groups received conventional therapy in addition to the stimulation. DC stimulation utilized a 600 µA current for two hours daily, whilst the AC group were treated with low-frequency pulsed currents two hours daily. The current was biphasic, charge-balanced pulses, with a pulse duration of 0.25 ms at a repetition rate of 40 Hz. The stimulation was delivered in four-second trains with a pause of the same duration. Current intensity was adjusted to achieve minimal muscle stimulation (15–25 µA). Electrodes were attached to the wound margin on 'normal' tissue for both stimulation groups, and the current was passed across the wound, rather than using one electrode in the wound bed as is the case with previously reported work. The groups were of different sizes and differing initial conditions. It was found that initial wound area and depth influenced the healing rate for all groups. For the control group, the pretreatment wound duration also affected the healing rate, though not so for the stimulation groups. The results to date suggest that the AC stimulation group achieved better results than the DC and control groups. The results are preliminary, with reservations expressed, particularly with regards to the DC stimulation protocol. Unlike other studies, neither electrode was placed in the wound, and it is difficult therefore to compare the results directly with other published work. The AC stimulation had a stronger effect on wound healing than all other parameters considered, and the authors conclude that an arbitrarily chosen wound has a chance of healing twice as fast when the AC treatment is applied. In addition, the stimulation appears to have its greatest effect on wounds where the natural healing mechanism is insufficient. Wounds of long duration appear to be strongly influenced by ES, whilst those that are healing without external assistance made a minimal response.

Brief Review of Electrical Stimulation for other Tissue

Although the main emphasis of this chapter has been related to the effects of ES on wound healing for skin lesions, there are several other areas in which ES has been applied. A large body of research is concerned with the effects of ES for stimulation of bone healing, so much so, that it is beyond the scope of this chapter to even outline the work. The interested reader should consult one of the more recent reviews identified previously. Similarly, the work on nerve regeneration is substantial (see Sisken, 1983; Borgens, 1988) but, in keeping with the general flavour of this review, two further pieces or work deserve mention, both of which concern patellar tendon repair, both in animal models.

Stanish et al. (1985) considered the effects of ES as a method of stimulating tendon healing in the dog. Using a controlled surgical lesion of the patellar tendon in nine dogs, this comparative study evaluated the effects of: immobilization alone, early mobilization alone, and early mobilization with ES using a constant current at 20 µA.

The control and treated tendons were tested for breaking strength eight weeks postoperatively and the results were reported as the percentage strength of the operated tendon compared with the control tendon from the opposite limb of the same animal. The results clearly favoured the group receiving the early mobilization combined with ES (92% normal strength at 8 weeks), with the immobilization group and the early mobilization group having reduced strength (47% and 49% respectively). The groups were small (N=3), but the results appear to suggest a strong combined effect of ES with early movement.

Akai *et al.* (1988) also conducted a study involving deliberate surgical insult to the patellar tendon, but this time from the rabbit. The study aimed to evaluate the effects of a constant direct current on healing from both a biomechanical and biochemical aspect. Forty-five rabbits were used for the two types of test and, in addition, samples from a further 16 rabbits who underwent no surgery were used as baseline controls.

A controlled lesion was produced bilaterally in the experimental animals. A treatment unit was implanted at the time of surgery with electrodes attached to both operated tendons, though only one was connected to the stimulator. The active stimulation consisted a cathodal (-ve) stainless steel electrode sutured at the tendon defect. The second electrode was implanted to the lateral aspect of the joint. A direct current of 10 µA was passed through the electrodes to one knee only. Animals were sacrificed at various times following the surgery, and the results show that the tensile stiffness of the treated tendons was significantly higher than that for the control (sham-treated) tendons at week five after surgery.

Differences in the collagen production showed a trend for different peaks, but these were not statistically significant. By week seven, both the treated and the control tendons had achieved the same collagen mass as the intact (non-operated) tendons. Considering the differences in the ratio of Type III collagen (which contributes to tissue elasticity) to Type I collagen (which contributes to tissue strength), there were marked differences between the groups. The non-operated tendons showed a negligible amount of Type III collagen, while both operated groups (treated and sham-

treated) showed an increased Type III percentage. The difference between the two operated groups was that the tendons which had been exposed to ES has significantly less Type III collagen at 3, 5, and 7 weeks. The dominant effect of ES under the conditions described appears to be to promote early remodeling of the repair, producing a more mature collagen type at an earlier stage.

Conclusions and Clinical Implications

The exact mechanism by which ES appears to enhance wound healing has not been established. Many components of the physiological response have been identified and are supported by the research to a greater or lesser extent. The clinical results support the use of ES in a variety of forms as a method which contributes to the management of chronic skin ulceration.

It would be inappropriate to suggest that ES alone would produce significant changes in chronic wound healing. In addition to ES, other wound management factors must be considered, such as elimination of detrimental forces acting at the wound site, prevention or elimination of infection, ensuring adequate tissue oxygenation, debridement and systemic well-being (Dayton, 1989). It remains possible that a proportion of the benefits reported in the literature may be attributed to the care and attention paid to the wound (and thereby of course, the patient). With the limited number of controlled trials, it is difficult to quantify the strength of this effect.

The effects and possible mechanisms of ES have been discussed in many of the publications cited in this chapter. Some of these effects are directly supported by the research, whilst some remain speculative.

Frank and Szeto (1983) suggest that electrical stimulation can affect soft tissue healing by inhibiting negative healing factors, by speeding normal healing processes, or by creating new and improved healing pathways, thus improving both the rate and the end-point of scar formation of tissue regeneration.

Dayton (1989) suggests the possible effects of ES to wounds includes reduction of bacteria (due to local pH changes, bactericidal ion release from the electrode, or phagocytic stimulation), increased rate of wound healing, increased wound strength, improved scar quality and pain relief.

Biedebach (1989) considers both local tissue response and general vasodilation response which may be neuronal or chemically mediated. Animal studies support the local tissue response together with DNA, ATP and protein (collagen) synthesis increases following the passage of current through the tissue. There is some evidence for this being a CNS mediated mechanism, supported by the demonstration that, in spinal injury patients, the response to ES is less marked than for other patients (Wolcott et al., 1979). Additionally, the effects might be due to a chemically mediated mechanism. Bourguinon (1987) demonstrated activation of fibroblasts on ES and in a separate study showed the effects of ES on T lymphocytes with increased Ca^{2+} levels, increased kinase activity, receptor clustering and increased DNA synthesis. It is suggested that calcium ions may act as the mediator for many of the cell activation changes which have been observed, with the ion acting as a second messenger. It is possible that increased cellular Ca^{2+} uptake not only results in increased cellular motility (via the actin any myosin in cytoskeleton) but

is also linked to cellular energy production (ATP) via mitochondrial mechanisms (see Chapter 2).

Dunn et al. (1988) have suggested that the accelerating effects of electrical stimulation on wound healing may be as a consequence of :

- Modification of endogenous bioelectricity;
- Activation or attraction of inflammatory cells;
- Presence of electrode-breakdown products;
- Attraction of connective tissue cells;
- Enhanced cell replication;
- Enhanced cell biosynthesis;
- Inhibition of infectious microorganisms.

Lundeberg et al. (1989) demonstrated significant changes in the capillary filling mechanisms in tissue with venous stasis, with subsequent reduction of oedema and stasis, whilst Griffin et al. (1991), in acknowledging the lack of a confirmed mode of action of ES in relation to wound healing, suggest that there are several attractive hypotheses. These include the attraction of connective tissue and inflammatory cells, modification of endogenous electrical potentials of tissue, stimulation of cellular biosynthesis and replication, bactericidal effects, enhanced circulation, and the generation of a cellular electrophysiological effect. Some changes at electrode sites (e.g. pH changes, ion release from electrodes) may be making a contribution during LIDC, but it is suggested from the available evidence that these reactions had not been demonstrated in a series of in vitro experiments with HVPC.

A wide range of ES applications have apparently been responsible for enhanced soft tissue (particularly skin) healing. Scepticism has often been voiced (quite reasonably) as many of these trials have lacked controls, have failed to report important stimulation parameters and often involve relatively small numbers of subjects. Confounding variables such as electrode contamination and the strength of the placebo effect could be responsible for a proportion of the results, but the accumulating evidence for the beneficial effects of electrical stimulation under a variety of applications suggests that a 'real' effect is likely. When the internal (endogenous) electrical activity of the body is considered, the electrical links between physiological processes and electrical activity is unlikely to be an epiphenomenon. This being the case, externally applied electrical and electromagnetic stimulation in its numerous guises could reasonably be responsible for an alteration in healing responses. The exact mechanisms remain unexplained, but the clinical results support the tenet that external energy intervention can have significant effects. Important questions remain and much further work is needed to identify the most important parameters. The stimulation could be used as a trigger to stimulate the process using amplitude or frequency windows. Alternatively, the energy input could force a chemical event or cascade, thereby stimulating natural events from an alternative start point.

This overview of one aspect of electrical stimulation is probably just the visible part of a substantial iceberg. Other chapters consider the effects of different energy forms (mechanical, electrical and electromagnetic), and the resultant picture should be one of excitement rather than dispair. The key to progress is research both in the laboratory and in the clinical field, providing the key(s) that will enable utilization of the endogenous bioelectric systems associated with healing and repair.

References

Akai, M, Oda, H, Shirasaki, Y, Tateishi, T (1988) Electrical stimulation of ligament healing; An experimental study of the patellar ligament of rabbits. *Clinical Orthopaedics* 235: 296–301.

Akers, TK, Gabrielson, AL (1984) The effect of high voltage galvanic stimulation on the rate of healing of decubitus ulcers. *Biomedical and Scientific Instrumentation* 20: 99–100.

Albert, SF, Wong, E (1991) Electrical stimulation of bone repair. *Clinics in Pediatric Medicine and Surgery* 8(4): 923–935.

Alvarez, OM, Mertz, PM, Smerbeck, RV, Eaglstein, WH (1983) The healing of superficial skin wounds is stimulated by external electrical current. *Journal of Investigations in Dermatology* 81: 144–148.

Assimacopoulos, D (1968) Wound healing promotion by the use of negative electric current. *American Surgery* 34: 423–431.

Bach, S, Bilgrav, K, Gottrup, F, Jorgensen, TE (1991) The effect of electrical current on skin incision. *European Journal of Surgery* 157: 171–174.

Barker, AT, Jaffe, LF, Vanable, JW (1982) The glabrous epidermis of cavies contains a powerful battery. *American Journal of Physiology* 242: R358–R366.

Barnes, TC (1945) Healing rate of human skin determined by measurement of the electrical potential of experimental abrasions. *American Journal of Surgery* 69: 82–88.

Bassett, C, Land, A, Herrmann, I (1968) The effect of electrostatic fields on macromolecular synthesis by fibroblasts *in vitro*. *Journal of Cell Biology* 39: 9A.

Becker, RO (1961) The bioelectric factors in amphibian limb regeneration. *Journal of Bone and Joint Surgery* 43A: 643–656.

Becker, RO (1962) Some observations indicating the possibility of longitudinal charge-carrier flow in the peripheral nerves. *Biol Prototypes Synthet Systems* 1: 31–37.

Becker, RO (1967) The electrical control of growth processes. *Medical Times* 95: 657–669.

Becker, RO (1974a) The basic biological data transmission and control system influenced by electrical forces. *Annals of the New York Academy of Sciences* 238: 236–241.

Becker, RO (1974b) The significance of bioelectric potentials. *Bioelectrochemistry and Bioenergetics* 1: 187–199.

Becker, RO (1982) Electrical control systems and regenerative growth. *Journal of Bioelectricity* 1(2): 239–264.

Becker, RO, Bachman, CG, Friedman, H (1962) The direct current control system: A link between environment and organism. *New York State Journal of Medicine* 62: 1169–1176.

Becker, RO, Bachman, CH and Slaughter, WH (1962) Longitudinal direct current gradients of spinal nerves. *Nature* 196: 675–676.

Becker, RO, Murray, DG (1967) A method for producing cellular dedifferentiation by means of very small electrical currents. *Transactions of the New York Academy of Sciences* 29: 606–615.

Becker, RO, Spadaro, JA (1972) Electrical stimulation of partial limb regeneration in mammals. *Bulletin of the New York Academy of Medicine* 48(4): 627–641.

Becker, RO, Spadaro, JA, Marino, AA (1977) Clinical experiences with low intensity direct current stimulation of bone growth. *Clinical Orthopedics and Related Research* 124: 75–83.

Biedebach, MC (1989) Accelerated healing of skin ulcers by electric stimulation and the intracellular physiological mechanisms involved. *Acupuncture and Electrotherapeutics* 14: 43–60.

Black, J (1987). *Electrical Stimulation: Its role in growth, repair and remodelling of the musculoskeletal system*. Praeger, New York.

Borgens, RB (1981). *Injury, Ionic Currents and Regeneration. Mechanisms of Growth Control*, pp. 107–136. Charles C Thomas, Springfield, Illinois.

Borgens, RB (1982) What is the role of naturally produced electric current in vertebrate regeneration and healing? *International Review of Cytology* **76**: 245–298.

Borgens, RB (1984) Endogenous ionic currents traverse intact and damaged bone. *Science* **225**: 478–482.

Borgens, RB (1988a) Stimulation of neuronal regeneration and development by steady electrical fields. *Advances in Neurology* **47**: 547–564.

Borgens, RB (1988b) Voltage gradients and ionic currents in injured and regenerating axons. *Advances in Neurology* **47**: 51–66.

Borgens, RB, McCaig, CD (1989). *Endogenous currents in nerve repair, regeneration and development. Electric Fields in Vertebrate Repair*, pp. 77–116. Alan R Liss Inc., New York.

Borgens, RB, Robinson, K, Vanable, JW, McGinnis, M (1989). *Electric Fields in Vertebrate Repair: Natural and Applied Voltages in Vertebrate Regeneration and Healing*. Alan R Liss Inc., New York.

Borgens, RB, Vanable, JW, Jaffe, LF (1977) Bioelectricity and regeneration: Large currents leave the stumps of regenerating newt limbs. *Proceeedings of the National Academy of Sciences, USA* **74**(10): 4528–4532.

Bourguignon, GJ, Bourguignon, LY (1987) Electric stimulation of protein and DNA synthesis in human fibroblasts. *FASEB Journal* **1**(8): 398–402.

Burr, HS, Harvey, SC, Taffel, M (1938) Bio-electric correlates of wound healing. *Yale Journal of Biology and Medicine* **11**: 103–107

Carey, LC, Lepley, D (1962) Effect of continuous direct electrical current on healing wounds. *Surgical Forum* **13**: 33–35.

Carley, PJ, Wainapel, SF (1985) Electrotherapy for acceleration of wound healing: Low intensity direct current. *Archives of Physical Medicine in Rehabilitation* **66**: 443–446.

Chakkalakal, DA, Wilson, RF, Connolly, JF (1988a) Epidermal and endosteal sources of endogenous electricity in injured canine limbs. *IEEE Transactions in Biomedical Engineering* **35**: 19–29.

Chakkalakal, DA, Wilson, RF, Connolly, JF (1988b) Electrophysiologic basis for prognosis in fracture healing. *Medical Instrumentation* **22**(6): 312–322.

Chang, KS, Snellen, JW (1982) Bioelectric activity in the rabbit ear regeneration. *Journal of Experimental Zoology* **221**: 193–203.

Charman, RA (1990a) Bioelectricity and Electrotherapy – Towards a new paradigm: Introduction. *Physiotherapy* **76**(9): 502–503.

Charman, RA (1990b) Bioelectricity and Electrotherapy – Towards a new paradigm: Part 1, The electric cell. *Physiotherapy* **76**(9): 503–508.

Charman, RA (1990c) Bioelectricity and Electrotherapy – Towards a new paradigm: Part 2, Cellular reception and emission of electromagnetic signals. *Physiotherapy* **76**(9): 509–516.

Charman, RA (1990d) Bioelectricity and Electrotherapy – Towards a new paradigm: Part 4, Strain generated potentials in bone and connective tissue. *Physiotherapy* **7**(11): 725–730.

Charman, RA (1990e) Bioelectricity and Electrotherapy – Towards a new paradigm: Part 5, Exogenous currents and fields – experimental and clinical applications. *Physiotherapy* **76**(12): 743–750.

Charman, RA (1991) Bioelectricity and Electrotherapy – Towards a new paradigm: Part 6, Environmental currents and fields – the natural background. *Physiotherapy* **77**(1): 8–14.

Cooper, MS, Schliwa, M (1985) Electrical and ionic controls of tissue cell locomotion in DC electric fields. *Journal of Neuroscience Research* **13**: 223–244.

Dayton, PD, Palladino, SJ (1989) Electrical stimulation of cutaneous ulcerations. *Journal of the American Podiatric Medical Association* **79**(7): 318–321.

Dunn, MG (1988) Wound healing using collagen matrix: Effect of DC electrical stimulation. *Journal of Biomedical and Material Research* **22**(A2 Suppl): 191–206.

Eaglstein, WH, Mertz, PM (1978) New method for assessing epidermal wound healing: The effects of triamcinolone acetonide and polyethylene film occlusion. *Journal of Investigations in Dermatology* **71**: 382–384.

Erickson, C, Nuccitelli, R (1984) Embryonic fibroblast motility and orientation can be influenced by physiological electric fields. *Journal of Cell Biology* **98**(1): 296–307.

Feedar, JA, Kloth, LC, Gentzkow, GD (1991) Chronic dermal ulcer healing enhanced with monophasic pulsed electrical stimulation. *Physical Therapy* **71**(9): 639–649.

Forrest, L (1983) Current concepts in soft connective tissue wound healing. *British Journal of Surgery* **70**: 133–140.

Foulds, IS, Barker, AT (1983) Human skin battery potentials and their possible role in wound healing. *British Journal of Dermatology* **109**: 515–522.

Frank, CB, Szeto, AY (1983) A review of electromagnetically enhanced soft tissue healing. *IEEE Engineering in Medicine and Biology* **2**: 27–32.

Friedenberg, Z, Brighton, CT (1966) Bioelectric potentials in bone. *Journal of Bone and Joint Surgery* **48**(A): 915–923.

Gault, WR, Gatens, PF (1976) Use of low intensity direct current in management of ischaemic skin ulcers. *Physical Therapy* **56**: 265–269.

Gentzkow, GD, Miller, KH (1991) Electrical stimulation for dermal wound healing. *Clinics in Podiatric Medicine and Surgery* **8**(4): 827–841.

Griffin, JW, Tooms, RE, Mendius, RA, Clifft, JK, Vander Zwaag, R, El-Zeky, F (1991) Efficacy of high voltage pulsed current for healing of pressure ulcers in patients with spinal cord injury. *Physical Therapy* **71**(6): 433–442.

Hinkle, L, McCaig, CD, Robinson, KR (1981) The direction of growth of differentiating neurones and myoblasts from frog embryos in an applied electric field. *Journal of Physiology* **314**: 121–135.

Illingworth, CM, Barker, AT (1980) Measurement of electrical currents emerging during the regeneration of amputated finger tips in children. *Clinical Physics and Physiological Measurement* **1**(1): 87–89.

Im, MJ, Lee, WPA, Hoopes, JE (1990) Effect of electrical stimulation on survival of skin flaps in pigs. *Physical Therapy* **70**(1): 37–40.

Jaffe, LF, Vanable, JW (1984) Electric fields and wound healing. *Clinics in Dermatology* **2**(3): 34–44.

Kincaid, CB (1989) Inhibition of bacterial growth in *vitro* following stimulation with high voltage, monophasic, pulsed current. *Physical Therapy* **69**: 651–655.

Kloth, LC, Feedar, JA (1988) Acceleration of wound healing with high voltage, monophasic pulsed current. *Physical Therapy* **68**: 503–508.

Konikoff, JJ (1976) Electrical promotion of soft tissue repairs. *Annals of Biomedical Engineering* **4**: 1–5.

Lundberg, T, Kiartansson, J, Samuelsson, U (1988) Effect of electrical nerve stimulation on healing of ischaemic skin flaps. *The Lancet* Sept 24: 712–714.

Mulder, GD (1991) Treatment of open skin wounds with electric stimulation. *Archives of Physical Medicine in Rehabilitation* **72**: 375–377.

Okihana, H, Uchida, A, Shimorura, Y (1985). Effects of direct current on the cultured growth of cartilage cells. *Bioelectrical Repair and Growth* Vol: 103–108.

Patel, NB (1986) Reversible inhibition of neurite growth by focal electric currents. *Progress in Clinical and Biological Research* **210**: 271–278.

Patel, NB, Poo, M-M (1982) Orientation of neurite growth by extracellular electric fields. *Journal of Neuroscience* **2**(4): 483–496.

Politis, MJ, Zanakis, MF, Miller, JE (1989) Enhanced survival of full thickness skin grafts following the application of DC electrical fields. *Plastic Reconstructive Surgery* **84**(2): 267–272.

Pomeranz, B (1986) Effects of applied DC fields on sensory nerve sprouting and motor nerve regeneration in adult rats. *Progress in Clinical and Biological Research* **210**: 251–260.

Reed, BV (1988) Effect of high voltage pulsed electrical stimulation on microvascular permeability to plasma proteins - A possible mechanism in minimising edema. *Physical Therapy* **68**: 491–495.

Reich, JD, Cazzaniga, AL, Mertz, PM, Kerdel, FA, Eaglstein, WH (1991) The effect of electrical stimulation on the number of mast cells in healing wounds. *Journal of the American Academy of Dermatology* **25**(1): 40–46.

Ross, SM, Ferrier, JM, Aubin, JE (1989) Studies on the alignment of fibroblasts in uniform applied electric fields. *Bioelectromagnetics* **10**: 371–384.

Rowley, BA (1985) Electrical enhancement of healing. Proceedings of the IEEE National Aerospace and Electronics Conference (NAECON). IEEE, Dayton, Ohio

Rowley, BA, McKenna, JM, Wolcott, LE (1974) The use of low level electrical current for enhancement of tissue healing. *Biomedical Scientific Instrumentation* **10**: 111–114.

Rubinacci, A, Black, J, Brighton, C, Friedenberg, Z (1988) Changes in bioelectric potentials on bone associated with direct current stimulation of osteogenesis. *Journal of Orthopaedic Research* **6**: 335–345.

Sisken, BF (1983) Nerve and limb regeneration. *IEEE Engineering in Medicine and Biology* **2**: 32–39.

Stanish, W, MacGillvary, G, Rubinovich, M, Kozey, J (1985). The effects of electrical stimulation on tendon healing. *Bioelectrical Repair and Growth* Vol: 311–318.

Stefanovska, A, Vodovnik, L, Benko, H, Turk, R (1993) Treatment of chronic wounds by means of electric and electromagnetic fields: Part 2: Value of FES parameters for pressure sore treatment. *Medical and Biological Engineering and Computing* **31**: 213–220.

Stromberg, BV (1988) Effects of electrical currents on wound contraction. *Annals of Plastic Surgery* **21**(2): 121–123.

Vanable, JW (1989) *Integumentary potentials and wound healing. Electric Fields in Vertebrate Repair,* pp. 171–224. Alan R Liss Inc., New York.

Vodovnik, L, Karba, R (1992) Treatment of chronic wounds by means of electric and electromagnetic fields. *Medical and Biological Engineering and Computing* **30**: 257–266.

Vodovnik, L, Miklavcic, D, Sersa, G (1992) Modified cell proliferation due to electrical currents. *Medical and Biological Engineering and Computing* **30**: CE21–CE28.

Watson, T (1995) *The Bioelectric Correlates of Musculoskeletal Injury and Repair.* PhD thesis, University of Surrey.

Weiss, DS, Eaglstein, WH, Falanga, V (1989) Exogenous electric current can reduce the formation of hypertrophic scars. *Journal of Dermatology, Surgery and Oncology* **15**: 1272–1275.

Weiss, DS, Kirsner, R, Eaglstein, WH (1990) Electrical stimulation and wound healing. *Archives of Dermatology* **126**: 222–225.

Wilber, MC (1978) Surface direct current bioelectric potentials in the normal and injured human thigh. *Texas Reports on Biology and Medicine* **36**: 197–204.

Wolcott, LE, Wheeler, PC, Hardwicke, HM, Rowley, BA (1969) Accelerated healing of skin ulcers by electrotherapy. *Southern Medical Journal* **62**: 795–801.

Wu, KT, Go, N, Dennis, C, Enquist, I, Sawyer, PN (1967) Effects of electric currents and interfacial potentials on wound healing. *Journal of Surgical Research* **7**: 122–128.

Appendix: *Safety in Practice*

Safe Application
•
Maintenance of Equipment
•
The Environment
•
Equipment Loan
•
Staff Exposure
•
Planned Replacement

Safety, including maintenance, is of paramount importance in the application of all electrophysical agents, and the general aspects are in this Appendix. Particular contraindications are addressed in the relevant chapters.

Safe Application

Irrespective of the mode of treatment used, physiotherapists have a duty of care to the patient. They should confine themselves to the use of electrophysical modalities in which they have been instructed and are competent, taking into account physiological and therapeutic effects, safe application, precautions and contraindica-

tions. They should also have access to relevant literature, equipment evaluation reports, safety information bulletins, hazard notices and clinical research papers.

It is most important that all treatment interactions are documented and signed. This should include assessment, indication for use, results of skin sensation tests, modality and machine used, time setting and treatment effects – beneficial or adverse – and outcome. Electrotherapy must never be used in the treatment programme for patients who are unable to understand warnings and instructions. As part of the assessment process, any drugs being taken by the patient must be identified as these could sensitize them or mask their condition and therefore alter their response to the intervention.

The patient is made comfortable and the area to be treated is exposed and inspected, before and after treatment. A visual check is made of the equipment in relation to plugs, cables, leads, electrodes, controls, dial and indicator lights, and the output is tested before use.

The patient must be able to contact the physiotherapist at all times during the treatment session. Patients should be advised not to move during treatment or touch the machine or controls, unless the equipment is fitted with a patient switch-off device, in which case they should be instructed in its use. It is important to ensure that the leads do not touch the patient or trail on the floor and or, that the machine is not in the near field of another modality that could distort the field and alter the effectiveness of treatment. Electrodes and cables should not be adjusted whilst the apparatus is in operation.

Maintenance of Equipment

Correct maintenance ensures that electrotherapy equipment is in the optimum condition for use. Visual checks must be made before using any electrotherapy equipment. Faults should be reported immediately and the machine or part must be removed from use until repaired.

Advice on the safe management of electromedical equipment are laid down in Health Equipment Information HEI 98 produced by the UK Department of Health.

Regular maintenance minimizes breakdown. When purchasing electrotherapy equipment for use in the UK National Health Service, MLQ request forms are sent out by Supplies Depart-

ments to suppliers, to reduce the risk of buying equipment which does not comply with BS 5724 and its supplements which are synonymous with the International Electrotechnical Commission Standard IEC 601. Their aim is to prevent faulty equipment being put into use and to ensure that correct equipment records are maintained.

Maintenance Contracts

Procedures for the testing of new machinery are outlined in HEI 95 and should be undertaken by the supplier before use. In the UK National Health Service the machine will also be checked for safety and function by the electromedical engineer.

Maintaining equipment in good working order is important, and a check should be made once a year at the minimum, though with heavy usage twice a year is desirable. This should be undertaken by a reputable company on a maintenance contract. The credentials of the company should be checked to ensure that it is appropriately licensed to maintain different manufacturers' equipment and to obtain and fit specialized spare parts. Maintenance contracts can be set up with individual suppliers to service their own equipment. The practitioner should check that the full maintenance contract includes planned preventative maintenance, all breakdown call-outs and the cost of labour, travel and spares. The cost of maintenance options varies widely, but the most comprehensive contract should cost less that 10% per annum of the capital cost of the equipment.

It is important to monitor the service contract, to check that visits are made, that all equipment is checked as agreed, and a report on its condition and the work done is received and kept. In the UK no-one other than the agreed contractor should repair equipment, as this may change liability under the Product Liability Act and the Consumer Protection Act. Maintenance service specifications should meet the needs of the service.

The Environment

It is important that there are facilities for the safe storage of eqipment. The area should be kept clean and dry and care should be taken over trailing leads.

Equipment Loan

In many cases equipment is loaned to patients on a trial basis. It is most important that the equipment is checked to be electrically safe. Patients must be well-instructed in its use, effects and maintenance, backed up by written instructions. These must include information concerning a contact point in case of problems. Regular contact must be kept with the patient during the loan period to ensure compliance. Records must be kept of each item loaned.

Indemnity

Where machinery is loaned by a company on a trial basis, an indemnity form must be completed by both the supplier and a representative of the trust or practice. This protects the practitioner / hospital from litigation or damage as a result of failure in any way of the loaned equipment.

Staff Exposure

In all cases, the operator must limit their exposure to the effects of the treatment being applied.

Planned Replacement

It is recommended that electrotherapy equipment is given a depreciation life of ten years. In a UK National survey much of the equipment held was many years older. Where possible, it is recommended that there should be a policy to ensure that equipment is replaced in a planned manner, though with financial restraints in both health premises and private practice, this is difficult to achieve.

Index